Encyclopedia of Colorectal Cancer: Genes and Tumor

Volume I

Encyclopedia of Colorectal Cancer: Genes and Tumor Volume I

Edited by **Teresa Young**

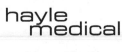

New York

Published by Hayle Medical,
30 West, 37th Street, Suite 612,
New York, NY 10018, USA
www.haylemedical.com

Encyclopedia of Colorectal Cancer: Genes and Tumor
Volume I
Edited by Teresa Young

International Standard Book Number: 978-1-63241-134-1 (Hardback)

Printed in the United States of America.

Contents

Preface

The cases of colorectal cancer are increasing worldwide. The researches and studies in this field would be helpful to provide some efficient therapeutic measures for colorectal cancer. This book presents some basic steps being taken in order to understand and diagnose this disease. This book discusses the analysis done by scientists on the data and evidences available related to genes, infections related to colorectal cancer and other factors. The escalating research and study into the aspects of genes and genetic background associated with colorectal cancer cellular, the molecular biochemical involved in colorectal carcinogenesis and tumor progression and its complexities have been described in the book. This text is a valuable account of information for scientists, researchers and medical professionals engaged in this field.

This book has been the outcome of endless efforts put in by authors and researchers on various issues and topics within the field. The book is a comprehensive collection of significant researches that are addressed in a variety of chapters. It will surely enhance the knowledge of the field among readers across the globe.

It is indeed an immense pleasure to thank our researchers and authors for their efforts to submit their piece of writing before the deadlines. Finally in the end, I would like to thank my family and colleagues who have been a great source of inspiration and support.

Editor

Part 1

Introduction

Colorectal Cancer: It Starts and It Runs

Rajunor Ettarh
Department of Structural and Cellular Biology,
Tulane University School of Medicine, New Orleans,
USA

1. Introduction

An automobile starts and runs. In much the same way, colorectal cancer starts and runs but our understanding of how this happens is incomplete. The disease affects millions of men and women around the world, and is responsible for significant morbidity and mortality in patients. Increasing numbers of new cases continue to appear worldwide and there is little evidence of a decline in incidence of the disease. The necessity for improved management and treatment of colorectal cancer in patients continues to drive studies and investigations towards a better understanding of the origins of the disease. Much of the evidence suggests that the origins of colorectal cancer are multifactorial: genetic and environmental factors intertwine with risk factors. Figure 1 lays out various aspects of colorectal cancer that provide broad focal points for studies and research investigations. In vitro studies have helped to define the scientific knowledge base regarding initiation of colorectal cancer and the mechanisms that sustain progression and encourage spread of the disease. Clinical studies and trials have provided insights into disease management and patient care. Animal modeling provides an important bridge between in vitro studies and investigations in patients. So what is the current state of the evidence regarding the causes and biological mechanisms involved in colorectal cancer? While the chapters in this volume of the book deliver detailed overviews of various aspects of the basic science involved in our understanding of the disease, this introductory chapter offers a summary outline of some of the evidence.

2. Genes and heredity

Genetic and hereditary mechanisms have a significant influence on colorectal cancer. Studies indicate that familial history plays a role in up to 25% of patients who are diagnosed with colorectal cancer (Gala & Chung, 2011) and this helps to explain the origins of their disease. Several genes have been implicated in the process of colorectal carcinogenesis including adenomatous polyposis coli (APC), rat sarcoma oncogene K-ras, tumor suppressor TP53, DNA glycosylase gene MUTYH, and murine sarcoma oncogene BRAF. In many patients, the most frequently mutated gene is the APC gene (Bettstetter et al, 2007; Vasovcak et al, 2011). Some of the methods by which these genes are affected include hypermethylation of promoter sequences for tumor suppressor genes as well as the induction of microsatellite instability. About 15% of colorectal cancers show microsatellite instability from mutated mismatch repair genes (Pino & Chung, 2011).

A majority of colorectal cancers are associated with colonic polyposis. Familial adenomatous polyposis (FAP) confers a genetic predisposition to developing multiple benign polyps in the large intestine, a reflection of the inherited mutation in the APC gene. Polyps eventually progress to malignant colorectal cancer. Patients with Lynch Syndrome have a genetic predisposition that confers a high risk for developing early onset, right-sided colorectal cancer (Bellizzi & Frankel, 2009). More recently recognized syndromes also include MUTYH-associated polyposis (MAP), and hyperplastic polyposis syndromes which show mutations of K-ras and microsatellite instability – changes similar to those associated with colorectal cancer (Hawkins et al, 2000; Jass et al, 2000; Liljegren et al, 2003).

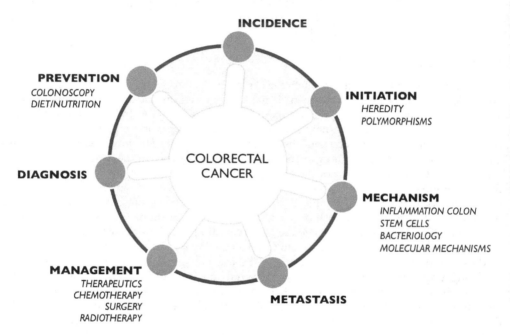

Fig. 1. The aspects of colorectal cancer that drive the quest for improved understanding, better management, effective therapies, and prevention. Aspects of initiation and mechanisms are considered in this volume of the book. Management, diagnosis and epidemiological considerations are dealt with in the second volume of the book.

Animal models of colorectal cancer have contributed to improving understanding of the disease. The APC min mouse model develops multiple intestinal polyps and illustrates the role of Wnt signaling and beta catenin regulation in the formation of these polyps (Kawahara et al, 2000; Senda et al, 2007). The model provides one avenue for testing and evaluating pharmacotherapeutic approaches in colorectal cancer.

3. Nutrition

The relationship between nutrition and colorectal cancer remains inconsistent and debatable. Some studies suggest variable colorectal cancer risk with ingestion of fruit and vegetables, other studies indicate a reduction in the risk (Millen et al, 2007; Koushik et al,

2007; Anemma et al, 2011). The evidence is just as conflicting even when specific food components such as folate are considered (Mason, 2011). Some of the published data supports the association between colorectal cancer and processed foods as well as with consumption of red meat: the risk of colorectal cancer increases in line with increasing intake (Fu et al, 2011; Gingras and Beliveau, 2011). In addition, the risk among heavy alcohol drinkers for developing colorectal cancer is considerably higher than the risk for those whose alcohol intake is low (Pelluchi et al, 2011).

4. Mechanisms

The role of inflammation in colorectal cancer is demonstrated by the increased risk of colorectal in patients with chronic inflammatory conditions: the risk in patients with ulcerative colitis is 2-fold higher than for the general population and up to 0.8% of patients with Crohn's disease develop colorectal cancer (Pohl et al, 2000; Rizzo et al, 2011). These inflammatory diseases also demonstrate genetic alterations in some of the same targets associated with colorectal cancer. In addition, anti-inflammatory therapy significantly reduces the risk of colorectal cancer (Trinchieri, 2011).

The intestine is colonized by great numbers of microbes in a symbiotic relationship with the gut epithelium, a relationship that affects digestion, absorption and nutrition. Nonetheless, there is increasing evidence of the association between intestinal streptococcal infection and colorectal cancer. However the precise mechanism by which these streptococcal strains are involved in the development or propagation of colorectal cancer remains unclear (Boleij et al, 2011). Enteric microbes are thought to alter normal regulatory mechanisms in epithelial cells to promote disruption and tumor growth (Wu et al, 2003; Sun et al, 2004; Franco et al, 2005; Ye et al, 2007; Suzuki et al, 2009; Gnad et al, 2010; Liu et al, 2010).

The idea that colorectal cancer is sustained by stem cells that continually supply new tumor cells continues to spur research investigations and generate new data. The idea however remains controversial despite several reports presenting data on putative cell surface markers for these stem cells. Isolated colorectal cancer stem cells (initiating cells) express a variety of cluster of differentiation proteins or markers that suggest a multipotent ability (Willis et al, 2008; Kemper et al, 2010; Davies et al, 2011; Zeki et al, 2011) but identification of a reliable stem cell biomarker is still elusive. These cells offer a potential target for cure of the disease in patients and for the control of metastatic spread that is thought to arise from residual stem cells that survive therapy for the primary tumor.

5. Conclusion

Our understanding of colorectal cancer in terms of origination, genesis, initiating causes and progression continues to improve. While multiple factors contribute to and influence the initiation and progression of the disease, the number of potential targets continues to increase. This targeting potential will ultimately lead to the development of effective strategies for management of the disease and translate into improved treatments for patients.

6. References

Annema N, Heyworth JS, McNaughton SA, Iacopetta B, Fritschi L. (2011). Fruit and vegetable consumption and the risk of proximal colon, distal colon, and rectal cancers in a case-control study in Western Australia. *J Am Diet Assoc*, Vol.111, No.10, pp. 1479-1490.

Bellizzi AM, Frankel WL. (2009). Colorectal cancer due to deficiency in DNA mismatch repair function: a review. *Adv Anat Pathol*, Vol.16, No.6, pp. 405-417.

Bettstetter M, Dechant S, Ruemmele P, Grabowski M, Keller G, Holinski-Feder E, Hartmann A, Hofstaedter F, Dietmaier W. (2007). Distinction of hereditary nonpolyposis colorectal cancer and sporadic microsatellite-unstable colorectal cancer through quantification of MLH1 methylation by real-time PCR. *Clin Cancer Res*, Vol.13. No.11, pp. 3221-3228.

Boleij A, van Gelder MM, Swinkels DW, Tjalsma H. (2011). Clinical Importance of Streptococcus gallolyticus Infection Among Colorectal Cancer Patients: Systematic Review and Meta-analysis. *Clin Infect Dis*, Vol.53, No.9, pp. 870-878.

Davies EJ, Marsh V, Clarke AR. (2011). Origin and maintenance of the intestinal cancer stem cell. *Mol Carcinog*, Vol.50, No.4, pp. 254-263.

Franco AT, Israel DA, Washington MK, Krishna U, Fox JG, Rogers AB, Neish AS, Collier-Hyams L, Perez-Perez GI, Hatakeyama M, Whitehead R, Gaus K, O'Brien DP, Romero-Gallo J, Peek RM Jr. (2005). Activation of beta-catenin by carcinogenic helicobacter pylori. *Proc Natl Acad Sci USA*, Vol.102, pp. 10646–10651.

Fu Z, Shrubsole MJ, Smalley WE, Wu H, Chen Z, Shyr Y, Ness RM, Zheng W. (2011) Association of meat intake and meat-derived mutagen exposure with the risk of colorectal polyps by histologic type. *Cancer Prev Res (Phila)*, Vol.4, No.10, pp. 1686-1697.

Gala M, Chung DC. (2011). Hereditary colon cancer syndromes. *Semin Oncol*, Vol.38, No.4, pp. 490-499.

Gingras D, Béliveau R. (2011) Colorectal cancer prevention through dietary and lifestyle modifications. *Cancer Microenviron*, Vol.4, No.2, pp. 133-139.

Gnad T, Feoktistova M, Leverkus M, Lendeckel U, Naumann M. (2010). Helicobacter pylori-induced activation of beta-catenin involves low density lipoprotein receptor-related protein 6 and dishevelled. *Mol Cancer*, Vol.9, pp.31

Hawkins NJ, Gorman P, Tomlinson IPM, Bullpitt P, Ward RL. (2000). Colorectal Carcinomas Arising in the Hyperplastic Polyposis Syndrome Progress through the Chromosomal Instability Pathway. *American Journal of Pathology*, Vol.157, pp. 385-392.

Jass JR, Lino H, Ruszkiewicz A, Painter D, Solomon MJ, Koorey DJ, Cohn D, Furlong KL, Walsh MD, Palazzo J, Edmonston TB, Fishel R, Young J, Leggett BA. (2000). Neoplastic progression occurs through mutator pathways in hyperplastic polyposis of the colorectum. *Gut*, Vol.47, pp. 43-49.

Kawahara K, Morishita T, Nakamura T, Hamada F, Toyoshima K, Akiyama T. (2000). Down-regulation of beta-catenin by the colorectal tumor suppressor APC requires association with Axin and beta-catenin. *J Biol Chem*, Vol.275, No.12, pp. 8369-8374.

Kemper K, Grandela C, Medema JP. (2010). Molecular identification and targeting of colorectal cancer stem cells. *Oncotarget*, Vol.1, No.6, pp. 387-395.

Koushik A, Hunter DJ, Spiegelman D, Beeson WL, van den Brandt PA, Buring JE, Calle EE, Cho E, Fraser GE, Freudenheim JL, Fuchs CS, Giovannucci EL, Goldbohm RA, Harnack L, Jacobs DR Jr, Kato I, Krogh V, Larsson SC, Leitzmann MF, Marshall JR,

McCullough ML, Miller AB, Pietinen P, Rohan TE, Schatzkin A, Sieri S, Virtanen MJ, Wolk A, Zeleniuch-Jacquotte A, Zhang SM, Smith-Warner SA. (2007). Fruits, vegetables, and colon cancer risk in a pooled analysis of 14 cohort studies. *J Natl Cancer Inst*, Vol.99, No.19, pp. 1471-1483.

Liljegren A, Lindblom A, Rotstein S, Nilsson B, Rubio C, Jaramillo E. (2003). Prevalence and incidence of hyperplastic polyps and adenomas in familial colorectal cancer: correlation between the two types of colon polyps. *Gut*, Vol.52, No.8, pp. 1140-1147.

Liu X, Lu R, Wu S, Sun J. (2010). Salmonella regulation of intestinal stem cells through the Wnt/beta-catenin pathway. *FEBS Lett*, Vol.584, pp. 911–916

Mason JB. (2011). Unraveling the complex relationship between folate and cancer risk. *Biofactors*, Vol.37, No.4, pp. 253-260.

Millen AE, Subar AF, Graubard BI, Peters U, Hayes RB, Weissfeld JL, Yokochi LA, Ziegler RG; PLCO Cancer Screening Trial Project Team. (2007). Fruit and vegetable intake and prevalence of colorectal adenoma in a cancer screening trial. *Am J Clin Nutr*, Vol.86, No.6, pp. 1754-1764.

Pelucchi C, Tramacere I, Boffetta P, Negri E, La Vecchia C. (2011) Alcohol consumption and cancer risk. *Nutr Cancer*, Vol.63, No.7, pp. 983-990.

Pino MS, Chung DC. (2011). Microsatellite instability in the management of colorectal cancer. *Expert Rev Gastroenterol Hepatol*, Vol.5, No.3, pp. 385-399.

Pohl C, Hombach A, Kruis W. (2000). Chronic inflammatory bowel disease and cancer. *Hepatogastroenterology*, Vol.47, No.31, pp. 57-70.

Rizzo A, Pallone F, Monteleone G, Fantini MC. (2011). Intestinal inflammation and colorectal cancer: A double-edged sword? World J Gastroenterol. 17(26):3092-100.

Senda T, Iizuka-Kogo A, Onouchi T, Shimomura A. (2007). Adenomatous polyposis coli (APC) plays multiple roles in the intestinal and colorectal epithelia. *Med Mol Morphol*, Vol.40, No.2, pp. 68-81.

Sun J, Hobert ME, Rao AS, Neish AS, Madara JL. (2004). Bacterial activation of beta-catenin signaling in human epithelia. *Am J Physiol Gastrointest Liver Physiol*, Vol.287, pp. G220–G227

Suzuki M, Mimuro H, Kiga K, Fukumatsu M, Ishijima N, Morikawa H, Nagai S, Koyasu S, Gilman RH, Kersulyte D, Berg DE, Sasakawa C. (2009). Helicobacter pylori CagA phosphorylation-independent function in epithelial proliferation and inflammation. *Cell Host Microbe*, Vol.5, pp. 23–34.

Trinchieri G. (2011) Innate inflammation and cancer: Is it time for cancer prevention? *F1000 Med Rep*, Vol.3, pp. 11.

Vasovcak P, Pavlikova K, Sedlacek Z, Skapa P, Kouda M, Hoch J, Krepelova A. (2011). Molecular genetic analysis of 103 sporadic colorectal tumours in czech patients. *PLoS One*, Vol.6, No.8, pp. e24114.

Willis ND, Przyborski SA, Hutchison CJ, Wilson RG. (2008) Colonic and colorectal cancer stem cells: progress in the search for putative biomarkers. *J Anat*, Vol.213, No.1, pp. 59-65.

Wu S, Morin PJ, Maouyo D, Sears CL. (2003). Bacteroides fragilis enterotoxin induces c-myc expression and cellular proliferation. *Gastroenterology*, Vol.124, pp. 392–400.

Ye Z, Petrof EO, Boone D, Claud EC, Sun J. (2007). Salmonella effector avra regulation of
    colonic epithelial cell inflammation by deubiquitination. *Am J Pathol*, Vol.171, pp.
    882–892
Zeki SS, Graham TA, Wright NA. (2011). Stem cells and their implications for colorectal
    cancer. *Nat Rev Gastroenterol Hepatol*, Vol.8, No.2, pp. 90-100

Part 2

Genes and Polymorphisms

2

Cytokine Gene Polymorphisms in Colorectal Cancer

Spaska Stanilova
Trakia University, Medical Faculty,
Department of Molecular Biology, Immunology and Medical Genetics,
Bulgaria

1. Introduction

Colorectal cancer is the second-leading cause of cancer-related deaths in Europe and the United States (Parkin DM, 2001). Although the primary therapy of CRC is surgical, the elucidation of different novel prognostic markers may prove to serve as future therapeutic options and contribute to the overall understanding of this cancer entity, as well as to improver disease outcome. Inflammation has been known to be a key factor of development and progression of cancer, and this is particularly notable in colorectal. At the cellular level, the colonic epithelium is exposed to a range of toxic and pathogenic challenges, including the balance between intestinal microflora. In turn, a shift can result in a change in immune response, leading to the induction of inflammation. Interactions between tumor and immune cells at the site of inflammation either enhance or inhibit cancer progression. The epidemiological data available are very impressive and show a clear association between chronic inflammatory conditions and subsequent malignant transformation in the inflamed tissue (Macarthur et al., 2004). New evidence suggests that up to 25% of all cancers are due to chronic infection or other types of chronic inflammation (Hussain SP, et al., 2007). Inflammation is mediated by an array of cytokines, which are synthesized by activated immune cells and exert their biological activities upon binding to specific receptors and activate the NF-κB transcription factor signal pathway in the epithelial cells. The ubiquitous transcription factor family NF-κB is a central regulator of the transcriptional activation of a number of genes involved in cell adhesion, immune and proinflammatory responses, apoptosis, differentiation, and growth. Induction of these genes in intestinal epithelial cells by activated NF-κB profoundly influences mucosal inflammation and repair (Jobin and Sartor, 2000).

There is strong evidence to suggest that cytokines are involved in the control of cancer development and also promote tumorigenesis, invasion, propagation, and metastasis of tumors, and that they may be relevant for gastrointestinal tumors. More recently, the molecular mechanism whereby the inflammation regulates the antitumor immune responses has been elucidated. In many tumors, signal transducers and activator of transcription (STAT)3 are activated, and thereby antitumor immune surveillance is suppressed (H. Yu and R. Jove, 2004).

In general the genes that encode cytokines involved in regulation of inflammatory conditions are genetically polymorphic and different genotypes are responsible for level of protein expression.

Genetic polymorphisms have emerged in recent years as important determinants of disease susceptibility and severity. Polymorphisms are naturally occurring DNA sequence variations, which differ from gene mutations in that they occur in the normal healthy population and have a frequency of at least 1%. Approximately 90% of DNA polymorphisms are single nucleotide polymorphisms (SNPs) due to single base substitutions. Others include insertion/deletion polymorphisms, minisatellite and microsatellite polymorphisms. Although most polymorphisms are functionally neutral, some have effects on regulation of gene expression or on the function of the coded protein. These functional polymorphisms, despite being of low penetrance, could contribute to the differences between individuals in susceptibility to and severity of disease. Many studies have examined the relationship between certain cytokine gene polymorphism, cytokine gene expression in vitro, and the susceptibility to and clinical severity of diseases (Bidwell et al., 1999; Hollegaard and Bidwell, 2006). SNPs are the most common sources of human genetic variation, and they may contribute to an individual's susceptibility to cancer. Cytokine gene polymorphisms have emerged in recent years as important determinants of susceptibility and severity of colorectal cancer. Cytokine polymorphisms directly influence interindividual variation in the magnitude of cytokine response, and this clearly contributes to an individual's ultimate clinical outcome. Dysregulation of cytokine production strongly influenced both tumor progression and host anti-tumor immunity. Cytokines secreted by activated immune and inflammatory cells can either promote tumor cell survival and growth or exert antitumor effects. In addition, some tumor cells may evade the immune system by secreting cytokines which may induce regulatory cells particularly the immunosuppressive CD4+CD25+ FoxP3+ T regulatory cells. In this chapter the polymorphisms of selected candidate genes for susceptibility to and/or severity of CRC are reviewed. Special attention is paid to studies concerning the genes of inflammatory related cytokines.

2. Cytokine gene polymorphisms of proinflammatory cytokines: IL-1; TNF-α and IL-6

The most compelling evidence for the role of inflammation in CRC comes from studies showing that proinflammatory cytokine gene polymorphisms increase the risk of cancer and its precursors.

IL-1β is a prominent proinflammatory cytokine, which together with tumor necrosis factor-α (TNF-α) serve as primary initiators of the complex inflammatory response and they are classical activators of NFkB signaling pathway. IL-1β and TNF-α genes have a number of functional polymorphisms. The IL-1B-31T/C and TNF-A-308G/A SNPs have been shown to be functionally significant with the C allele of IL-1B-31T/C and A allele of TNF-A-308G/A being associated with increased production of their respective cytokines (Hwang et al., 2002; Abraham and Kroeger, 1999). IL-1 gene cluster polymorphisms suspected of enhancing production of IL-1β have been shown to be relevant in the development of H. pylori-associated gastric adenocarcinoma. A study published in Nature showed for the first time that polymorphisms in interleukin-1B (IL-1B) were associated with gastric cancer risk (El Omar et al, 2000). Two of these polymorphisms are in near-complete linkage disequilibrium and one is a TATA-box polymorphism that markedly affects DNA–protein interactions in vitro. These linked IL-1B single nucleotide polymorphisms that increase IL-1β expression

(−511 C>T and −31 T>C) were associated with a 2- to 3-fold increased risk of gastric cancer. Heterozygosity at the IL1B −31T/C locus has also been associated with colorectal adenoma, a precursor of colorectal cancer (Gunter et al., 2006). However, Macarthur et al., 2005 did not reveal significant associations between the cytokine polymorphisms of IL-1B-31T/C and risk of colorectal cancer. In the same directions are results obtained by Ito et al., 2007 for the same SNP in IL-1B. Simultaneously they found that IL-1B-511 heterozygotes and T carriers had a significantly low risk for gastric and colorectal carcinoma in the Japanese population.

The TNF cytokines are well known for their cytotoxic and antitumor activity. TNF-α is a proinflammatory cytokine secreted mainly by activated monocytes/ macrophages. TNF-α mediates the early inflammatory response and regulates the production of other cytokines, including IL-1 and IL-6. TNF-α gene is transcriptionally silent in unstimulated monocytes and is rapidly transcribed in response to a variety of signals, such as bacterial endotoxin (LPS) and other stimuli. The signaling cascades leading to TNF-α production bifurcates to control both transcription of TNF-α gene and translation of TNF-α m RNA (Swantek et al., 1997). Transcriptional control of the TNF-α gene is mediated primarily by NF-kB binding sites present within the TNF-α gene promoter (Sweet and Hume, 1996; Yao et al., 1997). One microsatellite polymorphism in the vicinity of the TNF-α gene (TNF-A) has 14 different alleles (a1–a14). The a6 allele was associated with lower TNF-α secretion from activated monocytes (Pociot et al., 1993). For this TNF-α polymorphism, one allele was associated with an increased risk (a2 allele) and two other TNF-A alleles with decreased risks (a5 and a13 allele) of CRC (Gallagher, G et al., 1997; De Jong et al., 2002).

Among the other investigated polymorphisms of the TNF-α gene, the promoter -308G/A SNP was intensively studied. The presence of TNF-α -308A allele involved in gene transcription is associated with higher levels of TNF-α. Park et al., investigated TNF-A and Ncol RFLP of TNF-B genes and the risk of CRC (Park et al., 1998). The first intron of TNFB and the -308 promoter region of TNFA SNP polymorphisms were determined in 136 colorectal cancer patients and 325 healthy controls in an Asian population. Their results indicated that homozygous TNF-B*1/TNF-B*1 genotypes showed an increased risk for colorectal cancer, although no association in tumor susceptibility was found for the −308 G/A polymorphism of the TNF-α gene when comparing colorectal cancer patients and healthy controls. Landi et al., 2003 found a trend of reduced risk for CRC in TNF -308A allele carriers, but Theodoropoulos et al., 2006 found no effect of this SNP and the risk of CRC in Greek population.

For another SNP in TNF-α gene promoter, the −238 G > A site, has been reported that the A allele decreases the risk of developing colorectal cancer (Jang et al., 2001). Up to now, however, most studies have focused more on other cancer entities, such as melanoma and breast cancer, than on colorectal cancer.

The TNF-α pro-cancerous effect has recently been established. It's binding to specific receptors sets up signal transduction pathways, leading to cell apoptosis and gene regulation, via the MAPKinase and NF-kB pathways (Waterston A, and Bower, 2004).

Interleukin-6 (IL-6) is a pleiotropic cytokine that is participates in physiological and pathological processes for a variety of human malignancies including colorectal cancer. In particular, a preoperative IL-6 level is correlated with tumor stage, survival rate, and liver metastasis in CRC (Nakagoe et al., 2003). A significant association between serum IL-6 level and staging of the tumor (P<0.001), tumoral tissue IL-6 level (r=0.95, P<0.001) in the patients was founded (Esfandi F et al, 2006). IL-6 amount of the serum and tumoral tissue in the patients with colorectal cancer correlate significantly with the staging of the tumor and with each other. It has been demonstrated that IL-6 acts as a colorectal growth factor and as an autocrine growth factor for colorectal cancer cells (Chung and Chang, 2003).

A common G/C polymorphism located within the IL-6 gene promoter (chromosome 7p21) at position 174 bp, upstream from the start site of transcription (−174 G/C locus), has been reported (Fishman D et al, 1998). This promoter SNP affects the transcription of the gene, and altering the final levels of IL-6 released (Terry et al., 2000, Bonafe et al., 2001). The G allele increases IL-6 expression, both in stimulated and non stimulated conditions, the highest IL-6 levels being found in subjects homozygous for the G allele. In the same line are data of Belluco at al., 2003 for increased serum levels of IL-6 in colorectal cancer patients with genotype GG, regardless of the tumor stage, grade and location. Moreover, they also found a close correlation between high levels of circulating IL-6 and the presence of hepatic metastasis. The association between IL-6 serum level and CRC hepatic metastasis may depend on IL-6 properties to up-regulating the expression of adhesion receptors on endothelial cells and inducing the production of growth factors, such as hepatocyte growth factor and vascular endothelial growth factor, both of which may stimulate tumor metastasis. IL-6 promoter activation involves synergism between the transcription factors NF-IL-6 and NF-κB (Huang et al, 2000), and this may explain increased IL-6 serum levels in the CRC patients with hepatic metastasis. The first report, for investigation the promoter polymorphism in IL-6 gene with sporadic colorectal cancer risk has been the study of Landi et al., 2003. They found that the allele IL6 −174C is associated with increased risk of CRC. This association was seen both under a codominant model as well as when genotypes were grouped for both cancer of the colon and cancer of the rectum. A possible explanation of this effect is that the -174C allele could cause increased inflammation for colorectal cells in response to activated neutrophils (Nusrat et al., 2001). Slattery and colleagues reported that the GG genotype of the −174 G/C IL-6 polymorphism was associated with a significantly reduced risk of colon, but not rectal, cancers (Slattery et al., 2007). The IL6 −174C allele's role in CRC risk could not be replicated in the studies of others collectives (Theodopoulos et al., 2006; Cacev et al., 2010).

A possible cause for the conflicts and mismatches, like those observed here and the earlier study in allele and genotype distributions, may be the differences in racial or ethnical backgrounds. Duch et al. analyzed 52 patients with multiple myeloma and found that the G allele frequency was higher in the Brazilian population than in the European population (Duch C et al., 2007). Nowadays Yeh et al. observations on the allele and genotype distribution of the IL-6 −174 G/C polymorphism demonstrated that there are low frequencies of the G allele and GG genotype in the Taiwanese CRC population compared to the Western counterpart (Yeh et al., 2009).

Experimental data suggest that IL-6 plays an important role not only in developed but also in the progression of metastasis from colorectal cancer. In CRC patients, high expression of IL-6 has been correlated with poor survival and IL-6 -174 genotype CC was also significantly associated with shorter survival time when compared with the heterozygous genotype CG (Chung YC et al., 2006; Wilkening et al., 2008). Also, Belluco and colleagues analyzed 62 CRC patients and observed that patients with the C allele had lower serum IL-6 levels than those without the C allele, particularly in the presence of hepatic metastasis (Belluco C et al., 2003).

Specifically, IL-6/IL-6R complexes initiate homodimerization of gp 130, activate a cytoplasmic tyrosine kinase, and trigger signaling cascades through the JAK/STAT, Ras/MAPK and PI3-K/AKT pathways (Su et al., 2005; Chung YC et al., 2006). It has been shown that activation of signal transducers and activators of transcription 3 (STAT3) a member of a family of six different transcription factors is constitutively active in CRC cells (Corvinus et al., 2005). Ones of main activators of these signal transducers are proinflamatory cytokines such as IL-6, TNF-α and growth factors. STAT3 activity in CRC cells triggered through interleukins was found to be abundant in dedifferentiated cancer cells and infiltrating lymphocytes of CRC samples. These actions regulate inflammatory reactions, immune responses, and several other pathophysiological processes of malignancy including cell growth and survival, differentiation, cell mobility and angiogenesis. Thus, the presence of proinflammatory cytokine polymorphisms in colorectal cancer development remains a pertinent question and one that we are not aware of other investigators having considered.

3. Cytokine gene polymorphisms of antiinflamatory cytokines: TGF-β and IL-10

Anti-inflammatory cytokines play an important role in downregulation of inflammation and the prevention of neoplastic disorders. Genetic variations of anti-inflammatory cytokines are assumed to influence such responses. Typical anti-inflamatory cytokines (TGF-beta and IL-10) with immunosuppressive effect are secreted mainly from T regulatory cells (Tregs).

Transforming growth factor-beta (TGF-β or TGFB) is an immunoregulatory cytokine that plays an important role in tumor immune response within the gastrointestinal tract and this is shown in TGFB gene knockout mice, which proceed to develop uncontrolled inflammatory response and early death (Kulkarni et al., 1993). In mammalian cells, there are three isoforms described TGFB1, TGFB2, and TGFB3. Among them TGFB1 is the most abundant subtype.

TGF β1 is involved in many critical cellular processes, including cell growth, extracellular matrix formation, cell motility, angiogenesis, hematopoiesis, apoptosis, and immune function (Moustakas et al., 2002; Schuster & Krieglstein, 2002). All immune cell lineages, including B, T and dendritic cells as well as macrophages, secrete TGF-β, which negatively regulates their proliferation, differentiation and activation by other cytokines.

The TGF-β signaling pathway plays an important role in controlling cell proliferation and differentiation involved in colorectal carcinogenesis. Binding of cytokine to the TGF-β receptor complex leads to phosphorylation of Smad proteins and triggers Smads intracellular signaling mediators to modulate gene transcription, mainly by transcription factor Sp1. Xu and Pasche, 2007 shown that TGF-β signaling alterations have been implicated in susceptibility to colorectal cancer.

In normal intestinal epithelium TGF-β1 acts as a growth inhibitor, however loss of TGF-β1 - mediated growth restraint has been shown to be associated with the transformation of colorectal adenoma to cancer. In addition, there is evidence that excess production and/or activation of TGF-β by cancer cells can contributed to the tumor progression by paracrine mechanisms involving neoangiogenesis, production of stroma and proteases, and subversion of immune surveillance mechanisms in tumor hosts (Muraoka-Cook et al., 2005). Moreover, TGF-β is the most frequently up-regulated in tumor cells (Elliott and Blobe, 2005).

TGF-β1 is also a potent effector within the tumor microenvironment. It exerts a predominantly immunosuppressive effect on CD8+ cytotoxic T-lymphocytes and has been shown an active player in tumor immune evasion (Li et al., 2006). Friedman et al. reported that high levels of transforming growth factor β1 correlate with disease progression in human colon cancer (Friedman et al. 1995). In light of these finding TGF-β1 gene is a functional candidate gene for genetic predisposition in CRC.

The TGF-β1 gene is located on chromosome 19 and several SNPs were described in promoter region, in the non-translated region (introns), in the coding region (exons), and in the 3'-UTR region of the gene (Watanabe et al., 2002). Certain inherited variants in the promoter region of the TGF-β gene (-800G/A and -509C/T) have been associated with higher cytokine circulating concentrations. The -800G/A SNP is located in a consensus cyclic AMP response element binding protein (CREB) half site and may cause reduced affinity for CREB transcription factors whose binding is important for transcription control (Grainger D et al., 1999). The -509C/T is located within a YY1 consensus binding site and -509T allele has been associated with increased TGF-β1 plasma level (Grainger D et al., 1999) and reduced T-cell proliferation (Meng et al., 2005). Moreover these two SNPs of the TGF-β gene are in linkage disequilibrium. The 509 C/T polymorphism has been implicated in both colorectal adenoma and cancer risk. However, published data remains conflicting.

In the study of Macarthur et al., 2005 no association was found between -509C/T SNP in TGF-β1 promoter and colorectal cancer. Authors investigated also association between cytokine polymorphisms of IL-1, IL-10 and TNF-α genes in a population based case-control study of 264 CRC patients and 408 controls in the Northeast of Scotland and analyzed their interaction with regular aspirin use. The beneficial association between nonsteroidal anti-inflammatory drugs use, such as aspirin and decreased risk of colorectal cancer provided further evidence to suggest a role for chronic inflammation in the pathogenesis of sporadic colorectal cancer. Whereas a statistically significant association was not found between any of the SNPs and CRC alone, the authors observed a significant interaction between the IL-10-592 genotype and aspirin use. The effect of aspirin on CRC risk was limited to carriers of low producing A allele (AA and AC) compared with CC genotype. The authors postulated that individuals who are genetically prone to producing reduced levels of the anti-inflammatory IL-10 (i.e., carriers of the variant A allele) are more likely to benefit from the anti-inflammatory properties of aspirin in decreasing risk of CRC development.

Berndt et al., 2007 examined two SNPs in the promoter region of the TGFB1 (-800G/A; -509C/T) and two in exon 1 (Leu10Pro; Arg25Pro) and one in exon 5 (Thr263Ile) in association with advanced colorectal adenoma in population consisted primarily of Caucasians, living in the USA. The Leu10Pro and Arg25Pro SNPs encoded non synonymous amino acid substitution located in signal peptide sequence of the TGF-β1 pro-peptide.

Dunning et al., 2003 revealed that the 10Pro variant lead to increased TGF-β secretion compared with the 10Leu allele. Similarly, the 25Arg allele has been associated with increased TGF-β production upon stimulation in vitro (Awad MR et al., 1998).

Berndt et al., reported that the high TGF-β produced genotypes, −509TT and 10Pro/Pro genotypes were associated with an increased risk of advanced colorectal adenoma compared with other genotypes. These increased risks, particularly for -509TT association were greater for the subsets of participant with multiple adenomas and those with rectal adenomas. Risk factors for hyperplastic and adenomatous polyps were generally similar to those for colorectal cancer. Another study investigated the same Leu10Pro polymorphism in association with colorectal adenoma and hyperplastic polyps. In this study no association was found with this SNP and adenoma, but a lower risk of hyperplastic polyps was suggested for Pro allele carriers who were current or past smokers (Sparks et al, 2004).

Together these studies give support to the possible role of TGFB1 in the adenoma-carcinoma sequence and suggest that high TGFB1 produced genotypes may modulate the risk in this transformation.

To characterize association of genetic variation at the TGFB1 gene with circulating cytokine levels of TGF-β and risk of colorectal adenoma and adenocarcinoma, Saltzman et al., 2008 conducted two case-control studies (including 271 colorectal adenoma cases and 544 controls, and 535 colorectal adenocarcinoma cases and 656 controls) among Japanese Americans, Caucasians, and Native Hawaiians in Hawaii. The authors investigated 26 SNPs, spanning 39.8 kb region of the TGFB1 gene, distributed in two haplotype blocks of linkage disequilibrium named as tagSNPs, including all previously commented SNPs. They found that the variant A allele for tagSNP in 3'UTR A/G (rs6957) was associated with an increased serum level of TGF-β, and no association with promoter -509C/T and Leu10Pro polymorphisms was found. However, published data remains conflicting. In the recent study the association between -509 C/T and -800 G/A SNPs of the TGFB1 gene, and susceptibility to colorectal cancer in Iranian patients was investigated (Amighofran Z et al., 2009). They found a statistically significant lower frequency of 509T allele and TT genotype in patients than in control subjects. At position 800, no significant differences in genotype distribution and allele frequencies between the patients and healthy controls were found. The authors concluded that the genotype distributions and allele frequencies of the TGFB1 gene polymorphism at -509 C/T were significantly related to colorectal carcinoma in Iranian subjects. In the same directions are the results of Chung et al., 2007, that -509T variant allele reduced risk of colorectal cancer, but not adenoma in Koreans. A possible explanation for discrepancy in above commented results for involvement of -509 C/T SNP in colorectal cancer susceptibility occurs in the investigation of Fang et al., 2010. To derive a more precise estimation of the relationship, a meta-analysis of 994 colorectal cases and 2,335 controls from five published paper was performed. Overall, significantly increased colorectal cancer risks were found for CC versus TT in the subgroup analysis by ethnicity. Fang et al., 2010 concluded that TGFB1 -509 C/T substitution has a role in genetic predisposition for developing colorectal cancer in Asians, but no significant associations were found among Europeans.

Thus far, TGF-β1 −509 T/C gene polymorphisms have been also relevant to Crohn's disease development (Schulte et al., 2001). In the same time patients with Crohn's disease are at increased risk for developing colorectal cancer. Several lines of evidence implicate chronic inflammation in inflammatory bowel disease (ulcerative colitis and Crohn's disease) as a key predisposing factor to distinct subset of colorectal tumors. (Itzkowitz and Yio, 2004).

IL-10 is an immuno-regulatory cytokine that plays a crucial role in modulating gastrointestinal tract inflammation (Moore et al, 2001; Lin and Karin, 2007). IL-10 is produced mainly by regulatory T cell and antigen presenting cells. It is pivotal in inhibiting inflammation and interrupting carcinogenesis. In cancer patients, the production of immune suppressive cytokines: IL-10 and TGF is accelerated, and IL-10-producing type I T-regulatory (Tr1) cells are highly infiltrated in tumor microenvironment. Thus, tumor cells might escape from the immune surveillance. That is the way the IL-10 gene might be involved in genetically predisposition and severity of CRC.

Large interindividual differences in the IL-10 inducibility have been observed, which has shown to have a genetic component of over 70%. The IL-10 gene comprises 5 exons, and it has been mapped to chromosome 1q31-32. To date, at least 49 *IL10*–associated polymorphisms have been reported, and an even larger number of polymorphisms are recorded in SNP databases (Ensembl Genome Browser, 2006). Promoter polymorphisms have been subject to the most studies, particularly with regard to possible influences on gene transcription and protein production. Three SNPs at -1082(A/G), -819(C/T), -592(C/A) upstream from the transcription start site (D'Alfonso S et al., 1995; Turner D et al., 1997) have been described as well as additional two microsatellite (CA)n repeats, termed IL-10G and IL-10R and located at -1151 and -3978 respectively (Eskdale J and Galager G, 1995; Eskdale J et al., 1997). In particular, SNP at position -1082A/G of IL-10 gene was associated with IL-10 production alone or in haplotypes with other distal SNPs. Turner et al.,1997 have shown that -1082A allele is associated with lower in vitro IL-10 production by Con A-stimulated PBMC from normal subjects. Crawley et al., 1999 have reported that GCC haplotype was associated with higher IL-10 level compared to ATA in whole blood cultures after LPS stimulation. In our studies, the functional effect of -1082 A/G polymorphism was demonstrated among the Bulgarian population in both healthy volunteers and in patients with sepsis (Stanilova et al., 2006).

Positive associations between IL-10 genotype or haplotype and cancer susceptibility, progression, or both were reported (Howell and Rose-Zerilli, 2007). The IL-10-1082/-819/-592 genotype status was associated with an increased risk for gastric cancer in Japan. The presence of the ATA/GCC haplotype of IL-10-1082/-819/-592 polymorphisms significantly increased the risk of gastric cancer development compared with presence of the ATA/ATA haplotype. (Sugimoto et al, 2007). The AA genotype of the -1082 A/G polymorphism in the interleukin-10 gene promoter was associated with lower IL-10 production in LPS, PHA or PWM stimulated healthy PBMC (Stanilova et al, 2006). This cytokine possess anti-inflammatory and immunoregulatory role and it is no wonder that IL-10 play a dual role in tumor development and progression (Mocellin et al., 2003; Mocellin et al, 2004; Dranoff 2004; Lin and Karin, 2007). Contradictory results are present in the literature concerning IL-10 systemic or tissue levels and survival of cancer patients. For instance, Mocellin et al. found that IL-10 overexpression within the tumour microenvironment was implicated in cancer immune rejection.

Although IL-10 suppression of pro-inflammatory cytokines synthesis favors its anti-tumor immunity, it might also promote tumor growth by stimulating cell proliferation and inhibiting cell apoptosis. A high systemic level of IL-10 has been reported for advanced colorectal cancer patients (O'Hara et al., 1998; Galizia et al., 2002). Increased level of IL-10 might better control inflammatory responses and cancer development. Results from our study demonstrated a stage dependent association between IL-10 serum level and severity of CRC (Stanilov et al., 2010). The highest IL-10 serum level was found in stage-IV CRC patients, suggesting a pro-tumorigenic activity of systemic IL-10 in CRC progression and play a role in tumor-induced immunosupression in CRC patients. In addition, we determined a significantly increased mRNA in tumor tissue compared to normal mucosa (Stanilov et al., 2009). Moreover expression of IL-10 mRNA correlated positively with increased Foxp3 mRNA expression detected in tumor tissue. These results confirm the role of Foxp3 transcription factor in induction of IL-10 production and differentiation of Treg-1 cells in tumor microenvironment.

Cacev et al, 2008 reported a statistically significant decrease in IL-10 mRNA expression in tumor tissue then normal mucous depending on IL-10 SNPs. IL-10 promoter genotypes −819 TT and −592 AA associated with low IL-10 mRNA expression in tumor and corresponding normal mucosa. The 'low-producer genotypes' were present more frequently in colon cancer patients and this difference in genotype distribution was statistically significant. In the same study IL-10 -1082AA genotype was associated with lower IL-10 mRNA expression, whereas -1082GG genotype was associated with higher IL-10 mRNA expression in tumor tissue. In a group of colon cancer patients, an increased frequency of the -1082AA genotype compared with control group was observed without statistical significance. The authors conclude that IL-10-1082G/A SNP did not influence sporadic colon cancer susceptibility.

No associations were observed among colorectal cancer patients and controls for IL-10 -1082G/A and -592C/A genotype frequencies in a case-control study of 62 patients and 124 matched controls (Crivello et al., 2006). A possible reason for these contradictory results might be a small number of patients.

A recent study of Tsilidis K et al., 2009 investigated the association of 17 candidate SNPs in IL-10 with colorectal cancer in 208 patients. The authors established that -1082 promoter SNP is implicated. Compared with the AA genotype at the candidate IL10-1082 locus (rs1800896), carrying one or two G alleles, a known higher producer of the anti-inflammatory cytokine IL-10 was associated with lower risk of colorectal cancer (p = 0.03). Statistically significant associations with colorectal cancer were observed for three tagSNPs in IL10 (rs1800890, rs3024496, rs3024498) and one common haplotype, but these associations were due to high linkage disequilibrium with IL10-1082.

Associations between IL-10 genotypes and cancer chemopreventive strategies and survival were also published. Results of Macarthur et al. suggest that IL-10 SNPs may play a role in predicting response to chemopreventive strategies. Carriers of the IL-10-592A allele, had a statistically significant 50% reduced risk of colorectal cancer when taking regular aspirin, whereas risk was not reduced in carriers of the A allele who did not use aspirin, or among aspirin users with the CC genotype. It is possible that carriers of the IL-10-592C allele are more likely to derive chemopreventive benefits from aspirin in the presence of a lower production of their own endogenous anti-inflammatory interleukin-10 (Macarthur et al, 2005).

In particular proinflammatory genotypes characterized by a low IL-10 producer seem to be associated with a worse clinical outcome. Sharma et al. investigated the prognostic value of an inflammation-based Glasgow Prognostic Score in advanced colorectal cancer to explore a predictive pattern of cytokine gene polymorphisms for clinical outcome (Sharma et al., 2008). They found that IL-10-592A/C and IL-10 -1082A/G were predictive for overall survival. Patients homozygous for IL-10-592 CC had improved overall survival compared with those patients with ≥ 1 A allele (median survival, 12.2 ± 0.7 months vs. 8.6 ± 1.6 months). In contrast, patients homozygous for IL-10-1082 AA had poorer overall survival compared with patients with ≥ 1 G allele (median survival, 8.8 months ± 3.2 months vs. 11.2 ± 2.1 months).

Although the functional effects of polymorphisms in immunosuppressive genes TGFB and IL-10 have not yet been elucidated, obviously that they may play a significant role in modulating susceptibility, development and survival of colorectal cancer (Fig,1). The observation of increased circulating levels of IL-10 in colorectal cancer patients may have important implications for future investigations, immunological monitoring and therapeutic intervention on neoplastic patients, and suggests a mechanism for tumour cells escaping from immune surveillance.

Gene/ polymorphism	Genotype or allele associated with			
	Succeptibility - increased risk of CRC	Protection – decreased risk of CRC	Survival rate - Shorter survival	References
PROINFLAMMATORY				
IL-1B -511 C>T		TT ; CT		Ito et al., 2007
TNF-B	TNF-B*1/TNF-B*1			Park et al.,1998
TNF-A microsatellite	a2 allele	a5 and a13 allele		Gallager et al., 1997 ; DeJong et al, 2002
TNF-A- 238 G >A		AA and AG		Jang et al., 2001
IL6 −174G>C	C allele			Landi et al., 2003
			CC	Chung YC et al., 2006
		GG		Slattery M et al., 2007
ANTIINFLAMATORY				
TGFB1 -509C>T	−509TT			Berndt et al., 2007
TGFB1 Leu10Pro	10Pro/Pro			Berndt et al., 2007
TGFB1 -509C>T		−509TT		Amighofran Z et al., 2009
TGFB1 -509C>T		−509T allele		Chung et al., 2007
TGFB1 -509C>T		−509TT		Fang et al., 2010
IL-10 -1082 A>G		G allele		Tsilidis K et al., 2009
IL-10 -592 C> A	−592 AA			Cacev et al, 2008
IL-10 -819 C>T	−819 TT			Cacev et al, 2008
IL-10 -1082 A>G ; -592 C> A			IL-10 - 1082AA IL-10 - 592 AA	Sharma et al., 2008

Table 1. Involvement of IL-1; TNF, IL-6, IL-10 and TGF-β gene polymorphisms into colorectal cancer.

4. Role of IL-12-related cytokines

Human interleukin (IL)-12 (IL-12p70) is a disulfide-linked heterodimer composed of two subunits p40 and p35. IL-12p40 subunit can be secreted as monomer, which can also form IL-23, a heterodimeric pro-inflammatory cytokine composed of p40 and p19 subunits, and a homodimer, IL-12p80, which can act as an IL-12 and IL-23 antagonist by competing at their receptors (Hoelscher, 2004). The IL-12 family cytokines are produced by antigen-presenting cells such as macrophages and dendritic cells and play critical roles in the regulation of Th cell differentiation. IL-12 induces IFN-γ production by NK and T cells and differentiation to Th1 cells. IL-23 induces IL-17 production by memory T cells and expands and maintains inflammatory Th17 cells. IL-27 induces the early Th1 differentiation and generation of IL-10-producing regulatory T cells. Although IL-12p70 is one of the most powerful antitumor cytokine (Colombo and Trinchieri, 2002), accumulating evidence revealed that the individual members of the IL-12 family play distinct roles in the regulation of antitumor immune responses.

Several polymorphisms have been described in the IL12B gene, encoding IL-12p40 subunit, including a single-nucleotide polymorphism in 3'-untranslated region (UTR) of IL12B with number rs3212227 and a complex polymorphism in promoter region of the IL12B (IL12Bpro), resulting from 4bp microinsertion combined with an AA/GC transition (rs17860508). Moreover, several studies have demonstrated that these two polymorphisms affect gene expression and IL-12 production (Morahan et al., 2001; Seegers et al., 2002; Muller-Berghaus et al., 2004; Stanilova and Miteva, 2005; Stanilova et al., 2008; Dobreva et al., 2009) and consequently could influence the pathogenesis of CRC. To test this hypothesis, we performed a case-control study to investigate the association between these gene polymorphisms and the risk of colorectal cancer. The paper of Miteva et al., 2009 was the first study which investigated the distribution of IL12Bpro polymorphism and the +16974A/C SNP in 3'UTR of IL12B among 85 Bulgarian patients with colorectal cancer. No differences in genotype and allelic frequencies of the IL12B polymorphisms in the promoter and 3'UTR regions between patients with CRC and controls were found, either when patients were analyzed as a whole group or when they were separated according to the TNM classification or clinical characteristics such as tumor location, differentiation degree, lymph node and metastases status. These data are in principal agreement with other studies, where no association with SNP in 3'UTR of IL12B was found in pathogenesis of other related gastrointestinal diseases. Navaglia et al. have reported that none of the studied IL12B gene polymorphisms, including SNP in 3'UTR, was correlated with Helicobacter pylori infection and intestinal metaplasia (Navaglia et al., 2005). There was no statistically significant association between the SNPs investigated in IL-12A gene ((+7506 A>T, +8707 A>G, +9177 T>A, +9508 G>A) and colorectal cancer risk in the study of Landi et al., 2006. The lack of association suggests that the role of both investigated polymorphisms in IL12B in susceptibility of sporadic colorectal cancer can be excluded. However, these findings do not exclude a key role for IL-12p40 in development and progression of the CRC. In our investigations, we have demonstrated that serum levels for IL-12p40 and IL-23 were significantly higher in patients compared to healthy donors. Additionally, we found the highest level of IL-12p40 in sera from patients with I stage of CRC and significantly lower in patients with more advanced stages. (Miteva et al., 2009; Stanilov et al., 2009; Stanilov et al., 2010). In respect to recent findings regarding different proteins in IL-12 related family which share the p40 subunit, we could attribute the relationship of decreased serum level of IL-

12p40 and severity of CRC to the action of Th1-promoting form of IL-12, such as IL-12p70, or free IL-12p40 in monomeric and homodimeric form.

In a recent study there were significant differences in the genotype and allele frequencies of the IL-12 gene 16974 A/C polymorphism between the group of patients with glioma and the control group (Zhao et al., 2009). Moreover, genotypes carrying the IL-12 16974 C variant allele were associated with decreased serum IL-12p40 and IL-27p28 levels compared to the homozygous wild-type genotype in patients with glioma.

The promoter polymorphisms in the human IL12B gene could influence JNK and p38 MAPKs control of IL-12p40 expression in human PBMC in response to mitogens and proinflammatory stimuli. The study of Dobreva et al., revealed that JNK and p38 MAPK inhibition in PBMC stimulated with C3bgp and LPS, significantly upregulated the IL-12p40 production from IL12Bpro-1 homozygotes and did not influence the IL-12p40 production from 1.2/2.2 genotypes (Dobreva et al., 2009). Also, the p38 inhibition led to significant increase of IL-12p40 production in IL12Bpro-1 homozygous PBMC stimulated with PHA. IL-12p40 is secreted at a 50-fold excess compared with IL-12p70 in a murine shock model (Wysocka et al., 1995) and at a 10-20-fold excess by stimulated human peripheral blood mononuclear cells (D'Andrea et al., 1992). IL-12p40 chain may form also a homodimer IL-12p80 that serves as an IL-12p70 and IL-23 antagonist by competing for binding at the receptor complexes of both cytokines (Cooper & Khader, 2006). The proper balance between IL-12p40-related cytokines play a key immunoregulatory role and control the appearance of protective Th1-mediated immune response. Current results demonstrated an opposite effect of JNK and p38 MAPKs inhibition on the IL-12p70 and IL-23 production in LPS and C3bgp-stimulated PBMC (Dobreva et al., 2008).Our results demonstrated that p38 MAPK inhibition down regulates IL-23 and up regulates IL-12p40/p70 inducible expression suggesting the benefit of p38 control in the treatment of inflammatory conditions.

IL-12 related cytokines (IL-12p70; IL-12p40 and IL-23) produced locally or systemic exhibit a significant role in progression of CRC. Accumulating evidence revealed that the individual members of the IL-12 family play distinct roles in progression of CRC. Studies have defined IL-12p70 as an important factor for the differentiation of naive T cells into IFN-γ producing Th1 cells and exhibits anti-tumor activity (Brunda et al., 1995; Gri et al., 2002). Although the antitumor activities of IL-12p70 are well characterized, studies of the role of IL-23 in development of CRC in humans are contradictory. Some authors reported that IL-23, as well as IL-12p70, have anti-tumor activity in murine tumor models (Wang et al., 2003; Lo et al., 2003; Shan et al.,2006). Contradictory results have been reported in studies of Langowski et al., 2006 which showed data that IL-23 promotes tumor incidence and growth in various human cancers. In this respect our results for enhanced serum levels of IL-23 in cancer patients regardless of severity supported the hypothesis that IL-23 promotes tumor development unlike IL-12p70 (Stanilov et al., 2010). Besides, the highest increase in transcriptional activity in tumor samples for IL-23p19 mRNA has been also reported in our study (Stanilov et al., 2009). IL-23p19 mRNA was approximately 29 fold upregulated (p=0.0009), whereas IL-12p35 mRNA was not significantly upregulated, when compared to their adjacent normal tissue. This difference indicated that IL-23 could be synthesized many times more than IL-12p70 in tumor tissue. Based on our and others data, we could assume that increased serum and locally produced IL-23 indicates impaired anti-tumor immune response and could be associated with poor prognosis of CRC. A molecular mechanism involved in IL-23 activities includes STAT3 activation. STAT3 signaling within the tumor microenvironment was recently elucidated to induce a protumor cytokine, IL-17 and IL-22, while inhibiting a central antitumor cytokine, IL-12p70, thereby shifting the balance of tumor immunity toward tumorigenesis. Interestingly, unlike spleen Treg cells, tumor-associated Treg cells express IL-23R and activate STAT3 in response to IL-23, leading to upregulation of the Treg-specific transcription factor Foxp3 and the immunosuppressive cytokine IL-10 (Xu M et al., 2010). Collectively, IL-12 and IL-23 play critical roles in the regulation of antitumor or protumor response in respective situation.

5. Conclusion

In recent years, efforts have been made to identify genes involved in the genetic predisposition or progression of colorectal cancer. During the last two decades, many of the 'candidate' cytokine genes implicated in colorectal tumorigenesis have been identified and were summarized in this review. As cancer is a complex genetic disease, it is probable that besides oncogenes and tumor suppressor genes a number of cytokine genes also contribute to cancer susceptibility and development. Moreover cytokines are a key-player in inflammation, which have protumoral effect and mediated anti-tumor immune response. Cytokines present in tumor microenvironment have gained much attention due to their influence on cell activation, growth, differentiation or cell migration and they are increasingly recognized as potential cancer modifying genes. While numerous factors influence the inflammatory response in cancer, the role of an individual's genetic background has recently received increasing attention.

Cytokines and their receptors are often encoded by highly polymorphic genes. Single-nucleotide polymorphisms in cytokine genes potentially affect their production by either creating or eliminating key binding motifs within promoter and other regulatory sequences. In investigating disease–gene associations, there is a strong argument for focusing on polymorphisms of functional significance. Up to date contradictory results from case-control study have been published concerning cytokine gene polymorphisms and colorectal cancer development. Obviously reasons for such results included different numbers of patients; their ethnicity and differences in clinical and pathological data. In any case-control study, there are potential limitations. Despite the limitations of most published studies, the preliminary literature indicates that selected cytokine polymorphisms, particularly in IL-10; TGF-β; IL-6 and TNF-α are required in colorectal cancer. Data included in this review summarized in table1 suggest that functional cytokine polymorphisms participate more in the onset of colorectal cancer progression rather than in its initial development. Due to the strong evidence concerning the biological significance of these SNPs further studies and meta analysis are needed to evaluate the significance in the clinic. Careful selection of SNPs to cover the whole length of a candidate gene sequence so that areas of association can be defined and informative haplotypes constructed. Emerging genotyping technologies will facilitate such definitive, comprehensive studies.

The preliminary data indicate that larger studies are required to confirm or reject existing results, extend studies to include more detailed genotype and haplotype analysis, and combine genotype and gene expression studies in the same subjects. Even larger numbers of cases and controls would be required to demonstrate more modest odds ratios with higher statistical power. Collection of definitive clinical and pathological data for all cases must be an integral part of such an approach.

Such studies will contribute significantly to our understanding of the biological role of cytokine polymorphisms in colorectal cancer development.

6. References

Abraham LJ, & Kroeger KM. (1999) Impact of the −308 TNF promoter polymorphism on the transcriptional regulation of the TNF gene: relevance to disease. *J Leukoc Biol*, 66:pp562–566.

Amirghofran Z., Jalali SA, Ghaderi A, & Hosseini SV. (2009) Genetic polymorphism in the transforming growth factor β1 gene (-509 C/T and -800G/A) and colorectal cancer. *Cancer genetics and cytogenetics*, 190:pp21-25

Belluco C, Olivieri F, Bonafe M, Giovagnetti S, Mammano E, Scalerta R, Ambrosi A, Franceschi C, Nitti D, & Lise M. (2003) −174 G>C polymorphism of interleukin 6 gene promoter affects interleukin 6 serum level in patients with colorectal cancer. *Clin Cancer Res*; 9:pp2173–2176.

Berndt S, Huang WY, Chatterjee N, Yeager M, Welch R, Chanock S, Weissfeld J, Schoen R &. Hayes R. (2007) Transforming growth factor beta 1 (TGFB1) gene polymorphisms and risk of advanced colorectal adenoma, *Carcinogenesis*, 28 pp.1965–1970,

Bidwell J, Keen L, Gallagher G, Kimberly R, Huizinga T, McDermott MF, Oksenberg J, McNicholl J, Pociot F, Hardt C & D'Alfonso S. (1999) Cytokine gene polymorphism in human disease: on-line databases. *Genes and immunity* 1:3-19

Bonafe M., Olivieri F., & Cavallone L., Giovagnetti S., Marchegiani F., Cardelli M., Pieri C., Marra M., Antonicelli R., Lisa R., Rizzo M. R., Paolisso G., Monti D., Franceschi C. (2001) A. gender-dependent genetic predisposition to produce high levels of IL-6 is detrimental for longevity. Eur. J. Immunol., 31: pp2357-2361.

Brunda MJ, Luistro L, Hendrzak JA, Fountoulakis M, Garotta G, & Gately MK (1995) Role of interferon-γ in mediating the antitumor efficacy of interleukin-12. *J Immunother*, 17: pp71-77.

Cacev T, Jokić M, Loncar B, Krizanac S, & Kapitanović S. (2010) Interleukin-6-174 G/C polymorphism is not associated with IL-6 expression and susceptibility to sporadic colon cancer. *DNA Cell Biol.*; 29(4):177-82.

Cacev T, Radosevic S, Krizanac S, & Kapitanovic S. (2008) Influence of interleukin-8 and interleukin-10 on sporadic colon cancer development and progression. *Carcinogenesis*; 29:pp1572-1580

Chung Y.C. & Y.F. Chang, (2003), Serum interleukin-6 levels reflect the disease status of colorectal cancer, *J. Surg. Oncol.* 83: pp. 222–226.

Chung YC., Chaen YL & Hsu CP. (2006) Clinical significance of tissue expression of interleukin-6 in colorectal carcinoma. *Anticancer Res.* 26:pp3905-3911.

Chung SJ, Kim JS, Jung HC, & Song IS. (2007) Transforming growth factor-β1 509T reduces risk of colorectal cancer, but not adenoma in Koreans. *Cancer Sci.* 98:pp401–404

Colombo M. P. & G. Trinchieri. (2002) Interleukin-12 in anti-tumor immunity and immunotherapy. *Cytokine and growth factor Reviews*, 13: pp155-168,

Cooper, A.M. & Khader, S.A. (2006) IL-12p40: an inherently agonistic cytokine. Trends Immunol. 28, pp33-38.

Corvinus FM, Orth C, Moriggl R, Tsareva SA, Wagner S, Pfitzner EB, Baus D, Kaufmann R, Huber LA, Zatloukal K, Beug H, Ohlschläger P, Schütz A, Halbhuber KJ, & Friedrich K. (2005) Persistent STAT3 activation in colon cancer is associated with enhanced cell proliferation and tumor growth. *Neoplasia*. 7:pp545-55.

Crawley E, Kay R, Sillibourne J, Patel P, Hutchinson I, & Woo P. (1999) Polymorphic haplotypes of the interleukin-10 5'flanking region determine variable interleukin-10 transcription and are associated with particular phenotypes of juvenile rheumatoid arthritis. *Arthritis Rheum*; 42, pp1101-1108.

Crivello A, Giacalone A, Vaglica M, Scola L, Forte GI, Macaluso MC, Raimondi C, Di Noto L, Bongiovanni A, Accardo A, Candore G, Palmeri L, Verna R, Caruso C, Lio D, & Palmeri S. (2006) Regulatory cytokine gene polymorphisms and risk of colorectal carcinoma. *Ann N Y Acad Sci.*, 1089:pp98–103

D'Andrea, A., Rengaraju, M., Valiante, N.M., Chehimi, J., Kubin, M., Aste, M., Chan, S.H., Kobayashi, M., Young, D., Nickbarg, E., Chizzonite, R., Wolf, S.F., & Trinchieri, G. (1992) Production of natural killer cell stimulatory factor (NKSF/IL-12) by peripheral blood mononuclear cells. *J. Exp. Med.* 176,pp 1387-1398.

D'Alfonso S, Rampi M, Rolando V, Giordano M, & Momigliano-Richiardi P (2000) New polymorphisms in the IL-10 promoter region. *Genes Immun* 1:pp231-233.

De Jong MM, Nolte IM, te Meerman GJ, van der Graaf WT, de Vries EG, Sijmons RH, Hofstra RM, & Kleibeuker JH. (2002) Low-penetrance genes and their involvement in colorectal cancer susceptibility. *Cancer Epidemiol Biomarkers Prev* 11:pp1332-1352

Dobreva Z. Stanilova S. & Miteva L. (2008) Differences in the inducible gene expression and protein production of IL-12p40, Il-12p70 and IL-23: involvement of p38 and JNK kinase pathways. *Cytokine*, 43:pp76-82

Dobreva Z., Stanilova S, & Miteva L. (2009) Influence of JNK and p38 MAPKs inhibition on IL-12p40 and IL-23 production depending on IL12B promoter polymorphism. *Cell Mol Biol Lett,* , 14: pp609-621

Dranoff G (2004) Cytokines in cancer pathogenesis and cancer therapy. *Nat Rev Cancer*, 4: pp11-22.

Duch CR, Figueiredo MS, Ribas C, Almeida MS, Colleoni GW, & Bordin JO. (2007) Analysis of polymorphism at site −174 G/C of interleukin-6 promoter region in multiple myeloma. *Braz J Med Biol Res.* 40:pp265-267.

Elliott RL, Blobe GC. (2005) Role of transforming growth factor h in human cancer. *J Clin Oncol*; 23: pp2078–93.

El-Omar EM, Carrington M, Chow WH, McColl KE, Bream JH, Young HA, Herrera J, Lissowska J, Yuan CC, Rothman N, Lanyon G, Martin M, Fraumeni JF Jr, & Rabkin CS. (2000) Interleukin-1 polymorphisms associated with increased risk of gastric cancer. *Nature* 404: pp398-402,

El-Omar EM, Rabkin CS, Gammon MD, Vaughan TL, Risch HA, Schoenberg JB, Stanford JL, Mayne ST, Goedert J, Blot WJ, Fraumeni JF Jr, & Chow WH. (2003) Increased risk of noncardia gastric cancer associated with proinflammatory cytokine gene polymorphisms. *Gastroenterology*; 124: pp1193–1201.

Esfandi F, Mohammadzadeh Ghobadloo S, & Basati G. (2006) Interleukin-6 level in patients with colorectal cancer. *Cancer Lett.* 244: pp76-78

Eskdale J & Galager G (1995) A polymorphic dinucleotide repeat in the human IL- 10 promoter region. *Immunogenetics* 42: pp444-445.

Eskdale J, Kube D, Tesch H, & Gallagher G (1997) Mapping of the human IL10 gene and further characterization of the 5' flanking sequence. *Immunogenetics* 46:pp120-128

European Bioinformatics Institute, Sanger Institute. SNP database: Ensembl Genome Browser. 2006. Available at: http://www.ensembl.org/index.html.

Fang F, Yu L, Zhong Y, & Yao L. (2010) TGFB1 509 C/T polymorphism and colorectal cancer risk: a meta-analysis. *Med Oncol. Dec*; 27: pp1324-1328.

Fishman D, Faulds G, Jeffery R, Mohamed-Ali V, Yudkin JS, Humphries S, & Woo P. (1998) The effect of novel polymorphisms in the interleukin-6 (IL-6) gene on IL-6 transcription and plasma IL-6 levels, and an association with systemic-onset juvenile chronic arthritis. *J Clin Invest.*; 102:pp1369-1376

Friedman E, Gold LI, Klimstra D, Zeng ZS, Winawer S, & Cohen A. (1995) High levels of transforming growth factor β1 correlate with disease progression in human colon cancer. *Cancer Epidemiol Biomarkers Prev*, 4:pp549-554

Galizia G, Orditura M, Romano C, Lieto E, Castellano P, Pelosio L, Imperatore V, Catalano G, Pignatelli C, & De Vita F. (2002) Prognostic significance of circulating IL-10 and IL-6 serum levels in colon cancer patients undergoing surgery. *Clin Immunol*, 102: pp169-178,.

Gallagher, G., Lindemann, M., Oh, H. H., Ferencik, S., Walz, M. K.,Schmitz, A., Richards, S., Eskdale, J., Field, M., & Grosse-Wilde, H. (1997) Association of the TNFa2 microsatellite allele with the presence of colorectal cancer. *Tissue Antigens*, 50: pp47-51,.

Grainger DJ, Heathcote K, Chiano M, Snieder H, Kemp PR, Metcalfe JC, (1999) Genetic control of the circulating concentration of transforming growth factor type β1. *Hum Mol Genet.*; 8:pp93-97

Gri G, Chiodoni C, Gallo E, Stoppacciaro A, Liew F, & Colombo M (2002) Antitumor effect of Interleukin (IL)-12 in the absence of endogeneous IFN-γ: a role for intrinsic tumor immunogenicity and IL-15. *Cancer Res*, 62: pp4390-4397.

GunterM, Canzian F, Landi S, Chanock S, Sinha R, & Rothman N. (2006) Inflammation-Related Gene Polymorphisms and Colorectal Adenoma. *Cancer Epidemiol Biomarkers Prev*, 15: pp1126-1131

Hoelscher, C. (2004) The power of combinatorial immunology: IL-12 and IL-12-related dimeric cytokines in infectious diseases. *Med Microbiol Immunol.*, 193, pp1-17.

Hollegaard MV & Bidwell JL, (2006) Cytokine gene polymorphism in human disease: on-line databases, Supplement 3. *Genes Immun.*, 7:pp269-76.

Howell,W.M & Matthew J. Rose-Zerilli. (2007) Cytokine gene polymorphisms, cancer susceptibility, and prognosis. *J. Nutr.*, 137, pp194-199.

Huang 5., DeGuzman A., Bucana C. D., & Fidler I. J. (2000) Nuclear factor-kB activity correlates with growth, angiogenesis, and metastasis of human melanoma cells in nude mice. *Clin. Cancer. Res.*, 6: pp2573-2578.

Hussain SP, Harris CC, Inflammation and cancer: an ancient link with novel potentials. *Int. J. Cancer* 2007;121:pp2373-2380.

Hwang IR, Kodama T, Kikuchi S, Sakai K, Peterson LE, Graham DY, &Yamaoka Y. (2002) Effect of interleukin 1 polymorphisms on gastric mucosal interleukin 1β production in Helicobacter pylori infection. *Gastroenterology*; 123:pp1793-803.

Ito H, Kaneko K, Makino R, Konishi K, Kurahashi T, Yamamoto T, Katagiri A, Kumekawa Y, Kubota Y, Muramoto T, Mitamura K, & Imawari M (2007) Interleukin-1beta gene in esophageal, gastric and colorectal carcinomas. *Oncol Rep*. 18:pp473-81.

Jang WH, Yang YI, Yea SS et al (2001) The −238 tumor necrosis factor-alpha promoter polymorphism is associated with decreased susceptibility to cancers. *Cancer Lett* 166:pp41-46

Jobin C & Sartor B, (2000) The IκB/NF-κB system: a key determinant of mucosal inflammation and protection. *Am J Physiol Cell Physiol*, 278 ppC451-C462

Landi S, Gemignani F., Bottari F., Gioia-Patricola L, Guino E, Cambray M, Biondo S, Capella G, Boldrini L, Canzian F & Moreno V. (2006) Polymorphisms within inflammatory genes and colorectal cancer. *Journal of Negative Results in BioMedicine*, 5:pp5-15

Landi S, Moreno V, Gioia-Patricola L, Guino E, Navarro M, de Oca J, Capella G, & Canzian F; Bellvitge Colorectal Cancer Study Group (2003). Association of common polymorphisms in inflammatory genes interleukin (IL)6, IL8, tumor necrosis factor alpha, NFKB1, and peroxisome proliferator-activated receptor gamma with colorectal cancer. *Cancer Res*, 63:pp3560-3566.

Langowski JL, Zhang X, Wu L, Mattson JD, Chen T, Smith K, Basham B, McClanahan T, Kastelein RA, & Oft M (2006) IL-23 promotes tumor incidence and growth. *Nature*, 442: pp461-465.

Lin W, & Karin M (2007) A cytokine-mediated link between innate immunity, inflammation and cancer. *J Clin Invest*, 117: pp1175-1183.

Lo CH, Lee SC, Wu PY, Pan WY, Su J, Cheng CW, Roffler SR, Chiang BL, Lee CN, Wu CW, & Tao MH (2003) Antitumor and antimetastatic activity of IL-23. *J Immunol*, 171: pp600-607.

Macarthur M., Georgina L. Hold, & Emad M. El-Omar (2004) Inflammation and Cancer II. Role of chronic inflammation and cytokine gene polymorphisms in the pathogenesis of gastrointestinal malignancy. *Am J Physiol Gastrointest Liver Physiol* 286: ppG515-G520

Macarthur M, Sharp L, Hold GL, Little J, & El-Omar EM. (2005) The role of cytokine gene polymorphisms in colorectal cancer and their interaction with aspirin use in northeast of Scotland. *Cancer Epidemiol Biomarkers Prev.*;14:pp1623-1628.

Miteva L, Stanilov N, Deliysky T, Mintchev N, & Stanilova S. (2009) Association of polymorphisms in regulatory regions of interleukin-12p40 gene and cytokine serum level with colorectal cancer. *Cancer Investigation*, , 27:pp924-931

Mocellin S, Maricola FM, & Young HA: (2004) Interleukin-10 and the immune response against cancer: a counterpoint. *J Leukoc Biol*, 78: pp1043-1051.

Mocellin S, Panelli MC, Wang E, Nagorsen D, & Marincola FM (2003) The dual role of IL-10. *Trends Immunol*, 24: pp36-43.

Moore KW, de Waal MR, Coffman RL, & O'Garra A. (2001) Interleukin-10 and the interleukin-10 receptor. *Annu Rev Immunol*, 19:pp683-765.

Morahan, G.; Huang, D.; Wu, M.; Holt, B.J.; White, G.P.; Kendall, G.E.; Sly, P.D.; Holt, P.G. (2002) Association of IL12B promoter polymorphism with severity of atopic and non-atopic asthma in children. *Lancet.*, 360, pp455-459.

Morahan, G.; Huang, D.; Ymer, S.I.; Cancilla, M.R.; Stephen, K.; Dabadghao, P.; Werther, G.; Tait, B.D.; Harrison, L.C.; & Colman, P.G. (2001) Linkage disequilibrium of a type 1 diabetes susceptibility locus with a regulatory IL12B allele. *Nat Genet.*, 27, pp218-221.

Moustakas A, Pardali K, Gaal A, & Heldin CH. (2002) Mechanisms of TGF-β signaling in regulation of cell growth and differentiation. *Immunol Lett*, 82:pp85-91

Muller-Berghaus, J.; Kern, K.; Paschen, A.; Nguyen, X.D.; Klüter, H.; Morahan, G. & Schadendorf, D. (2004) Deficient IL-12p70 secretion by dendritic cells based on IL12B promoter genotype. *Genes Immun.*, 5, pp 431-434.

Nakagoe T., Tsuji T., Sawai T., Tanaka K., Hidaka S. & S. Shibasaki. (2003) Increased serum levels of interleukin-6 in malnourished patients with colorectal cancer, Cancer Lett. 202: pp. 109–115.

Navaglia, F.; Basso, D.; Zambon, C.F.; Ponzano, E.; Caenazzo, L.; Gallo, N.; Falda, A.; Belluco, C.; Fogar, P.; Greco, E.; Di Mario, F.; Rugge, M.; & Plebani, M. (2005) Interleukin 12 gene polymorphisms enhance gastric cancer risk in H pylori infected individuals. *J Med Genet.*, 42, pp 503-510.

Nusrat A., Sitaraman S. V., & Neish A. (2001) Interaction of bacteria and bacterial toxins with intestinal epithelial cells. *Curr. Gastroenterol. Rep.*, 3: pp392-398.

O'Hara RJ, Greenman J, MacDonald AW, Gaskell KM, Topping KP, Duthie GS, Kerin MJ, Lee PW, & Monson JR (1998) Advanced colorectal cancer is associated with impared interleukin 12 and enhanced interleukin 10 production. *Clin Cancer Res*, 4: pp1943-1948,.

Park KS, Mok JW, Rho SA & Kim JC (1998) Analysis of TNFB and TNFA NcoI RFLP in colorectal cancer. *Mol Cells* 8:pp246–249

Parkin DM (2001) Global cancer statistics in the year 2000. *Lancet Oncol* 2:533–543

Pociot, F., Briant, L., Jongeneel, C. V., Molvig, J., Worsaae, H., Abbal, M., Thomsen, M., Nerup, J., & Cambon-Thomsen, A. (1993) Association of tumor necrosis factor (TNF) and class II major histocompatibility complex alleles with the secretion of TNF-α and TNF-β by human mononuclear cells: a possible link to insulin-dependent diabetes mellitus. *Eur. J. Immunol.*, 23: pp224–231.

Schulte CM, Goebell H, & Roher HD (2001) C-509T polymorphism in the TGF-β1 gene promoter: impact on Crohn's disease susceptibility and clinical course? *Immunogenetics* 53:pp178–182

Schuster N, & Krieglstein K. (2002) Mechanisms of TGF-hmediated apoptosis. *Cell Tissue Res*; 307:pp1–14.

Seegers, D.; Zwiers, A.; Strober, W.; Pena, A.S.; & Bouma, G. (2002) A TaqI polymorphism in the 3′ UTR of the IL-12 p40 gene correlates with increased IL-12 secretion. Genes Immun., 3, pp 419-423.

Shan B, Hao J, & Li Q, & Tagawa M (2006) Antitumor activity and immune enhancement of murine interleukin-23 expressed in murine colon carcinoma cells. *Cell Mol Immunol*, 3: pp47-52.

Sharma R, Zucknick M, London R, Kacevska M, Liddle C, & Clarke SJ. (2008) Systemic inflammatory response predicts prognosis in patients with advanced-stage colorectal cancer. *Clin Colorectal Cancer.*, 7:pp331–337

Slattery ML, Wolff RK, Herrick JS, Caan BJ, & Potter JD (2007) IL6 genotypes and colon and rectal cancer. *Cancer Causes Control.*; 18:pp1095-1105.

Stanilov N, Miteva L, Mintchev N, & Stanilova S. (2009) High expression of Foxp3, IL-23p19 and surviving mRNA in colorectal carcinoma. *International Journal of Colorectal Disease*, 24: pp151-157.

Stanilov N., Miteva L, Deliyski T, Jovchev J, & Stanilova S. (2010) Advanced colorectal cancer is assosiated with enhanced Interleukin-23 and Interleukin -10 serum level. *LabMedicine*, 41 :pp 159-163

Stanilova, S. & Miteva, L. (2005) Taq-I polymorphism in 3′UTR of the IL-12 and association with IL-12p40 production from human PBMC. *Genes Immun.*, 6, pp364-366.

Stanilova, S.; Miteva, L.; & Prakova, G. (2008) IL-12Bpro and GSTP1 polymorphisms in association with silicosis. *Tissue Antigens.*, 71, pp 169-174.

Steven H. Itzkowitz & Xianyang Yio. (2004) Inflammation and Cancer IV. Colorectal cancer in inflammatory bowel disease: the role of inflammation . *Am J Physiol Gastrointest Liver Physiol* 287: ppG7–G17.

Su JL, Lai KP, Chen CA, Yang CY, Chen PS, Chang C, Chou CH, Hu CL, Kuo ML, Hsieh CY & Wei LH (2005) A novel peptide specifically binding to interleukin-6 receptor (gp 80) inhibits angiogenesis and tumor growth. *Cancer Res,* 65: pp 4827-4835.

Sugimoto M, Furuta T, Shira N, Nakamura A, Kajimura M, Sugimura H, & Hishida A. (2007) Effects of interleukin-10 gene polymorphism on the development of gastric cancer and peptic ulcer in Japanese subjects. *Journal of Gastroenterology and Hepatology.*, 22: pp1443-1449.

Swantek JL, Cobb MH, & Gepperd DT. (1997) Jun N-Terminal Kinase/Stress – Activated Protein Kinase (JNK/SAPK) Is Required for Lipopolysaccharide Stimulation of Tumor necrosis factor alpha (TNF-α) Translation: Glucocorticoids Inhibit TNF-α Translation by blocking JNK/SAPK. *Mol Cell Biol.*; 17: pp6274-6282.

Sweet MJ, & Hume DA. (1996) Endotoxin signal transduction in macrophages. *J. Leukoc. Biol.*; 60:8-26.

Terry C. F., Loukaci V., & Green F. R. (2000) Cooperative influence of genetic polymorphisms on interleukin 6 transcriptional regulation. *J. Biol. Chem.*, 275: pp18138-18144.

Theodoropoulos G, Papaconstantinou I, Felekouras E, Nikiteas N, Karakitsos P, Panoussopoulos D, Ch Lazaris A, Patsouris E, Bramis J, & Gazouli M. (2006) Relation between common polymorphisms in genes related to inflammatory response and colorectal cancer. *World J Gastroenterol*; 12: pp5037-5043

Tsilidis KK, Helzlsouer KJ, Smith MW, Grinberg V, Hoffman-Bolton J, Clipp SL, Visvanathan K, & Platz EA. (2009) Association of common polymorphisms in IL10, and in other genes related to inflammatory response and obesity with colorectal cancer. *Cancer Causes Control.* 20:pp1739-51.

Turner DM, Williams DM, Sankaran D, Lazarus M, Sinnott PJ, & Hutchinson IV. (1997) An investigation of polymorphism in the interleukin-10 gene promoter. *Eur J Immunogenetics*; 24:pp1-8.

Wang YQ, Ugai S, Shimozato O, Yu L, Kawamura K, Yamamoto H, Yamaguchi T, Saisho H, & Tagawa M (2003) Induction of systemic immunity by expression of interleukin-23 in murine colon carcinoma cells. *Int J Cancer*, 105: pp820-824.

Watanabe Y, Kinoshita A, Yamada T, Ohta T, Kishino T, Matsumoto N, Ishikawa M, Niikawa N, & Yoshiura K. (2002) A catalog of 106 single nucleotide polymorphisms (SNPs) and 11 other types of variations in genes for transforming growth factor- 1 (TGF- 1) and its signaling pathway. *J Hum Genet* 47:pp 478-483.

Waterston A, & Bower M. (2004) TNF and cancer: good or bad? *Cancer therapy*; 2: pp131-148.

Wilkening S, Tavelin B, Canzian F, Enquist K, Palmqvist R, Altieri A, Hallmans G, Hemminki K, Lenner P, & Försti A. (2008) Interleukin promoter polymorphisms and prognosis in colorectal cancer. *Carcinogenesis*; 29:pp1202 6.

Wong SF,& Lai LC. (2001) The role of TGFβ in human cancers. *Pathology*; 33:85–92

Wysocka, M., Kubin, M., Vieira, L.Q., Ozmen, L., Garotta, G., Scott, P. & Trinchieri, G. (1995) Interleukin 12 is required for interferon-γ production and lethality in lipopolysaccharide-induced shock in mice. *Eur. J. Immunol.* 25,pp 672-676

Xu M, Mizoguchi I, Morishima N, Chiba Y, Mizuguchi J, & Yoshimoto T, Regulation of Antitumor Immune Responses by the IL-12 Family Cytokines, IL-12, IL-23, and IL-27. (2010) *Clinical and Developmental Immunology.* Volume 2010, Article ID 832454, doi:10.1155/2010/832454

Xu Y, & Pasche B. (2007) TGF-β signaling alterations and susceptibility to colorectal cancer. *Hum Mol Genet,* 15:ppR14–R2016

Yao, J.; Mackman, N.; Edgington, T. S., & Fan, S. T. (1997) Lipopolysaccharide induction of the tumor necrosis factor - alpha promoter in human monocytic cells. Regulation by Egr-1, c-Jun and NF-kappa B transcription factors. *J. Biol. Chem.,* 272: pp17795-17801.

Yu H. & R. Jove. The stats of cancer—new molecular targets come of age, (2004) *Nature Reviews Cancer,* vol. 4, pp. 97–105.

Zhao B, Meng LQ, Huang HN, Pan Y & Xu Q. A (2009) Novel Functional Polymorphism, 16974 A/C, in the Interleukin-12-3' Untranslated Region Is Associated with Risk of Glioma. DNA and Cell Biology. 28: pp335-341.

3

Germline Genetics in Colorectal Cancer Susceptibility and Prognosis

Amanda Ewart Toland
*The Ohio State University,
USA*

1. Introduction

Population-based studies indicate that approximately 35% of an individual's risk of developing colorectal cancer (CRC) is due to inherited genetic factors (Lichtenstein et al. 2000). Indeed, approximately 50,000 individuals diagnosed with CRC in the United States each year will have at least one other family member with CRC (Kaz & Brenthall, 2006). Classically, genetic susceptibility to CRC is described as three types: Low, moderate and high risk. In reality, the risk of developing colorectal cancer due to genetic factors exists on a continuum from very low to very high risk (Figure 1). In addition to colon cancer susceptibility, genetic variants are likely to play a role in response to therapy and prognosis of colon cancer. This Chapter will provide an overview of the current knowledge in genetic susceptibility to hereditary and non-hereditary CRC, the complexities and issues around the identification of germline genetic risk factors, and the current and future use of genetic information in the clinic.

High penetrance risk includes inheritance of mutations in genes which segregate in a Mendelian fashion in families and confer a high lifetime risk of disease. Hereditary cancer syndromes are those in which a mutation confers a high lifetime risk of developing CRC. Several syndromes have been described. The two most familiar CRC syndromes are Familial Adenomatous Polyposis (FAP) and Lynch Syndrome (LS) (Table 1). Moderately-penetrant mutations are mutations or polymorphic variants which can manifest as colon cancer clustering in families but without a clear cancer syndrome or inheritance pattern. Low-penetrance variants are those which are present in a reasonably high frequency in the general population, but have small influences on risk and are not themselves sufficient for the development of colon cancer.

2. Hereditary colorectal cancer syndromes

Hereditary colorectal cancer syndromes are those in which an inherited or de novo germline mutation confers a high lifetime risk of developing CRC. Approximately 5% of all CRC diagnoses are thought to be due to highly penetrant mutations (Bodmer, 2006; de la Chapelle, 2004). These familial mutations were the first germline genetic alterations to be discovered to be important for CRC risk. Several syndromes have been described. They can be subdivided into syndromes with adenomatous polyps, those with hamartomatous polyps and syndromes with polyps of mixed histopathology (Table 1). Syndromes that present with a few or many adenomatous polyps include FAP, LS and MUTYH-associated polyposis (MAP) (Table 1). The hamartomatous polyp syndromes include Cowden Syndrome, Juvenile Polyposis and Peutz-Jeghers Syndrome. Not all genes contributing to hereditary CRC have been identified and characterized. It is likely as genome-wide and exonic sequencing become more common that additional rare mutations leading to hereditary colorectal cancer will be discovered.

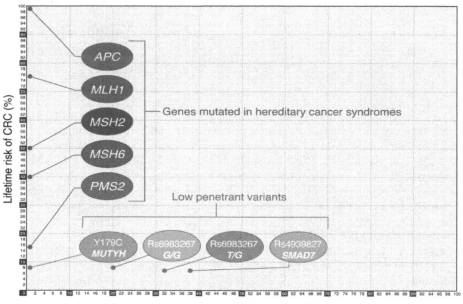

Frequency in the population (%)

Fig. 1. Genes and variants associated with CRC risk. The allele frequency and lifetime risk of genes associated with familial colorectal cancer (red) and variants associated with a small increase in lifetime risk of CRC (blue) are illustrated. (The Y179C variant is associated with a low risk of CRC when individuals only carry one mutated *MUTYH* allele.)

One common feature of all of these CRC syndromes is that the age of diagnosis of cancer tends to be much earlier than that in the general population. Typically colorectal cancer occurs 10-20 years earlier in individuals with these syndromes than in the general population. In individuals who carry a mutation in one of these hereditary CRC genes there is also considerable increased risk, up to 99%, of developing colon cancer. Individuals with most of these syndromes have detectable polyps prior to the onset of colorectal cancer; however many probands that were not undergoing regular screening are brought to attention following a diagnosis of CRC.

A clinical diagnosis of a specific cancer syndrome can be made based on an extensive family history in combination with histological and pathological information about the number and type of polyps. More definitive diagnoses are made by genetic testing coordinated through a genetic counsellor or medical geneticist of an affected proband, or, in the case of LS, analysis of tumours for loss of one of the LS-related proteins. Even though individually these syndrome are rare, proper management and diagnoses can impact the incidence and mortality related to CRC. Because mutations leading to these genes confer a high lifetime risk of CRC, knowledge of one's family history and mutation status influences medical management and can significantly reduce the incidence of CRC.

Syndrome	CRC Risk	Unique characteristics	Other features	Gene(s)
HNPCC	20-75%*	Microsatellite instability of tumors	Endometrial, gastric, ovarian, small bowel, biliary & urothelial ca	MSH1, MLH2, PMS2, MSH6 EPCAM
FAP	99%	Hundreds of polyps	Desmoids, hepatoblastoma & papillary thyroid ca, CHRPE	APC
Peutz-Jeghers	39%	Hamartomatous polyps	Gastric, breast, & ovarian ca, sex cord tumors, mucocutaneous hyperpigmentation	LKB1 (STK11)
MAP	80%	Recessive inheritance, many adenomatous polyps	Two common mutations in individuals with Northern European ancestry: Y179C and G396D	MUTYH (MYH)
Hereditary Mixed Polyposis	ND	Inflammatory & metaplastic polyps		BMPR1A
Cowden	None	Hamartomatous polyps	Macrocephaly, benign & malignant thryoid, breast & uterine neoplasms	PTEN
Juvenile Polyposis	39%	Hamartomatous polyps	GI polyps, gastric ca	SMAD4, BMPR1A,

Table 1. Hereditary Colon Cancer and Polyposis Syndromes. ca, cancer; CHRPE, congenital hypertrophy of the retinal pigment epithelium; ND, not determined; GI, gastrointestinal; *CRC risk depends on which gene is mutated.

2.1 Hereditary non-polyposis colorectal cancer/lynch syndrome

Hereditary non-polyposis colorectal cancer (HNPCC), also known as Lynch syndrome (LS), is the most common hereditary CRC syndrome associated with a strong family history of colon cancer. Approximately 2-4% of all colon cancers are due to LS (Hampel et al., 2008). Although individuals with LS frequently have adenomatous polyps, individuals with this syndrome do not have polyposis. In addition to a lifetime risk of approximately 50-80% for colorectal cancer, there is an increased risk of ovarian, endometrial and gastric cancers (Jasperson et al., 2010). Since the genes have been identified, some conditions which were once thought to be distinct (e.g. Muir-Torre syndrome which is characterized by familial

CRC with sebaceous neoplasms and Turcot syndrome which is characterized by CRC with glioblastomas) are variants of LS. LS is inherited in an autosomal dominant fashion and is associated with mutations in four genes important in mismatch repair (MMR): *MLH1*, *MSH2*, *PMS2* and *MSH6*. Tumours arising in individuals with germline mutations in these genes, which are important for DNA repair, typically exhibit microsatellite instability which is sometimes used clinically to aid in a diagnosis. The most commonly mutated genes in LS are *MLH1* and *MSH2*. Recently, deletions of the 3'end of *EPCAM*, a gene mapping 5' of the *MSH2* gene, have been found to give rise to LS by causing methylation of the *MSH2* gene in about 6% of LS cases (Niessen et al., 2009a).

Criteria based on family history, Amsterdam I, Amsterdam II and Bethesda criteria, were developed in order to identify families for further evaluation of Lynch syndrome. Amsterdam I criteria, the first described, includes three first degree relatives with CRC, two or more generations affected, one family member with CRC diagnosed under the age of 50 and FAP must be ruled out (Vasen et al., 1991). Amsterdam II criteria are the same as Amsterdam I except that endometrial, small bowel or other LS-related cancers can be substituted for CRC (Vasen et al., 1999). Revised Bethesda criteria include one CRC diagnosed under the age of 50, one CRC under the age of 60 with evidence of microsatellite instability, CRC or LS-related cancer in at least one first degree relative under the age of fifty or CRC or LS-related cancers in at least two first or second degree relatives at any age (Umar et al., 2004). In addition, three online prediction programs MMRpredict, PREMM, and MMRpro have been developed to identify families with LS. Sensitivities of the online models and revised Bethesda criteria are about 75% with a range of specificity from 50-60%; the Amsterdam II criteria have a lower sensitivity of 37.5%, but a better specificity of 99% (Tresallet et al., 2011). Many hospitals have begun to screen all colon cancer cases by immunohistochemistry for loss of the four MMR proteins or for microsatellite instability regardless of family history which has a higher sensitivity than the family history based models (Hampel et al., 2008). Individuals whose tumours show absence of MLH1, MSH2, PMS2 and MSH6 and/or microsatellite instability are referred for genetic evaluation of LS and, in some cases, additional testing to rule out somatic events specific to the tumours which lead to loss of the proteins.

The risk and spectrum of cancer depends on which LS gene is mutated. The lifetime colon cancer risk is 97% for males and 53% for females with germline *MLH1* mutations. Endometrial cancer risk associated with *MLH1* mutations ranges from 25 to 33% (Ramsoekh et al., 2009; Stoffel et al., 2009). The lifetime risk of CRC in male *MSH2* mutation carriers is 52% and is 40% for females. There is a 44-49% risk of endometrial cancer for female *MSH2* mutation carriers (Stoffel et al., 2009). About 10% of Lynch syndrome families have a mutation in *MSH6* (Talseth-Palmer et al., 2010). The estimated risk of colorectal cancer in individuals with a *MLH6* mutation is lower than some of the other mutations at 30-61% and the risk of endometrial cancer is higher with 65-70% of females developing endometrial cancer by the age of 70 (Talseth-Palmer et al., 2010; Ramsoekh et al., 2009). *PMS2* mutations are less frequently the cause of LS accounting for only 2 to 14% of LS cases (Senter et al., 2008; Niessen et al., 2009b; Talseth-Palmer et al., 2010). The cumulative risk by the age of 70 of developing a colon cancer in mono-allelic *PMS2* mutation carriers is 15-20%, endometrial cancer is 15% and other Lynch-related cancers is from 25-32% (Senter et al., 2008). Bi-allelic mutations in the MMR genes have been observed and lead to a severe phenotype with childhood brain tumours, leukaemia, and LS-associated tumors known as Constitutional MMR Deficiency (Senter et al., 2008; Felton et al., 2007; Wimmer & Kratz, 2010). *EPCAM* deletions show a comparable risk of colon cancer to *MLH1* and *MSH2* mutation carriers, but a decreased risk of endometrial cancer. In families with *EPCAM* deletions there is a 75% risk of developing cancer by the age of 70 and a 12% risk of endometrial cancer (Kempers et al., 2011). As the risks of colon, endometrial and other cancers are high, regardless of the gene, individuals with LS are recommended to follow more intensive cancer screening guidelines.

2.2 Familial adenomatous polyposis

Familial adenomatous polyposis (FAP) is an autosomal dominant CRC syndrome that accounts for less than 1% of all CRC diagnoses (Burt, 2000). In classic FAP, individuals develop hundreds to thousands of adenomatous polyps beginning in the early to mid-teen years. By age 35, 95% of individuals with FAP have polyps and the penetrance of colorectal cancer associated with this disease is over 90% (Petersen et al., 1991) which is why prophylactic colectomy is recommended in individuals who have this syndrome. FAP is caused by mutations in the adenomatous polyposis coli (*APC*) gene, although a high percentage (12-20%) of individuals with a clinical diagnosis of classical FAP do not have identifiable mutations in *APC* or another polyposis gene, *MUTYH*, (de la Chapelle, 2004; Filipe et al., 2009). Other features of FAP include small bowel adenomas, gastric polyposis, congenital hypertrophy of the retinal pigment epithelium (CHRPE), and desmoids (Allen & Terdiman, 2003). Desmoids cause significant mortality in FAP despite their non-malignant nature. Attenuated FAP is a milder form of this disease in which there are fewer polyps and a later onset of disease. Two other variants of FAP are Turcot syndrome which includes FAP and central nervous syndrome tumors, primarily medulloblastomas, and Gardner syndrome which includes soft-tissue tumours, osteomas and dental abnormalities.

2.3 *MUTYH*-associated polyposis

MUTYH-associated polyposis (MAP) is an autosomal recessive syndrome conferring a 43 to nearly 100% lifetime risk of CRC (Farrington et al., 2005; Lubbe et al., 2009). Penetrance for cancer in bi-allelic mutation carriers is estimated to be 20% at 40 years and 43% at 50 years of age (Lubbe et al., 2009). Individuals typically present with 10-100 adenomatous polyps, although some bi-allelic mutation carriers do not have any polyps on screening (Farrington et al, 2005; Nielsen et al., 2007). Polyposis of the duodenum can also be observed. Between 24 and 56% of FAP and attenuated-FAP families lacking mutations in APC have been found to carry bi-allelic mutations in *MUTYH*, suggesting that mutations in the two genes account for a significant proportion of familial polyposis (Nielsen et al., 2007; Gomez-Fernandez et al., 2009). Two common *MUTYH* mutations comprising 80-85% of disease causing mutations in Caucasians of Northern European ancestry are Tyr179Cys and Gly396Asp (previously known as Y165C and G382D; Al-Tassan et al., 2002). Importantly, 4% of bi-allelic mutation carriers will not have either of the two common mutations (Goodenberger et al., 2011). The mutation frequency of these mutations varies between populations and other founder and relatively frequent mutations have been identified (Gomez-Fernandez et al., 2009).

2.4 Other adenomatous polyposis syndromes

A handful of case reports of mutations leading to unique or rare familial presentation of CRC exist which may explain a small proportion of polyposis families that do not have *APC* or *MUTYH* germline mutations. One recent description is of homozygous mutations in *BUB1B* leading to CRC (Rio Frio et al., 2010). This gene has not been extensively tested in polyposis families so it is unknown if it will contribute much to the overall risk of familial adenomatous polyposis. Mutations in the *AXIN2* gene are associated with tooth agenesis-colorectal cancer syndrome in a large Finnish family (Lammi et al., 2004), but mutations in this gene do not appear to account for a large proportion of hereditary CRC.

2.5 Familial Colorectal Cancer Type X

About half of the families that have a strong-family history of colorectal cancer suggestive of LS by Amsterdam or Bethesda criteria have no evidence of mismatch repair deficiency or loss of any of the HNPCC related proteins in tumours (de la Chapelle & Lynch, 2003). To be classified as Familial Colorectal Cancer Type X, families must meet Amsterdam I criteria and have no evidence of MMR deficiency. A closer look at these pedigrees shows that they tend to have fewer individuals diagnosed with cancer, their cancers are less likely to look like those in LS and their average age of diagnosis is older than those in families with MMR mutations (Jass et al., 1995; Lindor et al. 2005). The genes contributing to Familial Colorectal Cancer Type X are as yet unknown.

2.6 Peutz-Jeghers syndrome

Peutz-Jeghers syndrome is a rare autosomal dominant condition with an estimated incidence of 1 in 200,000 births first described by Peutz in 1921. It is characterized by childhood onset of hamartomatous polyps in the gastrointestinal tract and by mucocutaneous pigmentation of the lips and buccal mucosa. Mutations in *LKB1* (*STK11*) are the only known cause of Peutz-Jeghers syndrome. *LKB1* mutations have been found in 50-94% of individuals with classic features of this disorder indicating that there may be locus heterogeneity (Boardman et al. 2000; Volikos et al., 2006; Aretz et al., 2005). The penetrance for GI polyps in this syndrome is 100%. There is also a 76-85% lifetime risk of cancer which includes lifetime risks of 40% for colon cancer, 30-60% for gastric cancer, 15-30% for small intestinal cancer and 11-35% for pancreatic cancer (Hearle et al., 2006, van Lier et al., 2010; van Lier et al., 2011). Breast and gynaecological cancers can be seen at high frequencies. There is a high mortality associated with this syndrome with a median age of death at 45 years of life, mostly due to cancer or bowel intussusceptions (van Lier et al., 2011).

2.7 Cowden syndrome

Cowden syndrome is an autosomal dominant syndrome with features of skin lesions, macrocephaly, thyroid manifestations and hamartomatous polyps of the GI tract. It is caused by mutations in the *PTEN* gene. Although this disorder and an allelic disorder Bannayan-Ruvalcaba-Riley Syndrome are both characterized by many hamartomatous polyps, there is no clear increased risk of colon cancer associated with Cowden syndrome.

2.8 Juvenile Polyposis

Hereditary juvenile polyposis (JP) is defined as the presence of 10 or more juvenile polyps. These polyps are primarily hamartomatous. The typical age of diagnosis is between the ages of 5 and 15 years (Merg & Howe, 2004). Most children are brought to medical attention because of colorectal bleeding. The risk of CRC associated with JP varies from 20-50% depending on the study and the gene which is mutated. (Handra-Luca et al., 2005). In addition to CRC, there is a significant risk of upper GI cancers. JP is inherited as an autosomal dominant syndrome. Multiple genes have been implicated in this disorder. The majority of mutations in individuals with JP have been found in *SMAD4* and *BMPR1A*. Individuals with *BMPR1A* mutations have a higher risk of cancers including those of the stomach, pancreas and small bowel. Mutations have also been found in *PTEN*, but these may be misdiagnosed cases of Cowden syndrome. There have been reports of *SMAD4* mutations in families with features of both juvenile polyposis and hereditary hemorrhagic telangiectasia (Gallione et al., 2004). Not all individuals with features of JP have identifiable mutations implicating additional as yet unidentified genes (Handra-Luca et al., 2005).

2.9 Hereditary mixed polyposis

Hereditary mixed polyposis (HMP) is an autosomal dominant condition characterized by polyps of mixed histology including adenomatous, hyperplastic and atypical juvenile types. Mutations in *BMPR1A* have been found in a proportion of families presenting with polyps of mixed type (Cheah et al., 2009). Despite the observation that families with both juvenile polyps and hereditary mixed polyposis can have mutations in *BMPR1A*, families with HMP are less likely to have juvenile type polyps and have an older age of diagnosis in adulthood (Merg & Howe, 2004). A locus for HMP, called *CRAC1* or *HMPS*, has been mapped to chromosome 15q13 q14 in multiple in several Ashkenazi Jewish families, but the gene has not yet been identified (Jaeger et al., 2008).

2.10 Hyperplastic polyposis (HPP)

Hyperplastic polyposis syndrome (HPP) is not yet well defined, but is characterized by multiple or large hyperplastic or serrated polyps and an association with an increased risk of CRC. The range of polyps has been described from 5 to over 100 and the pathology of the polyps can be diverse. HPP is often diagnosed in the fifth through seventh decade of life. The frequency of CRC in individuals with HPP ranges from 25-50% (Lage et al., 2004; Kalady et al., 2011). About 30% of individuals with HPP have a family history of CRC. The inheritance pattern of HPP is not well defined, but a few characterized families show possible recessive inheritance (Young & Jass, 2006). A germline mutation in *EPHB2* was identified in an individual who had more than 100 hyperplastic polyps, but *EPHB2* mutations have not been observed in other HPP cases (Kokko et al., 2006). Thus, the causal genes for most individuals with HPP have yet to be identified.

2.11 Rare cancer predisposition syndromes and risk of colon cancer

Whereas many hereditary cancer syndromes have specific cancers which occur at greater frequency than the general population, a few syndromes have elevated risks of many different types of cancer. Li-Fraumeni syndrome (LFS) is a rare autosomal dominant inherited condition caused by germline mutations in *TP53*. The classical types of cancer seen in individuals with LFS include breast cancer, sarcomas, brain tumors, leukemia and adrenal cortical tumours; however, there is also an increased risk of colon cancer of 2.8-fold over the general population (Ruijs et al., 2010).

3. Moderate risk alleles

Familial clusters of colon cancer account for approximately 20% of all CRC cases, however, most of these cases will not be due to the known CRC syndromes (Burt et al., 1990). A familial cluster is multiple individuals within families who have a similar presentation, but no clear inheritance pattern of disease transmission. The risk of colon cancer is increased to individuals who have a relative with CRC or adenomas; first-degree relatives of affected individuals have a two- to three-fold increase in risk and when more than one first-degree relative is affected the risk increases to nearly four-fold (Butterworth et al., 2006; Taylor et al. 2010). To date, moderate-risk alleles (ORs of 3-5) have not been identified. It is possible that some families exhibiting clustering of CRC may have multiple low-penetrance alleles which work synergistically to increase risk.

4. Low-penetrance risk alleles

The majority of genetic risk for CRC in the population is likely to be due to low-penetrance susceptibility alleles which act with other low-pentrance variants and the environment. A debate in the field is whether most of the genetic risk will be due to common variants with low effects and allele frequencies greater than 1% or rare or unique variants with low to moderate effects (Bodmer, 2006). Historically, variants conferring an increased risk of CRC in the general population have been identified through cohort or population-based case/control studies looking at candidate genes, but recent genome-wide association studies (GWAS) have been quite successful in identifying well-replicated variants conferring risk. Whereas a great many studies have identified positive associations with some of these genes, the vast majority have not been consistently replicated. Lack of replication does not mean in all cases that the initial association is faulty, but could be due to differences in populations leading to differences in allele frequencies or linkage disequilibrium, environmental exposures, study design or underpowered replicate studies.

Whereas the low-penetrance variants identified to date are not particularly predictive for CRC risk on their own, several direct-to-consumer genetic testing companies include some of these variants in their analysis of genomic risks of common disease. We will highlight some of the different types of variants which have been identified through multiple types of studies as showing evidence of contribution to CRC risk.

4.1 Candidate-gene studies

The studies to assess the risk of DNA variants, mainly single nucleotide polymorphisms (SNPs), have been association case/control studies or cohort studies testing SNPs in genes with relevant biological function for CRC. Many such candidate gene studies for CRC risk have been completed. Some of these have been replicated in one or two studies, but few have stood up to repeated replication studies or meta-analyses. A meta-analysis of 50 published CRC association studies for common alleles in 13 genes found three variants: *APC* I1307K, a *HRAS1* repeat variant and *MTHFR* 677V were convincingly associated with modest CRC risk in the general population (Houlston & Tomlinson, 2001). Other genes with variants showing CRC risk in multiple studies include *NAT1*, *NAT2* and *TGFBRII* (Burt, 2010). It is possible that some of these are real associations, but are population-specific or depend upon gene-environment interactions present only in certain individuals.

Candidate genes for CRC case/control studies have been chosen in a variety of ways. Variants and genes studied include common variants in high-risk genes, genes in pathways believed to be important in CRC and genes in pathways linked to environmental factors associated with CRC. One strategy which has been under-utilized is to map loci for cancer susceptibility in the mouse and then test these genes/loci for cancer risk in human populations (Ruivenkamp et al., 2002; Ewart-Toland et al., 2005; Toland et al., 2008). A large number of cancer susceptibility and resistance loci for cancers of the lung, colon, skin, liver, and the hematopoetic system have been identified using mouse models. Two putative CRC susceptibility genes, *PTPRJ* and *AURKA*, were first identified from mouse studies (Ruivenkamp et al., 2002; Ewart-Toland et al., 2003). Variants in these genes show evidence of modest CRC risk in some human studies (Ewart-Toland et al., 2005; Toland et al., 2008).

4.2 Variants of high-risk genes
Once genes for hereditary cancer syndromes began to be identified, researchers hypothesized that common variants in these genes contribute to cancer risk in the general population. Studies on common variants of almost all hereditary CRC predisposition genes have been assessed, but only a handful of variants in these high risk genes have been determined to contribute to sporadic CRC risk.

4.2.1 Carriers of *MUTYH* mutations
Bi-allelic mutations in *MUTYH* lead to MAP as described above. Several studies have looked at the cancer risks associated with mono-allelic mutations in *MUTYH*. The range of cancer incidence associated with the Y179C allele is between 1.27 to 2-fold (Table 2, Jones et al., 2009; Tenesa et al., 2006; Theodoratou et al., 2010). As a result, colon adenomas or cancer cancer may be seen in multiple generations in families with MAP.

4.2.2 APC I1307K
One frequently described modest-risk allele is the I1307K variant in the *APC* gene. This variant is seen in approximately 6% of individuals of Ashkenazi jewish (AJ) ancestry and 28% of AJ individuals with a family history of CRC (Laken et al., 1997). Carriers of the I1307K allele have 1.5 to 2-fold increased risk of CRC compared to individuals who are non-carriers (Table 2, Dundar et al., 2007; Gryfe et al., 1999). The variant itself is not thought to change function of the APC gene, however, the change results in a stretch of eight consecutive adenosines. During replication this polyadenosine track is thought to have increased risk of somatic mutation due to polymerase slippage. Addition or loss of a single nucleotide then results in a frame-shift and non-functional *APC* gene (Laken et al., 1997). As the age of onset of CRC related to this polymorphism does not appear to differ from sporadic CRC, cancer screening beyond general population recommendations is not typically done (Petersen et al., 1999).

4.2.3 Bloom's syndrome mutation carriers
Bloom's syndrome is a rare autosomal recessive condition characterized by abnormal rates of sister chromatid exchange, growth deficiency and an increased incidence of multiple types of cancer. One in 107 individuals of AJ ancestry carries a founder mutation, designated as *Blm^Ash*, in the Bloom's syndrome gene, *BLM* (Li et al., 1998). Early studies suggested a 2-fold increase in colon cancer risk in *Blm^Ash* carriers, but this has not held up in subsequent studies (Gruber et al, 2002; Cleary et al., 2003).

4.2.4 *CHEK2*
CHEK2 is a gene important in response to DNA damage. Studies have demonstrated increased risk of breast cancer with an 1100delC polymorphism but have been inconclusive

for the role of the 1100del C variant in CRC risk. However, another variant, I157T, has been associated with Lynch-syndrome like cancers and confers an increased risk of 1.4 to 2-fold of CRC (Kilpivaara et al., 2006).

4.3 Genome-wide association studies (GWAS)

With technological advances allowing the genotyping of up to millions of SNPs, the ability to interrogate the entire genome without bias has led to the identification of SNPs with reproducible, but small associations with cancer risk. The strength of these studies is that that very large numbers of samples were used, large independent replication studies have been completed and very low p-values were required to meet genome-wide significance. About 18 SNPs have been identified to date (Table 2). Interestingly, although many map near genes, none of them fall within coding regions of genes suggesting that these SNPs may play a role in gene regulation. Despite the confidence that these are "real", the variants identified through GWAS to date explain a very small percentage of the overall risk of CRC ascribed to genetics. One computational assessment estimates that there may be as many as 170 low-penetrance variants which contribute to CRC risk (Tenesa and Dunlop, 2009).

4.3.1 8q24 and rs6983267

Two of the first GWAS studies for CRC identified a variant, rs6983267, on chromosome 8q24 which was significantly associated with CRC risk (Tomlinson et al. 2007; Haiman et al. 2007). The effects were modest with ORs ranging from of 1.14 to 1.24. Additional variants on 8q24 including rs7014346, rs783728, and rs10505477 were also identified in subsequent screens (Tenesa et al. 2008; Poynter et al. 2007). Several groups have replicated these findings and show a consistent effect of the rs6983267 variant. This SNP falls into a gene-poor region on 8q24 with the closest gene, *cMYC*, 335 kb away. One study showed that the rs6983267 variant falls within an enhancer element and alleles differentially bind a WNT-related transcription-factor 7-like 2 (TCF7L2). However, correlation with expression of *MYC* has not been detected, and the exact role of this SNP in colon cancer development has yet to be definitively determined (Pomerantz et al. 2009; Tuupanen et al. 2009).

4.3.2 GWAS variants in the Bone Morphogenic Protein (BMP)/Transforming Growth Factor Beta (TGFβ) pathway

Multiple variants identified by GWAS (rs4444235, rs4939827, rs4779584, rs961253 rs10411210, rs4925386) are located near genes involved in BMP and/or TGFβ signalling (Tenesa & Dunlop, 2009). BMP proteins are positive regulators of the Wnt pathway which have long been known to be important in CRC tumorigenesis. TGFβ is a master signalling molecule controlling many processes important in cancer and cancer suppression. There is considerable overlap and interaction between the BMP and TGFβ pathways. Germline mutations in *SMAD4*, *BMPR1A* and *APC* are associated with specific hereditary colon cancer syndromes. Whereas the exact effect of these SNPs on the nearby BMP/TGFβ signalling genes is not determined, location and number of these SNPs suggest that perturbation of these pathways may be critical for CRC risk in the general population.

4.4 Population specific risk factors

One of the caveats to many of the candidate gene and GWAS studies for CRC risk to date is that they have been predominantly completed in Caucasian populations. The rs6983267

SNP	Locus	Nearby genes	OR	Type of Study	Reference
Rs6691170	1q41	DUSP10	1.06	GWAS	Houlston et al., 2010
Rs6687758	1q41	DUSP10	1.09	GWAS	Houlston et al., 2010
Rs10936599	3q26.2	MYNN	0.93	GWAS	Houlston et al., 2010
Rs16892766	8q23.3	EIF3H	1.27	GWAS	Tomlinson et al., 2008
Rs6983267	8q24	Gene desert	1.21-1.23	GWAS	Tomlinson et al. 2007; Xiong et al. 2011
Rs7014346	8q24	POU5F1P1, DQ515897	1.19	GWAS	Tenesa et al., 2008
Rs719725	9p24	Several	1.46	GWAS	Poynter et al. 2007
Rs10795668	10p14	FLJ3802842	1.23	GWAS	Tomlinson et al., 2008; Xiong et al., 2011
Rs3802842	11q23	Several	1.11-1.29	GWAS	Pittman et al., 2008; Tenesa et al., 2008; Xing et al., 2011
Rs11169552	12q13.13	LARP4, DIP2B	0.92*	GWAS	Houlston et al., 2010
Rs7136702	12q13.13	LARP4, DIP2B	1.06	GWAS	Houlston et al., 2010
Rs4444235	14q22.2	BMP4	1.11	GWAS	Houlston et al. 2008
Rs4779584	15q13.3	CRAC1/ GREM1	1.23	GWAS	Jaeger et al., 2008
Rs9929218	16q22.1	CDH1	0.91*	GWAS	Houlston et al. 2008
Rs4939827	18q21	SMAD7	1.17	GWAS	Tenesa et al., 2008; Xiong et al., 2011
Rs10411210	19q13.1	RHPN2	0.87*	GWAS	Houlston et al. 2008
Rs961253	20p12.3	BMP2	1.12-1.37	GWAS	Xiong et al., 2011
Rs4925386	20q13.3	LAMA5	0.93	GWAS	Houlston et al., 2010
I1307K	5q21-22	APC	1.5-2.0	Candidate	Dundar et al., 2007; Gryfe et al., 1999
Y179C (mono-allelic)	1p34.1	MUTYH	1.27-2.0	Candidate	Tenesa et al., 2006 Theodoratou et al., 2010

Table 2. Low-penetrance variants associated with CRC Risk
OR, odds ratio; *The common allele is the risk allele.

variant has been replicated in multiple ethnic groups including African-American and Chinese populations with fairly consistent results (Xiong et al., 2011; He et al. 2011). However, rs3802842 on chromosome 11q23 is associated with no increased risk in Japanese populations. A GWAS performed in Japanese CRC cases identified a novel variant, rs7758229 on chromosome 6 which has not been linked with risk in Caucasians (Cui et al.,

2011). These examples illustrate that specific variants identified by GWAS are often markers for the causal, as yet unidentified variant, which may be absent or in different linkage disquilibrium patterns with the identified SNP in other populations. Additional possibilities for the differential risk effects include different frequencies of important interacting variants or population specific gene-environment interactions. When low-penetrance variants become a part of determination of cancer risk, care should be taken to ensure that only variants which have been validated in the ethnic background of the patient be utilized.

4.5 Missing heritability: Additive effects, gene-gene and gene-environmental factors

When GWAS were first utilized they were hailed as the tool by which all low-penetrance variants for disease risk would be identified. While these screens have been successful, the variants identified to date explain less than 10% of the estimated genetic contributions to CRC which makes use of known variants for risk prediction difficult. Several possible explanations for the "missing heritability" exist. One is that much of the genetic risk of CRC will be due to rare or unique low-penetrance variants which are not detectible by population-based GWAS. A second is that synergistic or epistatic gene-gene interactions which are only detectible when taking into account interacting loci will account for the missing heritability. Gene-environmental interactions in which risk is dependent on both a variant and exposure to the environmental risk factor may also play a role. Transgenerational epigenetic effects, epigenetic alterations which are inherited through the germline and/or observed through multiple generations, may also account for some of the missing heritability (Fleming et al., 2008).

As the effects of single variants identified by candidate gene or genome-wide studies have been low, it is important to determine if there are combined effects of carrying multiple risk alleles. One study assessed three SNPs identified through GWAS (rs3802842, rs7014346, rs4939827) and found that carrying all six risk alleles confers a 2.6-fold increased risk of CRC (Tenesa et al., 2008). It is likely that CRC risk could increase if all 18 identified GWAS variants were included in the analysis. Animal models have been instrumental for demonstrating synergistic and epistatic interactions between genetic risk factors (Nagase et al. 2001). Mouse models led to the identification of several CRC susceptibility loci that interact synergistically or epistatically (van Wezel et al., 1996; van Wezel et al. 1999). Thus far, no synergistic or epistatic interactions for CRC risk have been definitively identified in human populations. As computational tools for assessing the data from GWAS studies improve, genetic interactions are likely to be identified as important factors for CRC risk in humans.

Several environmental factors including cigarette smoking, body mass index, polycyclic aromatic hydrocarbons, N-nitroso compounds, and diets high in red meat which increase exposure to heterocyclic amines have been associated with increased risk of CRC (Botteri et al. 2008; Norat et al. 2002; Pischon et al. 2006). Although many studies show contradictory results, interactions between genetic variations and environmental exposures can modify CRC risk. mEH is an enzyme important in xenobiotic activation of tobacco carcinogens. Two variants have been identified in the *mEH* gene which lead to low or high activity. A meta-analysis of several studies showed that smokers with the *mEH3* low metabolizer genotype had lower risk of colon cancer compared to smokers with a *mEH3* high metabolizer genotype suggesting that genetic variants can modify the cancer risk associated with smoking (Raimondi et al. 2009). Interactions between dietary factors and genotypes have also been observed for CRC. In one study, individuals who consumed browned red meat and had the 751Lys/Lys and 312 Asp/Asp genotypes in the *XPD* gene were at highest risk of developing CRC (Joshi et al., 2009). Much work remains to be done to fully assess gene-environment interactions for CRC.

4.6 Modifier genes for penetrance in high-risk syndromes
The risk of cancer does not reach 100% even for individuals with mutations leading to high-penetrance CRC syndromes like LS. Thus, it has been proposed that even in the context of a mutation, environmental factors and low-penetrance variants may impact cancer risk. To this end, modifier genes, alleles that modify the risk of a mutation, have been sought. Most of the studies to date have been for LS. A variant in *CHEK2*, 1100delC, has been established as a moderate risk allele for breast cancer. Some families with 1100delC mutations have CRC in addition to breast cancer. Several studies have tested this variant for risk in LS families and some found modest increases in risk in LS carriers who also have the 1100delC variant (Wasielewski et al., 2008) while others have found no increase in risk (Sanchez et al., 2005). Genes with variants conferring suggestive effects in some studies for age of diagnosis in HNPCC carriers include *CCND1*, *CDKN2A*, *AURKA*, *TP53*, *E2F2*, and *IGF1* (Talseth et al. 2008; Jones et al., 2004; Chen et al. 2009).

5. The use of genetic information for CRC treatment and prognosis
Currently, the use of germline genetic variants is not used routinely for making clinical decisions regarding colorectal cancer therapy. The bulk of research and clinical application has been with somatic tumour mutations. Despite this, germline mutations and variants have been associated with different tumor histopathology and survival outcomes.

5.1 Low-penetrance risk alleles and tumor histopathology
In addition to playing a role in overall CRC risk, studies indicate that SNPs may impact morphology and type of colon cancer. Some of the low-penetrance SNPs identified through GWAS (rs3802842, rs4939827) have higher risks for rectal cancer than colon cancer (Tanesa et al., 2008). Preliminary studies also suggest differences in risk of necrosis (rs719725), mucin production (rs96153), desmoplastic reaction (rs10411210), Crohn-like lymphocytic reaction (rs6983267, rs4444235) and moderate/well-differentiated histology (rs10795668)(Ghazi et al., 2010). The SNP rs4779584 is associated with reduced risk of death in a Chinese cohort (Xing et al. 2011), but thus far, none of the GWAS-identified variants assessed show an effect on overall survival in Caucasian populations (Tenesa et al., 2010). These studies suggest that variants may impact the development of certain subtypes of colon cancer which provide possible mechanistic insights into colon tumorigenesis and new therapeutic targets.

5.2 Variants to predict response to and off-target effects of cancer therapy
Targeted therapies for colorectal cancer have been developed based on somatic mutations occurring during tumorigenesis. In addition to targeted therapies to somatic mutations, germline variations in enzymes which process more standard chemotherapeutic agents impact prognosis and treatment response. Standard therapies for CRC include 5-fluorouracil and oxaliplatin (FOLFOX). One study looked at the role of germline variants of DNA repair pathways on metastatic CRC patients' response to FOLFOX (Lamas et al., 2011). One variant in *XPD*, Lys751Gln, was associated with longer survival, but the numbers in this study were

small. Variants in *TS* and *GSTT1* have been found to be associated with response to both LV5FU2 and FOLFOX (Boige et al. 2010), and two variants in *MTHFR* (677C>T and 1298 C>A) were associated with better response to FOLFOX (Etienne-Grimaldi et al. 2010). A variant in *ERCC2*, K751Q was associated with FOLFOX-induced hematologic toxicity (Boige et al. 2010), suggesting that germline variations may also predict CRC treatment side-effects. Since the field of colon cancer pharmacogenomics is still new, it is likely that other variants important in metabolism of CRC therapeutics will be identified.

5.3 Prognosis in tumors with mismatch instability mutations

Colorectal cancers can be divided into different subtypes depending on histology and the presence or absence of specific molecular markers. Treatment and prognosis of these subtypes varies. About 15% of all CRC tumours show evidence of microsatellite instability of which a small proportion are germline mutations (Murphy et al., 2006; Salovaara et al., 2000). A meta-analysis of 32 studies correlating MSI status with clinical outcomes included patients with both germline LS mutations and sporadic MMR defects. Individuals with no evidence of MSI or with MSI-low tumours showed decreased survival (HR=0.67, 95%CI 0.53-0.83) compared to individuals with MSI-high tumours. Polymorphisms in MMR genes are also associated with specific phenotypes. In one study, individuals who carried one or more G alleles of the *MLH1* 655A>G SNP had a better outcome and less risk of vascular invasion, distant metastasis or recurrence (Nejda et al., 2009). Some studies have documented better survival in individuals with MUTYH-associated colorectal cancer compared to matched controls with colon cancer (Nielsen et al., 2010). Together these data suggest that tumours that have deficits in DNA repair capabilities through germline or somatic mutations show better survival than tumours competent in DNA repair.

6. Conclusion

In summary, just over a third of colorectal cancer risk is thought to be due to inherited genetic factors. A number of mutations in genes have been found to increase CRC in individuals with hereditary cancer syndromes. These syndromes confer a vastly increased risk of CRC over the general population and an earlier age of diagnosis. Individuals with a family history of CRC should be referred to genetics for evaluation of a genetic syndrome and for guidelines for risk-reducing strategies. In addition to highly-penetrant mutations, many variants of small effect sizes have been identified through family-based and genome-wide association based studies. Whereas many of the variants identified through GWAS have been replicated in many studies, the effect size is small, only a small part of the total genetic risk has been identified, and the clinical utility is not established. The use of germline genetic information may be of clinical utility in the prevention and treatment of CRC; yet there is much that remains to be discovered. Technological advances are yielding new insights into genetic susceptibility to CRC on the population level, but we have yet to find the aetiology of most of the genetic risk contributing to CRC.

7. Acknowledgments

This work was funded by the National Institutes of Health/National Cancer Institute (R01 CA-134461-01) and the Ohio State University Comprehensive Cancer Center. We thank Heather Hampel for thoughtful review of this manuscript.

8. References

Al-Tassan, N.; Chmiel, N.H.; Maynard, J.; Fleming, N.; Livingston, Al.L.; Williams, G.T.; Hodges, A,K.; Davies, D.R.; David, S.S.; Sampson, J.R. & Cheadle, J.P. (2002).Inherited mutations of MYH associated with somatic G:C>T:A mutations in colorectal tumors. *Nature Genetics*, Vol.30, No.2, pp.227-32, ISSN 1061-4036.

Allen, B. & Terdiman, J.P. (2003). Hereditary polyposis syndromes and hereditary non-polyposis colorectal cancer. *Best Practice & Research Clinical Gastroenterology*, Vol.17, No.2, pp.237-58, ISSN 1521-6981.

Aretz, S.; Stienen, D.; Uhlhaas, S.; Loff, S.; Back, W.; Pagenstecher, C.; McLeod, D.R.; Graham, G.E.; Mangold, E.; Santer, R.; Propping, P. & Friedl, W. (2005). High propotion of large genomic STK11 deletions in Peutz-Jeghers syndrome. *Human Mutation*, Vol.26, No.6, pp.513-9, ISSN 1098-1004.

Boardman, L.A.; Couch, F.J.; Burgart, L.J.; Schwartz, D.; Berry, R.; McDonnell, S.K.; Schaid, D.J.; Hartmann, L.C.; Schroeder, J.J.; Stratakis, C.A. & Thibodeau, S.N. (2000). Genetic heterogeneity in Peutz-Jeghers syndrome. *Human Mutation*, Vol.16, No.1, pp.23-30, ISSN 1098-1004.

Bodmer, W.F. (2006). Cancer genetics: colorectal cancer as a model. *Journal of Human Genetics*, Vol.51, No.5, pp.391-6, ISSN 1434-5161.

Boige, V.; Mendiboure, J.; Pignon, J.P, Loriot,M.A. Castaing, M.; Barrois, M.; Malka, D.; Tregouet, D.A.; Bouche, O.; Le Corre, D.; Miran, I.; Mulot, C.; Ducreux, M.; Beaune, P. & Laurent-Puig, P. (2010). Pharmacogenetic assessment of toxicity and outcome in patients with metastatic colorectal cancer treated with LV5FU2, FOLFOX and FOLFIR: FFDC 2000-05. *Journal of Clinical Oncology*, Vol.28, No.15, pp.2556-64. ISSN 0732-183X.

Botteri, E.; Iodice, S.; Bagnardi, V.; Raimondi, S.; Lowenfels, A.B. & Maisonneuve, P. (2008). Smokijng and colorectal cancer: a meta-analysis. *JAMA*, Vol.300, No.23, pp.2765-78, ISSN 0098-7484.

Burt, R.W., Bishop, D.T.; Lynch, H.T.; Rozen, P. & Winawer, S.J. (1990). Risk and surveillance of individuals with heritable factors for colorectal cancer: WHO collaborating centre for the prevention of colorectal cancer, *Bulletin of the World Health Organization*, Vol.68, No.5, pp.655-65, ISSN 0042-9686.

Burt, R.W. (2000). Colon cancer screening. *Gastoenterology*, Vol.119, No.3, pp.837-53, ISSN 0016-5085.

Butterworth, A.S.; Higgins, J.P. & Pharoah, P. (2006). Relative and absolute risk of colorectal cancer for individuals with a family history: a meta-analysis. *European Journal of Cancer*. Vol.42, No.2, pp.216-27, ISSN 0959-8049.

Cheah, P.Y.; Wong, Y.H.; Chau, Y.P.; Loi, C.; Lim, K.H.; Lim, J.F.; Koh, P.K. & Eu, K.W. (2009). Germline bone morphogenesis protein receptor 1A mutation causes colorectal tumorigenesis in hereditary mixed polyposis syndrome. *American Journal of Gastroenterology*, Vol.104, No.12, pp.3027-33, ISSN 0002-9270.

Cleary, S.P.; Zhang, W.; Di Nicola, N.; Aronson, M.; Aube, J.; Steinman, A.; Haddad, R.; Redston, M.; Gallinger, S.; Narod, S.A. & Gryfe, R. (2003). Heterozygosity for the BLM(Ash) mutation and cancer risk. *Cancer Research*, Vol.63, No.8, pp.1769-71, ISSN 1538-7445.

Chen, J.; Etzel, C.J.; Amos, C.I.; Zhang, Q.; Viscofsky, N.; Lindor, N.M.; Lynch, P.M. & Frazier, M.L. (2009). *Cancer Causes and Control*, Vol.20, No.9, pp.1769-77, ISSN 1573-7225.

Cui, R.; Okada, Y.; Jang, S.G.; Ku, J.L.; Park, J.G.; Kamatani, Y.; Hosono, N.; Tsunoda, T.; Kumar, V.; Tanikawa, C.; Kamatani, N.; Yamada, R.; Kubo, M.; Nakamura, Y.; Matsuda, K. (2011). Common variant in 6q26-q27 is associated with distal colon cancer in an Asian population. *Gut*, Vol.60, No.6, pp.799-805, ISSN 1468-3288.

de la Chapelle, A. (2004). Genetic predisposition to colorectal cancer. *Nature Reviews Cancer*, Vol.4, No.10, pp769-80, ISSN 1474-175X.

Des Guetz, G.; Mariani, P.; Cucherousset, J.; Benamoun, M.; Lagorce, C.; Sastre, X.; Le Toumelin, P.; Uzzan, B.; Perret, G.Y.; Morere, J.F.; Breau, J.L.; Fagard, R.; Schischmanoff, P.O. (2007). Microsatellite instability and sensitivitiy to FOLFOX treatment in metastatic colorectal cancer. *Anticancer Research*, Vol.27, No.4, pp.2715-9, ISSN 1791-7530.

Dundar, M.; Caglayan, A.O.; Saatci, C.; Karaca, H.; Baskol, M.; Tahiri, S. & Ozkul, Y. (2007). How the I1307K adenomatous polyposis coli gene variant contributes in the assessment of risk of colorectal cancer, but not stomach cancer in a Turkish population. *Cancer Genetics & Cytogenetics*, Vol.177, No.2, pp.95-77, ISSN 0165-4608.

Etienne-Grimaldi, M.C.; Milano, G.; Maindrault-Goebel, F.; Chibaudel, B.; Formento, J.L.; Francoual, M.; Lledo, G.; Andre, T.; Mabro, M.; Mineur, L.; Flesch, M.; Carola, E. & de Gramont, A. (2010). Methylenetetrahydrofolate reductase (MTHFR) gene polymorphisms and FOLFOX response in colorectal cancer patients. *British Journal of Clinical Pharmacology*, Vol.69, No.1, pp.58-66, ISSN 1365-2125.

Ewart-Toland, A.; Briassouli, P.; de Koning, J.P.; Mao, J.H.; Yuan, J.; Chan, F.; MacCarthy-Morrogh, L.; Ponder, B.A.; Nagase, H.; Burn, J.; Ball, S.; Almeida, M.; Linardopoulous, S. & Balmain, A. (2003). *Nature Genetics*, Vol.34, No.4, pp.403-12, ISSN 1061-4036.

Ewart-Toland, A.; Dai, Q.; Gao, Y.T.; Nagase, H.; Dunlop, M.G.; Farrington, S.M.; Barnetson, R.A.; Anton-Culver, H.; Peel, D.; Ziogas, A.; Lin, D.; Miao, X.; Sun, T.; Ostrander, E.A.; Stanford, J.L.; Langlois, M.; Chan, J.M.; Yuan, J.; Harris, C.C.; Bowman, E.D.; Clayman, G.L.; Lippman, S.M.; Lee, J.J.; Zheng, W. & Balmain, A. (2005). Aurora-A/STK15 T+91A is a general low penetrance cancer susceptibility gene: a meta-analysis of multiple cancer types. *Carcinogenesis*, Vol.26, No.8, pp1368-73, ISSN 1460-2180.

Farrington, S.M. Tenesa, A.; Barnetson, R.; Wiltshire, A.; Prendergast J.; Porteous, M.; Campbell, H. & Dunlop, M.G. (2005). Germline susceptibility to colorectal cancer due to base-excision repair gene defects. *American Journal of Human Genetics*, Vol.77, No.1, pp.112-9, ISSN 0002-9297.

Felton, K.E.; Gilchrist, D.M.; & Andrew, S.E. (2007). Constitutive deficiency in DNA mismatch repair: is it time for Lynch III? *Clinical Genetics*, Vol.71, No.6, pp.499-500, ISSN 1339-0004.

Filipe, B.; Baltazar, C.; Albuquerque, C.; Fragosi, S.; Lage, P.; Vitoriano, I.; Mao de Ferro, S.; Claro, I.; Rodrigues, P.; Fidalgo, P.; Chaves, P.; Cravo, M. & Nobre Leitao, C. (2009). APC or MUTYH mutations account for the majority of clinically well-characterized families with FAP or AFAP phenotype and patients with more than 30 adenomas. *Clinical Genetics*, Vol.76, No.3, pp.242-55. ISSN 1399-0004.

Fleming, J.L.; Huang, T.H. & Toland, A.E. (2008). The role of parental and grandparental epigenetic alterations in familial cancer risk. *Cancer Research*, Vol.68, No.22, pp.9116-21, ISSN 1538-7445.

Gallione, C.; Aylsworth, A.S.; Beis, J.; Berk, T.; Bernhardt, B.; Clark, R.D.; Clericuzio, C.; Danesino, C.; Drautz, J.; Fahl, J.; Fan, Z.; Faughman, M.E.; Ganguly, A.; Garvie, J.; Henderson, K.; Kini, U.; Leedom, T.; Ludman, M.; Luz, A.; Maisenbacher, M.; Mazzucco, S.; Olivieri, C.; van Amstel, J.K.Pl; Prigoda-Lee, N.; Pyeritz, R.E.; Reardon, W.; Vandezande, K.; Waldman, J.D.; White, R.I.; Williams, C.A. & Marchuck, D.A. (2010). Overlapping spectra of *SMAD4* mutations in juvenile polyposis (JP) and JP-HHT syndrome. *American Journal of Medical Genetics Part A*, Vol.152A, No.2, pp333-9, ISSN 1552-4833.

Ghazi, S.; von Holst, S.; Picelli, S.; Linforss, U.; Tenesa, A.; Farrington, S.M.; Campbell, H.; Dunlop, M.G.; Papadogiannakis, N.; Lindblom, A.; Low-Risk Colorectal Cancer Study Group. (2010). Colorectal cancer susceptibility loci in a population-based study:Associations with morphological parameters. *American Journal of Pathology*, Vol.177, No.6, pp.2688-93, ISSN 0002-9440.

Gomez-Fernandez, N.; Castellvi-Bel, S.; Fernandez-Rozadilla, C., Balaguer, F.; Muñoz, J.; Madrigal, I.; Mila, M.; Grana, B.; Vega, A.; Castells, A.; Carracedo, A. & Ruiz-Ponte, C. (2009). Molecular analysis of the APC and MUTYH genes in Galician and Catalonian FAP families: a different spectrum of mutations? *BMC Medical Genetics*, Vol.10, pp.57, ISSN 1471-2350.

Goodenberger, M. & Lindor, N. (2011). Lynch syndrome and MYH-associated polyposis: review and testing strategy. *Journal of Clinical Gastroenterology*, Vol.45, No.6, pp.488-500, ISSN 0192-0790.

Gruber, S.B.; Ellis, N.A.; Scott, K.K.; Almog, R.; Kolachana, P.; Bonner, J.D.; Kirchoff, T.; Tomsho, L.P; Nafa, K.; Pierce, H.; Low, M.; Satagopah, J.; Rennert, H.; Huang, H.; Greenson, J.K.; Groden, J.; Rapaport, B.; Shia, J.; Johnson, S.; Gergersen, P.K.; Harris, C.C.; Boyd, J.; Rennert, G. & Offit, K. (2002). BLM heterozygosity and the risk of colorectal cancer. *Science*, Vol.297, No.5589, ISSN 1095-9203.

Gryfe, R.; Di Nicola, N.; Lal, G.; Gallinger, S. & Redston, M. (1999). Inherited colorectal polyposis and cancer risk of the APC I1307K polymorphism. *American Journal of Human Genetics*, Vol.64, No.2, pp.378-84, ISSN 0002-9297.

Haiman, C.A.; Le Marchand, L.; Yamamato, J.; Stram, D.O.; Sheng, X.; Kolonel, L.N.; Wu, A.H.; Reich, D. & Henderson, B.E. (2007). A common genetic risk factor for colorectal and prostate cancer. *Nature Genetics*, Vol.39, No.8, pp.954-6, ISSN 1061-4036.

Hampel H.; Frankel, W.L.; Martin, E.; Arnold, M.; Khanduja, K.; Kuebler, P.; Clendenning, M.; Sotamaa, K.; Prior, T.; Westman, J.A.; Panescu, J.; Fix, D.; Lockman, J.; LaJeunesse, J, Comeras, I. & de la Chapelle, A. (2008). Feasibility of screening for Lynch syndrome among patients with colorectal cancer. *Journal of Clinical Oncology*, Vol.26, No.35 , pp.5783-8, ISSN 1527-7755.

Handra-Luca, A.; Condroyer, C.; de Moncuit, C.; Tepper, M.; Flejou, J.-F.; Thomas, G. & Olschwang, S. (2005). Vessels' morphology in SMAD4 and BMPR1A related juvenile polyposis. *American Journal of Medical Genetics Part A*, Vol.138A, No.2, pp.113-117, ISSN 1552-4833.

He, J.; Wilkens, L.R.; Stram, D.O.; Kolonel, L.N.; Henderson, B.E.; Wu, A.H.; Le Marchand, L. & Haiman, C.A. (2011). Generalizability and epidemiologic characterization of eleven colorectal cancer GWAS hits in multiple populations. *Cancer Epidemiology, Biomarkers & Prevention*, Vol.20, No.1, pp.70-81, ISSN 1055-9965.

Hearle, N.; Schumacher, V.; Menko, F.H.; Olschwang, S.; Boardman, L.A.; Gille, J.J.P.; Keller, J.J.; Westerman, A.M.; Scott, R.J.; Lim, W.; Trimbath, J.D.; Giardiello, F.M.; Gruber, S.B.; Offerhaus, G.J.A.; de Rooij, F.W.M.; Wilson, J.H.P.; Hansmann, A.; Moslein, G.; Royer-Polora, B.; Voget, T.; Phillips, R.K.S.; Spigelman, A.D. & Houlston, R.S. (2006). Frequency and sprectrum of cancers in the Peutz-Jeghers syndrome. *Clinical Cancer Research*, Vol.12, No.10, pp.3209-15, ISSN 1557-3265.

Houlston, R.S; Webb, E.; Broderick, P.; Pittman, A.M.; Di Bernardo, M.C.; Lubbe, S.; Chandler, I.; Vijayakrishnan, J.; Sullivan, K.; Penegar, S.; Colorectal Cancer Association Study Consortium, Carvajal-Carmona, L.; Howarth, K.; Jaeger, E.; Spain, S.L.; Walther, A.; Barclay, E.; Martin, L.; Gorman, M.; Domingo, E.; Teixeira, A.S.; CoRGI Consortium, Kerr, D.; Cazier, J.B.; Nittymaki, I.; Tuupanen, S.; Karhu, A.; Aaltonen, L.A.; Tomlinson, I.P.; Farrington, S.M.; Tenesa, A.; Prendergast, J.G.; Barnetson, R.A.; Cetnarskyj, R.; Poretous, M.E.; Paroah, P.D.; Koessler, T.; Hampe, J.; Buch, S.; Schafmayer, C.; Tepel, J.; Schreiber, S.; Volzke, H.; Chang-Claude, J.; Hoffmeister, M.; Brenner, H.; Zanke, B.W.; Montpetit, A.; Hudson, T.J.; Gallinger, S.; International Colorectal Cancer Genetic Association Consortium, Campbell, H.; Dunlop, M.G. (2008). Meta-analysis of genome-wide association data identifies four new susceptibility loci for colorectal cancer. *Nature Genetics*, Vol. 40, No.12, pp.1426-35, ISSN 1061-4036.

Houlston, R.S.; Cheadle, J.; Dobbins, S.E.; Tenesa, A.; Jones, A.M.; Howarth, K.; Spain, S.L; Broderick, P.; Domingo, E.; Farrington, S.; Prendergast, J.G.; Pittman, A.M. Theodoratou, E.; Smith, C.G.; Olver, B.; Walther, A.; Barnetson, R.A.; Churchman, M.; Jaeger, E.E.; Penegar, S.; Barclay, E.; Martin, L.; Gorman, M.; Mager, R.; Johnstone, E.; Midgley, R.; Nittymaki, I. Tuupanen, S.; Colley, J.; Idziaszczyk, S.; COGENT Consortium; Thomas, H.J.; Lucassen, A.M.; Evans, D.G.; Maher, E.R.; CORGI Consortium; COIN Collaborative Group; COINB Collaborative Group, Maughan, T.; Dimas, A. Dermitzakis, E.; Cazier, J.B.; Aaltonen, L.A.; Pharoah, P.; Kerr, D.J.; Carvajal-Carmona, L.G.; Campbell, H.; Dunlop, M.G. & Tomlinson, I.P. (2010). Meta-analysis of three genome-wide association studies identifies loci for colorectal cancer at 1q41, 3q26.2, 12q13.13 and 20q13.33. *Nature Genetics*, Vol.42, No.11, pp.973-7, ISSN 1061-4036.

Houlston, R.S. & Tomlinson, I.P.M. (2001). Polymorphisms and colorectal cancer risk. *Gastroenterology*, Vol.121, No.2, pp.282-301, ISSN 0016-5085.

Jaeger, E.; Webb, E.; Howarth, K.; Carvajal-Carmona, L.; Rowan, A.; Broderick, P.; Walther, A.; Spain, S.; Pittman, A.; Kemp, Z.; Sullivan, K.; Heinimann, K.; Lubbe, S.; Domingo, E.; Barclay, E.; Martin, L.; Gorman, M.; Chandler, I.; Vijayakrishnan, J.; Wood, W.; Papaemmanuil, E.; Penegar, S.; Qureshi, M.; CORGI Consortium; Farrington, S.; Tenesa, A.; Cazier, J.B.; Kerr, D.; Gray, R.; Peto, J.; Dunlop, M.; Campbell, H.; Thomas, H.; Houlston, R.; & Tomlinson, I. (2008). Common genetic variants at the CRAC1 (HMPS) locus on chromosome 15q13.3 influence colorectal cancer risk. *Nature Genetics*, Vol.40, No.1, pp.26-8, ISSN 1061-4036.

Jasperson, K.W.; Tuohy, T.M.; Neklason, D.W. & Burt, R.W. (2010). Hereditary and familial colon cancer. *Gastroenterology*, Vol.138, No.6, pp.2044-58, ISSN 0016-5085.

Jass, J.R.; Cottier, D.S.; Jeevaratnam, P.; Pokos, V.; Holdaway, K.M.; Bowden, Ml.L. Van de Water, N.S. & Browett, P.J. (1995). Diagnostic use of microsatellite instability in hereditary non-polyposis colorectal cancer. *Lancet*, Vol.346, No.8984, pp.1200-1, ISSN 0140-6736.

Jones, J.S.; Chi, X.; Gu, X.; Lynch, P.M.; Amos, C.I. & Frazier, M.L. (2004). P53 polymorphism and age of onset of hereditary nonpolyposis colorectal cancer in a Caucasian population. *Clinical Cancer Research*, Vol.10, No.17, pp.5845-9, ISSN 1557-3265.

Jones, N.; Vogt, S.; Nielsen, M.; Christian, D.; Wark, P.A.; Ecceles, D.; Edwards, E.; Evans, D.G.; Maher, E.R.; Vasen, H.F.; Hes, F.J.; Aretz, S. & Sampson, J.R. (2009). Increeased colorectal cancer incidence in obligate carriers of heterozygous mutations in MUTYH. *Gastroenterology*, Vol.137, No.2, pp.489-94, ISSN 0016-5085.

Joshi, A.D.; Corral, R.; Siegmund, K.D.; Hailc, R.W.; Le Marchard, L.; Martinez, M.E.; Ahnen, D.J.; Sandler, R.S.; Lance, P. & Stern, M.C. (2009). Red meat and poultry intake, polymorphisms in the nucleotide excision repair and mismatch repair pathways and colorectal cancer risk. *Carcinogenesis*, Vol.30, No.3, pp.472-9, ISSN 1460-2180.

Kalady, M.; Jarrar, A.; Leach, B.; LaGuardia, L.; O'Malley, M.; Eng, C. & Church, J. (2011). Defining phenotypes and cancer risk in hyperplastic polyposis syndrome. *Diseases of the Colon & Rectum*, Vol.54, No.2, ISSN 0012-3706.

Kaz, A.M. & Brentnall, T.A. (2006). Genetic testing for colon cancer. *Nature Clinical Practice Gastroenterology and Hepatology*, Vol.3, No.12, pp.670-9, ISSN 1743-4378.

Kempers, M.J.; Kuiper, R.P.; Ockeloen, C.W.; Chappuis, P.O.; Hutter, P.; Raner, N.; Schackert, II.K.; Steinke, V.; Holinski-Feder, E.; Morak, M.; Kloor, M.; Buttner, R.; Verwiel, E.T.; van Krieken, J.H.; Nagtegaal, I.D.; Goossens, M.; van der Post, R.S.; Niessen, R.C.; Sijmons, R.H.; Kluijt, I.; Hogervorst, F.B.; Leter, E.M.; Gille, J.J.; Aalfs, C.M.; Redkerc, E.J.; Hes, F.J.; Tops, C.M.; van Nesselrooij, B.P.; van Gijn, M.E.; Gomez Garcia, E.B.; Eccles, D.M.; Bunyan, D.J.; Syngal, S.; Stoffel, E.M.; Culber, J.O.; Palomares, M.R.; Garham, T.; Velsher, L.; Papp, J.; Olah, E.; Chan, T.L.; Leung, S.Y.; van Kessel, A.G.; Kiemeney, L.A.; Hoogerbrugge, N. & Ligtenberg, M.J. (2011). Risk of colorectal and endometrial cancers in EPCAM deletion-positive Lynch syndrome: a cohort study. *Lancet Oncology*, Vol.12, No.1, pp.49-55, ISSN 1470-2045.

Kilpivaara, O.; Alhopuro, P.; Vaheristo, P.; Aaltonen, L.A. & Nevanlinna, H. (2006). CHEK2 I157T associates with familial and sporadic colorectal cancers. *Journal of Medical Genetics*, Vol.43, No.7, p.e34, ISSN 1468-6244.

Kokko, A.; Laiho, P.; Lehtonen, R.; Korja, S.; Carvajal-Carmona, L.G.; Jarvinen, H.; Mecklin, J.P.; Eng, C.; Schleutker, J.; Tomlinson, I.; Vahteristo, P. & Aaltonen, L.A. (2006). EPHB2 germline variants in patients with colorectal cancer or hyperplastic polyposis. *BMC Cancer*, Vol.6, pp.145. ISSN 1471-2407.

Lage, P.; Cravo, M.; Sousa, R.; Chaves, P.; Salazar, M.; Fonseca, R.; Claro, I.; Suspiro, A.; Rodrigues, P.; Raposo, H.; Fidalgo, P. & Nobre-Leitao, C. (2004). Management of Portugese patients with hyperplastic polyposis and screening of at-risk first-degree relatives: a contribution for future guidelines based on a clinical study. *American Journal of Gastroenterology*, Vol.99, No.9, pp.1779-84, ISSN 0002-9270.

Laken, S.J.; Petersen, G.M.; Gruber, S.B.; Oddoux, C.; Ostrer, H.; Giardiello, F.M.; Hamilton, S.R.; Hampel, H.; Markowitz, A.; Klimstra, D.; Jhanwar, S.; Winawer, S.; Offit, K.;Luce, M.C.; Kinzler, K.W. & Vogelstein, B. (1997). Familial colorectal cancer in Ashkenazim due to a hypermutable tract in APC. *Nature Genetics*, Vol.17, No., pp.79-83, ISSN 1061-4036.

Lamas, M.J.; Duran, G.; Balboa, E.; Bernardez, B.; Touris, M.; Vidal, Y.; Gallardo, E.; Lopez, R.; Carracedo, A. & Barros, F. (2011). Use of a comprehensive panel of biomarkers to predict response to a fluorouracil-oxaliplatin regimen in patients with metastatic colorectal cancer. *Pharmacogenomics*, Vol.12, No.3, pp. 433-442, ISSN 1462-2416.

Lammi, L.; Arte, S.; Somer, M.; Jarvinen, H.; Lahermo, P.; Thesleff, I.; Pirinen, S.; Nieminen, P. (2004). Mutations in AXIN2 cause familial tooth agenesis and predispose to colorectal cancer. *American Journal of Human Genetics*, Vol.74, No.5, pp.1043-50, ISSN 0002-9297.

Li, L.; Eng, C.; Desnick, R.J.; German, J. & Ellis, N.A. (1998). Carrier frequency of the Bloom syndrome blmAsh mutation in the Ashkenazi Jewish population. *Molecular Genetics and Metabolism*, Vol.64, No.4, pp.286-90, ISSN 1096-7192.

Lichtenstein, P.; Holm, N.V.; Verkasalo, N.V.; Iliadou, A. Kaprio, J.; Koskenvuo, M.; Pukkala, E.; Skytthe, A. & Hemminki, K. (2000). Environmental and heritablefactors in the causation of cancer: analyses of cohorts of twins from Sweden, Denmark, and Finland. *New England Journal of Medicine*, Vol.343, No.2, pp.78-84, ISSN 1533-4406.

Lim, W.; Hearle, N.; Shah, B.; Murday, V.; Hodgson, S.V.; Lucassen, A.; Eccles, D.; Talbot, I.; Neale, K.; Lim, A.G.; O'Donohue, J.; Donaldson, A.; Macdonald, R.C.; Young, I.D.; Robinson, M.H.; Lee, P.W.; Stoodley, B.J.; Tomlinson, I.; Alderson, D.; Holbrook, A.Gl.; Vyas, S.; Swarbrick, E.T.; Lewis, A.A.; Phillips, R.K. & Houlston, R.S. (2003). Further observations on LKB1/STK11 status and cancer risk in Peutz-Jeghers syndrome. *British Journal of Cancer*, Vol.98, No.2, pp.308-13, ISSN 0007-0920.

Lindor, N.M.; Rabe, K.; Petersen, G.M.; Haile, R.; Casey, G.; Baron, J.; Gallinger, S.; Bapat, S.; Aronson, M.; Hopper, J.; Jass, J.; LeMarchand, L.; Grove, J.; Potter, J.; Newcomb, P.; Terdiman, J.P.; Conrad, P.; Moslein, G.; Goldberg, R.; Ziogas, A.; Anton-Culver, H.; de Andrade, M.; Siegmund, K.; Thibodeau, S.N.; Boardman, L.A. & Seminara, D. (2005).Lower cancer incidence in Amsterdam-I criteria families without mismatch repair deficiency: familial colorectal cancer type X. *JAMA*, Vol.293, No.16, pp.1979-85, ISSN 0098-7484.

Lubbe, S.J.; Di Bernardo, M.C.; Chandler, I.P. & Houlston, R.S. (2009). Clinical implications of the colorectal cancer risk associated with MUTYH mutation. *Journal of Clinical Oncology*, Vol.27, No.23, pp.3975-80, ISSN 1527-7755.

Lynch, H. & de la Chapelle, A. (2003). Hereditary colorectal cancer, *New England Journal of Medicine*, Vol.348, No.10, pp.919-32, ISSN 1533-4406.

Merg, A. & Howe, J.R. (2004). Genetic conditions associated with intestinal juvenile polyps. *American Journal of Medical Genetics*, Vol.129c, No. 1, pp.44-55, ISSN 1552-4825.

Murphy, K.M.; Zhang, S.; Geiger, T.; Hafez, M.J.; Bacher, J.; Berg, K.D. & Eshleman, J.R. (2006). *Journal of Molecular Diagnostics*, Vol.8, No.3, pp.305-11, ISSN 1525-1578.

Nagase, H.; Mao, J.H.; de Koning, J.P. Minami, T. & Balmain. A. (2001). Epistatic interactions between skin tumor modifier loci in interspecific (spretus/musculus) backcross mice. *Cancer Research*, Vol.61, No.4, pp.1305-8, ISSN 1538-7445.

Nejda, N.; Iglesias, D.; Moreno Azcoita, M.; Medina Arana, V.; Gonzalez-Aguilera, J.J. & Prenandez-Peralta, A.M. (2009). A *MLH1* polymorphism that increase cancer risk is associated with better outcome in sporadic cancer. *Cancer Genetics & Cytogenetics*, Vol.193, No.2, pp.71-7, ISSN 0165-4608.

Nielsen, M.; Hes, F.J.; Nagengast, F.M.; Weiss, M.M.; Mathus-Vliegen, E.M.; Morreau, H.; Breuning, M.H.; Wijnen, J.T.; Tops, C.M.J.; Vasen, H.F.A. (2007). Germline mutations in APC and MUTYH are responsible for the majority of families with attenuated familial adenomatous polyposis. *Clinical Genetics*, Vol. 71, No.5, pp.427-33. ISSN 1399-0004.

Nielsen, M.; van Steenbergen, L.N.; Jones, N.; Vogt, S.; Vasen, H.F.A.; Morreau, H.; Aretz, S.; Sampson, J.R.; Dekkers, O.M.; Janssen-Heijnen, M.L.G. & Hes, F.J. (2010). Survival of MUTYH-associated polyposis patients with colorectal cancer and matched control colorectal cancer patients. *Journal of the National Cancer Institute*, Vol.102, No.22, pp.1724-1730, ISSN 1460-2105.

Niessen, R.C.; Hofstra, R.M.; Westers, H.; Ligtenberg, M.J.; Kooi, K.; Jager, P.O.; de Groote, M.L.; Dijkhuizen, T.; Olderode-Berends, M.J.; Hollema, H.; Kleibeuker, J.H.& Sijmons, R.H. (2009a). Germline hypermethylation of *MLH1* and *EPCAM* deletions are a frequent cause of Lynch syndrome. *Genes Chromosomes Cancer*, Vol.48, No.8, pp.737-44, ISSN 1098-2264.

Niessen, R.C.; Kleibeuker, J.H.; Westers, H.; Jager, P.O.; Roseveld, D.; Bos, K.K.; Boersma-van Ek, W.; Hollema, H.; Sijmons, R.H. & Hofstra, R.M. (2009b). PMS2 involement in patients suspected of Lynch syndrome. *Genes Chromosomes Cancer*, Vol.48, No.4, pp.322-9, ISSN 1098-2264.

Norat, T.; Lukanova, A.; Ferrari, P. & Riboli, E. (2002). Meat consumption and colorectal cancer risk: dose-dependent meta-analysis of epidemiological studies. *International Journal of Cancer*, Vol.98, No.2, pp.241-56, ISSN 1097-0215.

Peterson, G.M.; Slack, J.; Nakamura, Y. (1991). Screening guidelines and premorbid diagnosis of familial adenomatous polyposis using linkage. *Gastroenterology*, Vol.100, No.6, pp. 1658-64, ISSN 0016-5085.

Petersen, G.M.; Brensinger, J.D.; Johnson, K.A. & Giardiello, F.M. (1999). Genetic testing and counseling for hereditary forms of colorectal cancer. *Cancer*, Vol.86, No. 11Suppl, pp.2450-50, ISSN 1097-0142.

Pischon, T.; Lahmann, P.H.; Boening, H.; Friedenreich, C.; Norat, T, Tjonneland, A.; Halkjaer, J.; Overvad, K.; Clavel-Chapelon, F.; Boutron-Rualut, M.C.; Guernec, G.; Bergmann, M.M.; Linseisen, J.; Becker, N.; Trichopoulou, A.; Trichopoulos, D.; Sieri, S.; Palli, D.; Tumino, R.; Vineis, P., Panico, S.; Peeters, P.H.; Bueno-de-Mesquita, H.B.; Boshuizen, H.C.; Van Guelpen, B.; Palmqvist, R.; Berglund, G.; Gonzalez, C.A.; Dorronsoro, M.; Barricarte, A.; Navarro, C.; Martinez, C.; Quiros, J.R.; roddam, A.; Allen, N.; Bingham, S.; Khaw, K.T.; Ferrari, P.; Kaaks, R.; Slimani, N. & Riboli, E. (2006). Body size and risk of colon and rectal cancer in the European Prospective Investigation into cancer and nutrition (EPIC). *Journal of the National Cancer Institute*, Vol.98, No.13, pp.320-31, ISSN 1460-2105.

Pittman, A.M.; Webb, E.; Carvajal-Carmona, L.; Howarth, K.; Di Bernardo, M.C., Broderlck, P.; Spain, S.; Walther, A.; Price, A.; Sullivan, K.; Twiss, P.; Fielding, S.; Rowan, A.; Jaeger, E.; Vijayakrishnan, J.; Chandler, I.; Penegar, S.; Qureshi, M.; Lubbe, S.; Domingo, E.; Kemp, Z.; Barclay, E.; Wood, W.; Martin, L.; Gorman, M.; Thomas,

H.; Peto, J.; Bishop, T.; Gray, R.; Maher, E.R.; Lucassen, A.; Kerr, D.; Evans, G.R.; CORGI Consortium; van Wezel, T.; Morreau, H.; Wijnen, J.T.; Hopper, J.L.; Southey, M.C.; Giles, G.G.; Severi, G.; Castellví-Bel, S.; Ruiz-Ponte, C.; Carracedo, A.; Castells, A.; EPICOLON Consortium; Försti, A.; Hemminki, K.; Vodicka, P.; Naccarati, A.; Lipton, L.; Ho, J.W.; Cheng, K.K.; Sham, P.C.; Luk, J.; Agúndez, J.A.; Ladero, J.M.; de la Hoya, M.; Caldés, T.; Niittymäki, I.; Tuupanen, S.; Karhu, A.; Aaltonen, L.A.; Cazier, J.B.; Tomlinson, I.P. & Houlston, R.S. (2008). Refinement of the basis and impact of common 11q23.1 variation to the risk of developing colorectal cancer. *Human Molecular Genetics*, Vol.17, No.23, pp.3720-7, ISSN 1460-2083.

Pomerantz, M.M., Ahmadiyeh, N.; Jia, L.; Herman, P.; Verzi, M.P.; Doddapaneni, H.; Beckwith, C.A.; Chan, J.A.; Hills, A.; Davis, M.; Yao, K.; Kehoe, S.M.; Lenz, H.J.; Haiman, C.A.; Yan, C.; Henderson, B.E.; Frenkel, B.; Barretina, J.; Bass, A.; Tabernero, J.; Baselga, J.; Regan, M.M.; Manak, J.R.; Shivdasani, R.; Coetzee, G.A. & Freedman, M.L. (2009). The 8q24 cancer risk variant rs6983267 shows long-range interaction with MYC in colorectal cancer. *Nature Genetics*, Vol.41, No.8, pp.882-4, ISSN 1061-4036.

Poynter, J.N.; Figueiredo, J.C.; Conti, D.V.; Kennedy, K.; Gallinger, S.; Siegmund, K.D.; Casey, G.; Thibodeau, S.N.; Jenkins, M.A.; Hopper, J.L.; Byrnes, G.B.; Baron, J.A.; Goode, E.L.; Tiirikainen, M.; Lindor, N.; Grove, J.; Newcomb, P.; Jass, J.; Young, J.; Potter, J.D.; Haile, R.W.; Duggan, D.J.; Le Marchand, L. & Colon C.F.R. (2007). Variants on 9p24 and 8q24 are associated with risk of colorectal cancer: results from the Colon Cancer Family Registry. *Cancer Research*, Vol.63, No.23, pp.11128-32, ISSN 1538-7445.

Raimondi, S.; Botteri, E.; Iodice, S.; Lowenfels, A.B.; & Maisonneuve, P. (2009). Gene-smoking interaction on colorectal adenoma and cancer risk: review and meta-analysis. *Mutation Research*, Vol.670, No.1-2, pp.6-14, ISSN 0921-8262.

Ramsoekh, D.; Wagner, A.; van Leerdam, M.E.; Dooijes, D.; Tops, C.M>; Steyerberg, E.W.; Kuipers, E.J. (2009). Cancer risk in MLH1, MSH2, and MSH6 mutation carriers; different risk profiles may influence clinical management. *Hereditary Cancer in Clinical Practice*, Vol.23, No.1, pp.17, ISSN 1897-4287.

Ribic, C.M.; Sargent, D.J.; Moore, M.J.; Thibodeau, S.N.; French, A.J.; Goldberg, R.M.; Hamilton, S.R.; Laurent-Puig, P.; Gryfe, R.; Shepherd, L.E.; Tu, D.; Redston, M. & Gallinger, S. (2003). Tumor microsatellite-instability status as a predictor of benefit from flurouracil-based adjuvant chemotherapy for colon cancer. *New England Journal of Medicine*, Vol.349, No.3, pp.247-57, ISSN 1533-4406.

Rio Frio, T.; Lavoie, J.; Hamel, N.; Geyer, F.C.; Kushner, Y.B.; Novak, D.J.; Wark, L.: Capelli, C.; Reis-Filho, J.S.; Mai, S.; Pastinen, T.; Tischlowitz, M.D.; Marcus, V.A.& Foulkes, W.D. (2010). Homozygous BUB1B Mutation and Susceptibility to Gastrointestinal Neoplasia. *New England Journal of Medicine*, Vol.363, No.27, pp.2628-37, ISSN 1533-4406.

Ruijs, M.W.G.; Verhoef, S.; Rookus, M.A.; Pruntel, R.; van der Hout, A.H.; Hogervorst, F.B.L.; Kluijt, I.; Sijmons, R.H.; Aalfs, C.M.; Wagner, A.; Ausems, M.G.E.M.; Hoogerbrugge, N.; van Asperen, C.J.; Gomez Garcia, E.B.; Meijers-Heijboer, H.; ten Kate, L.P.; Menko, F.H. & van't Veer, L. (2010). TP53 germline mutation testing in 180 families suspected of Li-Fraumeni syndrome: mutation detection rate and relative frequency of cancers in different familial phenotypes. *Journal of Medical Genetics*, Vol. 47, No.6, pp.421-428, ISSN 1468-6244.

Ruivenkamp, C.A.; van Wezel, T.; Zanon, C.; Stassen, A.P.; Vlcek, C.; Csikos, T.; Klous, A.M.; Tripodis, N.; Perrakis, A.; Beorrigter, L.; Groot, P.C.; Lindeman, J.; Mooi, W.J.; Meijer, G.A.; Scholten, G.; Dauwerse, H.; Paces, V.; van Zandwijk, N.; van Ommen, G.J. & Demant, P. (2002). Ptprj is a candidate for the mosue colon-cancer susceptibility locus Scc1 and is frequently deleted in human cancers. *Nature Genetics*, Vol.31, No.3, pp.295-300, ISSN 1061-4036.

Salovaara, R.; Loukola, A.; Kristo, P.; Kaariainen, H.; Ahtola, H.; Eskelinen, M.; Harkonen, N.; Julkunen, R.; Kangas, E.; Ojala, S.; Tulikoura, J.; Valkamo, E.; Jarvinen, H.; Mecklin, J.P.; Aaltonen, L.A. & de la Chapelle, A. (2000). Population-based molecular detection of hereditary nonpolyposis colorectal cancer. *Journal of Clinical Oncology*, Vol.18, No.11, pp.2193-200, ISSN 1527-7755.

Sanchez de Abajo, A.; de la Hoya, M.; Fodrino, J.; Furio, V.; Tosar, A.; Perez-Segura, P.; Diaz-Ruibo, E. & Caldes T. (2005). The CHEK2 1100delC allele is not relevant for risk assessment in HNPCC and HBCC Spanish Families. *Familial Cancer*, Vol.4, No.2., pp.183-6, ISSN 1573-7292.

Senter, L.; Clendenning, M.; Sotamaa, K.; Hampel, H.; Green, J.; Potter, J.D.; Lindblom, A.; Lagerstedt, K.; Thibodeau, S.N.; Lindor, N.M.; Young, J.; Winship, I.; Dowty, J.G.; White, D.M.; Hopper, J.L.; Baglietto, L.; Jenkins, M.A. & de la Chapelle, A. (2008). The clinical phenotype of Lynch syndrome due to germl-line PMS mutations. *Gastroenterology*, Vol.135, No.2, pp.419-28, ISSN 0016-5085.

Talseth, B.A.; Ashton, K.A.; Meldrum, C.; Suchy, J.; Kurzawski, G.; Lubinski, J. & Scott, R.J. (2008). Aurora-A and Cyclin D1 polymorphisms and the age of onset of colorectal cancer in hereditary nonpolyposis colorectal cancer. *International Journal of Cancer*, Vol.122, No.6, pp.1273-7, ISSN 1097-0215.

Talseth-Palmer, B.A.; McPhillips, M.; Groombridge, C.; Spigelman, A. & Scott, R.J. (2010). MSH6 and PMS2 mutation positive Australian Lynch syndrome families: novel mutations, cancer risk and age of diagnosis of colorectal cancer. *Hereditary Cancer in Clinical Practice*, Vol.8, No.1, p.5. ISSN 1897-4287.

Tenesa, A.; Campbell, H.; Barnetson, R.; Porteous, M.; Dunlop, M. & Farrington, S.M. (2006). Association of MUTYH and colorectal cancer. *British Journal of Cancer*, Vol.95, No.2, pp.239-42, ISSN 0007-0920.

Taylor, D.P.; Burt, R.W.; Williams, M.S.; Haug, P.J. & Cannon-Albright, L.A. (2010). Population-based family history specific risks for colorectal cancer: a constellation approach. *Gastroenterology*, Vol.138, No.3, pp.877-85, ISSN 0016-5085.

Tenesa, A.; Farrington, S.M.; Prendergast, J.G.; Porteous, M.E.; Walker, M.; Haq, N.; Barnetson, R.A.; Theodoratou, E.; Cetnarskyj, R.; Cartwright, N.;, Semple, C.; Clark, A.J.; Reid, F.J.; Smith, L.A.; Kavoussanakis, K.; Koessler, T.; Pharoah, P.D.; Buch, S.; Schafmayer, C.; Tepel, J., Schreiber, S; Völzke, H.; Schmidt, C.O.;Hampe, J.; Chang-Claude, J.; Hoffmeister, M.; Brenner, H.; Wilkening, S.; Canzian, F.; Capella, G.; Moreno, V.; Deary, I.J.; Starr, J.M.; Tomlinson, I.P.; Kemp, Z.; Howarth, K.; Carvajal-Carmona, L.; Webb, E.; Broderick, P.; Vijayakrishnan, J.; Houlston, R.S.; Rennert, G.; Ballinger, D.; Rozek, L.; Gruber, S.B.; Matsuda, K.; Kidokoro, T.; Nakamura, Y.; Zanke, B.W.; Greenwood, C.M.; Rangrej, J.; Kustra, R.; Montpetit, A.; Hudson, T.J.; Gallinger, S.; Campbell, H. & Dunlop, M.G. (2008). Genome-wide association scan identifies a colorectal cancer susceptibility locus on 11q23 and replicates risk loci at 8q24 and 18q21. *Nature Genetics*, Vol.40, No.5, pp.631-7, ISSN 1061-4036.

Tenesa, A. & Dunlop, M.G. (2009). New insights into the aetiology of colorectal cancer from genome-wide association studies. *Nature Reviews in Genetics*, Vol.10, No.6, pp.353-8, ISSN 1471-0056.

Tenesa, A.; Theodoratou, E.; Din, F.V.N.; Farrington, S.M.; Cetnarskyj, R.; Barnetson, R.A.; Porteous, M.E.; Campbell, H. & Dunlop, M.G. (2010). Ten common genetic variants associated with colorectal cancer risk are not associated with survival after diagnosis. *Clinical Cancer Research*, Vol.16, No.10, pp.3754-9, ISSN 1557-3265.

Theodoratou, E.; Campbell, H.; Tenesa, A.; Houlston, R.; Webb, E.; Lubbe, S.; Broderick, P.; Gallinger, S.; Croitoru, E.M.; Jenkins, M.A.; Win, A.K.; Cleary, S.P.; Koessler, T.; Pharoah, P.D.; Küry, S.; Bézieau, S.; Buecher, B.; Ellis, N.A.; Peterlongo, P.; Offit, K.; Aaltonen, L.A.; Enholm, S; Lindblom, A.; Zhou, X.L.; Tomlinson, I.P.; Moreno, V.; Blanco, I.; Capellà, G.; Barnetson, R.; Porteous, M.E.; Dunlop, M.G. & Farrington, S.M. (2010). A large-scale meta-analysis to refine colorectal cancer risk associated with MUTHY variants. *British Journal of Cancer*, Vol.103, No.12, pp.1875-84, ISSN 0007-0920.

Toland, A.E.; Rozek, L.S.; Presswala, S.; Rennert, G.; Gruber, S.B. PTPRJ haplotypes and colorectal cancer risk. (2008). *Cancer Epidemiology, Biomarkers & Prevention*, Vol.17, No.10, pp.2782-5, ISSN 1055-9965.

Tomlinson, I.; Webb, E.; Carvajal-Carmona, L.; Broderick, P.; Kemp, Z., Spain, S.; Penegar, S.; Chandler, I.; Gorman, M.; Wood, W.; Barclay, E.; Lubbe, S.; Martin, L.; Sellick, G.; Jaeger, E.; Hubner, R.; Wild, R.; Rowan, A.; Fielding, S.; Howarth, K.; CORGI Consortium; Silver, A.; Atkin, W.; Muir, K.; Logan, R.; Kerr, D.; Johnstone, E.; Sieber, O.; Gray, R.; Thomas, H.; Peto, J.; Cazier, J.B. & Houlston, R. (2007). A genome-wide association scan of tag SNPs identifies a susceptibility variant for colorectal cancer at 8q24.21. *Nature Genetics*, Vol.39, No.8, pp.984-8, ISSN 1061-4036.

Tomlinson, I.P.; Webb, E.; Carvajal-Carmona, L.; Broderick, P.; Howarth, K.; Pittman, A.M.; Spain, S.; Lubbe, S.; Walther, A.; Sullivan, K.; Jaeger, E.; Fielding, S.; Rowan, A.; Vijayakrishnan, J.; Domingo, E.; Chandler, I.; Kemp, Z.; Qureshi, M.; Farrington, S.M.; Tenesa, A.; Prendergast, J.G.; Barnetson, R.A.; Penegar, S.; Barclay, E.; Wood, W.; Martin, L.; Gorman, M.; Thomas, H.; Peto, J.; Bishop, D.T.; Gray, R.; Maher, E.R.; Lucassen, A.; Kerr, D.; Evans, D.G.; CORGI Consortium; Schafmayer, C.; Buch, S.; Völzke, H.; Hampe, J.; Schreiber, S.; John, U.; Koessler, T.; Pharoah, P.; van Wezel, T.; Morreau, H.; Wijnen, J.T.; Hopper, J.L.; Southey, M.C.; Giles, G.G.; Severi, G.; Castellví-Bel, S.; Ruiz-Ponte, C.; Carracedo, A.; Castells, A.; EPICOLON Consortium; Försti, A.; Hemminki, K.; Vodicka, P.; Naccarati, A.; Lipton, L.; Ho, J.W.; Cheng, K.K.; Sham, P.C.; Luk, J.; Agúndez, J.A.; Ladero, J.M.; de la Hoya, M.; Caldés, T.; Niittymäki, I.; Tuupanen, S.; Karhu, A.; Aaltonen, L.; Cazier, J.B.; Campbell, H.; Dunlop, M.G. & Houlston, R.S. (2008). A genome-wide association study identifies colorectal cancer susceptibility loci on chromosomes 10p14 and 8q23.3. *Nature Genetics*, Vol.40, No.5, pp.623-30, ISSN 1061-4036.

Tresallet C.; Brouquet, A.; Julie, C.; Beauchet, A.; Vallot, C.; Menegaux, F.; Mitry, E.; Radvanyi, F.; Malafosse, R.; Rougier, P.; Nordlinger, B.; Laurent-Puig, P.; Boileau, C.; Emile, J.-F.; Muti, C.; Penna, C.; Hofmann-Radvanyi, H. (2011). Evaluation of predictive models for the identification in daily practice of patients with Lynch syndrome. *International Journal of Cancer*, E-pub ahead of print, ISSN 1097-0215.

Tuupanen, S.; Turunen, M.; Lehtonen, R.; Hallikas, O.; Vanharanta, S.; Kivioja, T.; Bjorklund, M.; Wei, G.; Yan, J.; Nittymaki, I.; Mecklin, J.P.; Jarvinen, H.; Ristimaki, A.; Di-Bernardo, M.; East, P.; Carvajal-Carmona, L.; Houlston, R.S.; Tomlinson, I.; Palin, K.; Ukkonen, E.; Karhu, A.; Taipale, J.; Aaltonen, L.A. (2009). The common colorectal cancer predisposition SNP rs6983267 at chromosome 8q24 confers potential to enhanced Wnt signaling. *Nature Genetics*, Vol.41, No.8, pp.885-90, ISSN 1061-4036.

Umar, A.; Boland, C.R.; Terdiman, J.P.; Syngal, S.; de la Chapelle, A.; Ruschoff, J.; Fishel, R.; Lindor, N.M.; Burgart, L.J.; Hamelin, R.; Hamilton, S.R.; Hiatt, R.A.; Jass, J.;Lindblom, A.; Lynch, H.T.; Peltomaki, P.; Ramsey, S.D.; Rodriguez-Bigas, M.A.; Vasen, H.F.; Hawk, E.T.; Barrett, J.C.; Freedman, A.N. & Srivastava, S. (2004). Revised Bethesda guidelines for hereditary nonpolyposis colorectal cancer (Lynch syndrome) and microsatellite instability. *Journal of the National Cancer Institute*, Vol.96, No.4, pp.261-8, ISSN 1460-2105.

Van Lier, M.G.; Wagner, A.; Mathus-Vliegen, E.M.; Kuipers, E.J.; Steyerberg, E.W.; van Leerdam, M.E. (2010). High cancer risk in Peutz-Jeghers syndrome: a systematic review and surveillance recommendations. *American Journal of Gastroenterology*, Vol.105, No.6, pp.1258-1264, ISSN 0002-9270.

Van Lier, M.G.F.; Westerman, A.M.; Wagner, A.; Looman, C.W.N.; Wilson, J.H.P. de Rooij, F.W.M.; Lemmens, V.E.P.P.; Kuipers, E.J.; Mathus-Vliegen, E.M.H. & van Leerdam, M.E. (2011). High cancer risk and increased mortality in patients with Peutz-Jeghers syndrome. *Gut*, Vol. 60, No. pp.141-7, ISSN 1468-3288.

Van Wezel, T.; Stassen, A.P.; Moen, C.J.; Hart, A.A. van der Val, M.A. & Demant, P. (1996). Gene interaction and single gene effects in colon tumour susceptibility in mice. *Nature Genetics*, Vol.14, No.4, pp.468-70, ISSN 1061-4036.

Van Wezel, T.; Ruivenkamp, C.A.; Stassen, A.P.; Moen, C.J. & Demant, P. (1999). Four new colon cancer susceptibility loci, Scc6 to Scc9 in the mouse. *Cancer Research*, Vol.59, No.17, pp.4216-8, ISSN 1538-7445.

Vasen, H.F.; Mecklin, J.P.; Khan, P.M. & Lynch, H.T. (1991). The international collaborative group on Hereditary Non-Polyposis Colorectal Cancer (ICG-HNPCC). *Diseases of the Colon & Rectum*, Vol.34, No.5, pp.424-5, ISSN 1530-0358.

Vasen, H.F.; Watson, P.; Mecklin, J.P.; Lynch, H.T. (1999). New clinical criteria for hereditary nonpolyposis colorectal cancer (HNPCC, Lynch syndrome) proposed by the International Collaborative group on HNPCC. *Gastroenterology*, Vol.116, No.15, pp.1453-6, ISSN 0016-5085.

Volikos, E.; Robinson, J.; Aittomaki, K.; Mecklin, J.P.; Jarvinen, H.; Westerman, A.M.; de Rooji, F.W.; Vogel, T.; Moeslein, G.; Launonen, V.; Tomlinson, I.P.; Silver, A.R. & Aaltonen, L.A. (2006). LKB1 exonic and whole gene deletions are a common cause of Peutz-Jeghers syndrome. *Journal of Medical Genetics*, Vol.43, No.5, pp.e18, ISSN 1468-6244.

Wasielelewski, M.; Vasen, H.; Wijnen, J.; Hooning, M.; Dooijes, D.; Topa, C., Klign, J.G.; Meijers-Heijboer, H. & Schutte, M. (2008). CHEK2 1100delC is a susceptibility allele for HNPCC-related colorectal cancer. *Clinical Cancer Research*, Vol.14, No.15, pp. 4989-94, ISSN 1557-3265.

Wimmer, K. & Kratz, C.P. (2010). Constitutional mismatch repair-deficiency syndrome. *Haematologica*, Vol.95, No.5, pp.699-701, ISSN 1592-8721.

Xing, J.; Myers, R.; He, X.; Qu, F.; Zhou, F.; Ma, X.; Hylsop, T.; Bao, G.; Wan, S.; Yang, H.; Chen, Z. (2011). GWAS-identified colorectal cancer susceptibility locus associates with disease prognosis. *European Journal of Cancer*, Vol.47, No.11, pp.1699-707, ISSN 0959-8049.

Xiong, F.; Wu, C.; Bi, X.; Yu, D.; Huang, L.; Xu, J.; Zhang, T.; Zhai, K.; Chang, J.; Tan, W.; Cai, J. & Lin D. (2011). Risk of Genome-Wide Association Study-Identified Genetic Variants for Colorectal Cancer in a Chinese Population. *Cancer Epidemiology, Biomarkers &Prevention*, Vol.19, No.7, pp.1855-61, ISSN 1538-775.

Young, J. & Jass, J.R. (2006). The case for a genetic predisposition to serrated neoplasia in the colorectum: hypothesis and review of the literature. *Cancer Epidemiology, Biomarkers & Prevention*, Vol.15, No.10, pp.1778-84, ISSN 1538-7755.

4

The Role of Modifier Genes in Lynch Syndrome

Rodney J. Scott[1,2,3], Stuart Reeves[1] and Bente Talseth-Palmer[1,3]
[1]The Centre for Information Based Medicine,
The School of Biomedical Sciences
and Pharmacy, University of Newcastle,
[2]Division of Genetics, Hunter Area Pathology Service,
[3]Hunter Medical Research Institute,
United Kingdom

1. Introduction

There are a number of inherited predispositions to colorectal cancer (CRC) which can be broadly categorized into two groups; those with associated polyposis, such as familial adenomatous polyposis and the hamartomatous polyposis syndromes; and those that are linked to the non-polyposis syndromes, such as hereditary non polyposis colorectal cancer (HNPCC). The genetic basis of both the polyposis and non-polyposis syndromes are reflected in the CRC population who have no apparent family history of disease. Approximately 80% of all cases of CRC are associated with chromosomal instability [1] and are likely to have mutations in the Adenomatous Polyposis Coli (APC) gene whereas the remaining 20% with microsatellite instability appears to be due primarily to epigenetic inactivation of the DNA mismatch repair (MMR) gene *MLH1* [2].

The disease HNPCC accounts for somewhere between 2% and 5% of all CRCs diagnosed and is associated with a younger age of disease onset compared to the general population [3,4]. HNPCC is a disease by definition based on the Amsterdam Criteria where there need to be three cases of CRC, one of which must be diagnosed under the age of 50 years, one patient must be a first degree relative of the other two, span two generations and familial adenomatous polyposis should be excluded [5]. Modification of the Amsterdam Criteria has been ongoing since its original inception due to an increasing awareness of what constitutes this disease. HNPCC used to be known as either the Cancer Family Syndrome or Lynch Syndrome [6]. It is now accepted that families where a mutation in the DNA mismatch repair genes (MMR) *MSH2, MLH1, MSH6* or *PMS2* has been identified are now termed Lynch Syndrome families whereas those with no mutation are termed HNPCC [7]. The primary function of MMR genes is to eliminate base-base mismatches and insertion-deletion loops which arise as a consequence of DNA polymerase slippage during DNA replication [8]. MMR confers several genetic stabilisation functions; it corrects DNA biosynthesis errors, ensures the fidelity of genetic recombination and participates in the earliest steps of cell cycle checkpoint control and apoptotic responses [9,10]. MMR gene defects increases the risk of malignant transformation of cells, which ultimately results in the disruption of one or several genes associated with epithelial integrity. The identification of germline mutations in families with Lynch Syndrome accounts for only ~50% of all families that fulfil the clinical diagnosis defined by the Amsterdam criteria [11]. The remaining families have no identifiable genetic predisposition yet fulfil the diagnostic criteria for the disease and are referred to as HNPCC families.

DNA MMR is a housekeeping function of all nucleated cells and as such any breakdown in the fidelity of this process is likely to result in disease irrespective of which gene is affected. Unlike other predispositions to colorectal cancer such as familial adenomatous polyposis, there are no obvious genotype/phenotype correlations in Lynch syndrome. Mutations that result in the loss of MSH2 or MLH1 irrespective of where they occur in the respective gene alter the risk of developing malignancy. Furthermore, mutations in DNA MMR genes do not predict a phenotype since any breakdown in the fidelity of this process results in a "mutator phenotype". It has been obvious from the first MSH2 and MLH1 mutation reports that differences in the ages of cancer diagnosis in patients harbouring germline mutations in DNA MMR genes do occur both within and between families. Furthermore, unrelated families harbouring the same mutation present with different disease profiles as do patients from within the same family [12-14]. The differences in disease expression both within and between families harbouring the same mutation are most likely a result of environmental, genetic or a mixture of both influences.

Identification of environmental factors that could account for differences in the age of colorectal cancer diagnosis of Lynch Syndrome is almost intractable when undertaken as a retrospective study and is best undertaken prospectively to include as many environmental variables as possible. Notwithstanding, knowledge about environmental factors and disease risk in Lynch Syndrome is important and studies are required to identify those which protect or promote disease.

Conversely, as genetic factors can be assessed after the fact they lend themselves more readily to retrospective interrogation and consequently identification. Identifying genetic factors that could explain differential disease expression in Lynch syndrome is now achievable due to the development of appropriate technology that allows for the rapid screening of large numbers of patients in conjunction with the accumulation of large cohorts of patients that allow for robust statistical analysis.

The search for modifier genes has been ongoing ever since the first groups of Lynch syndrome families were identified. Initial studies focused on genes associated with xenobiotic metabolism which have been followed by genes involved in the immune response, DNA repair, cell cycle control and as yet undefined genomic regions identified as a result of large genome wide association studies searching for genetic risk factors for colorectal cancer. This review will focus on "modifiable" (those that can be altered by manipulation) candidate modifier genes and those that have been chosen as a result of biological plausibility (which may or may not be modifiable), as shown in Table 1.

Biological plausibility and pathways of published "positive" results have been questioned [15], indicating that the functional significance of single nucleotide polymorphisms (SNPs) should be known before they are linked to disease [16]. A few published reports linking SNPs without known functional significance [17,18] or studies have failed to confirm a reported associations [19]. Known genetic variation has significantly impacted on the early detection and diagnosis of inherited cancer [20, 21], indicating that the search for genetic variation in cancer should continue.

Modifier Genes and polymorphisms studied in Lynch Syndrome			
Candidate Genes	Type of Polymorphisms	Effect	Publication indicating association or not
IGF1	CA-repeat	promoter function	[22, 23]
MTHFR	SNP	enzyme activity	[24]
HFE	SNP	protein function	[25]
NAT2	SNP	enzyme activity	[26, 27]
GSTM1	null allele	enzyme activity	[26, 27]
GSTT1	null allele	enzyme activity	[26, 27]
ATM	SNP	protein function	[28]
IL6	SNP	cytokine activity	[29]
IL4	SNP	cytokine activity	[29]
IL1β	SNP	receptor binding	[29]
IL10	SNP	cytokine activity	[29]
IL1Rn	SNP	null receptor	[29]
TNF-α	SNP	cytokine activity	[29]
IFN-γ	SNP	cytokine activity	[29]
TP53	SNP	protein function	[32, 39, 40]
MDM2	SNP	promoter function	[42]
Aurora-A	SNP	protein function	[44, 45, 48]
Cyclin D1	SNP	protein function	[44, 45, 48]

Table. 1. Candidate modifier genes and their respective types of polymorphism that have been studied in cohorts of Lynch syndrome patients.

2. Cell cycle control gene polymorphisms: TP53. MDM2, Aurora-A and CyclinD1

The TP53 gene isa tumour suppressor gene that regulates the transcription of genes necessary for the maintenance of genomic integrity by blocking cell proliferation after DNA damage and initiating apoptosis if it is too extensive [30, 31]. In 2004 the R72P polymorphism in TP53 was found to be associated with age of diagnosis of colorectal cancer (CRC) in an American Lynch syndrome study [32]. The R72P SNP in TP53 has been shown to result in two forms of the protein, which are not functionally equivalent [33, 34], and has been widely studied in a variety of malignancies [35 - 38]. Subsequent studies, including one Finnish and a collaborative Australian and Polish study, of the TP53 polymorphism and age of diagnosis of CRC in Lynch syndrome failed to confirm the reported association [39, 40]. The lack of an association was suggested to be related to a polymorphism in MDM2, which results in increased levels of MDM2 that culminates in the inability to properly stabilise TP53's response to cellular stress [40]. Evidence supporting this notion in HNPCC however, could not be found in other studies [39, 41]. The failure to corroborate the role of TP53 as a modifier gene between the different studies could be due to differences in the mutation spectrum of the various study populations; number of relatives included, population stratification and/or type 1 statistical error. Population stratification is unlikely to account for differences between the study populations as it has been shown that for most of the common disease associated polymorphisms, ethnicity is likely to be a poor predictor of an individuals' genotype [43]. Type 1 statistical error seems to be the most likely explanation since the population sizes differ significantly in size with a range between 86 cases through to a maximum number of 220. In the larger studies reported to date (encompassing 193 and 220 patients, respectively), no association was observed thereby providing evidence against an association.

Aurora-A and Cyclin D1, genes both involved in cell cycle control, have also been associated with the age of onset of CRC in Lynch syndrome patients from North America [44, 45]. After the initial studies suggesting Aurora-A polymorphisms were linked to the average age of disease diagnosis follow-up reports in larger patient populations consistently failed to replicate this finding. In contrast, studies of Cyclin D1 polymorphisms and their association with the age of disease onset in Lynch syndrome resulted in contradictory results when studied in populations from North America, Germany, Finland and a combined study of Australian and Polish patients [44, 46 – 48]. A potential explanation for the association between Cyclin D1 and hMSH2 mutation carriers observed in the Australian and Polish Lynch syndrome patients was the relative paucity of MSH2 mutation carriers in the German and Finnish populations [47]. With the expansion of the study population from the Australian/Polish patient cohort the original report of an association with Cyclin D1 could not be replicated (See Fig. 1). In conclusion, the evidence now suggests that there is no association between Cyclin D1, MSH2 and disease risk in Lynch syndrome, such that overall Cyclin D1 does not appear to be associated with the age of disease diagnosis.

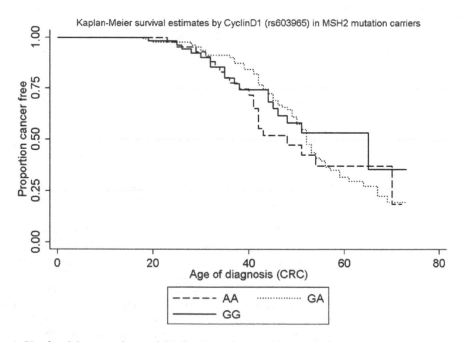

Fig. 1. Kaplan-Meier analysis of Cyclin D1 polymorphism and the age of disease onset in Australian and Polish Lynch syndrome patients. 276 MSH2 mutation positive patients were included in this study of which 107 were diagnosed with colorectal cancer. Log-rank, Wilcoxon and Tarone-Ware tests were not significant.

3. Xenobiotic clearance gene polymorphisms: NAT1, NAT2, GST, CYP1A1

Genes involved in xenobiotic metabolism, which include N-acetyl transferase 1 (NAT1), N-acetyl transferase 2 (NAT2), glutathione-S-transferase (GST) and cytochrome P450, have the ability to influence an individual's susceptibility to environmental and occupational carcinogens and predisposition to cancer [49]. The detoxification and elimination of foreign chemicals is controlled by complex mechanisms involving phase I enzymes that include cytochrome P450, and phase II enzymes such as GSTs and NATs [50]. Because of the significance of xenobiotics in the environment, perturbations in the ability to remove them are likely to alter disease risk. Polymorphisms in the genes mentioned above have been associated with colorectal cancer but the roles that the different SNPs have on cancer risk are controversial [26, 27, 51 – 61].

In 1999 an association between polymorphisms in NAT2 and the age of diagnosis of CRC in Lynch syndrome patients was reported, and the association was later replicated in a second independent report [26, 54]. Both studies had relatively small sample sizes (78 and 86 cases). Re-investigation of the association in a smaller study (69 cases) and a more appropriately sized one (220 cases) failed to confirm the association [58, 26]. The failure to confirm the association could be due to population stratification, but this is unlikely since if there is a functional difference in the gene in question,so its effects should be observed in all subjects, although not necessarily statistically significant in all populations. The most likely explanation for the failure to replicate initial findings is the small study population sizes that were used in assessing the potential association. This is further confirmed in a review by Brockton *et al.* 2000 [62] concluding that in 10 of 11 studies of invasive CRC and NAT2 acetylator genotype, no association was observed.

Similar results are reported for the polymorphisms in GST and cytochrome p450 genes and Lynch syndrome. Several research groups reported an association, while others failed to confirm them [25, 26, 51, 52, 53, 53, 63]. In on study the Msp1 wildtype allele of cytochrome P450 1A1 gene (CYP1A1) was associated with a decreased risk of CRC [26] which could have been due to it not being in Hardy-Weinberg equilibrium. The identification of an allele that is not in Hardy-Weinberg equilibrium suggests that either a genotyping error has occurred thereby skewing the results or it can be taken as supporting evidence for a correlation with disease [64]. The CYP1A1 gene has previously been associated with CRC and two SNPs in the CYP1A1 gene have been associated with CRC [65], which taken together with the report of Talseth et al. 2006 [26] supports the notion that variation in this gene is involved in the some aspect of CRC development.

Studies examining variation in xenobiotic clearance are likely to be subject to strong environmental influence and this is supported by findings from different countries. Studies examining patients of European descent for polymorphisms in GST genes seems to find no obvious relationship between the SNPs and cancer risk, while a study from Korea reports an association [25, 26, 63]. Taken together, these results suggest a complex relationship between the environment and individual genotypes that add to other more obvious problems associated with searching for modifier genes. Additional studies are required to determine the relationship between GST and CYP1A1 polymorphisms and disease risk in Lynch syndrome.

4. Immune response gene polymorphisms: IL6, IL4, IL1β, IL10, IL1Rn, TNF-α, IFN-γ

Cytokine mediated events may play a role in tumour development within inflammatory cells by producing an environment that supports tumour growth by promoting angiogenesis and facilitating genomic instability. The quintessential example is that of Crohn's disease where there is an increased risk of developing CRC if left untreated [66]. Inflammatory responses can also increase DNA damage, growth stimulation and enhanced survival of damaged cells [66, 67]. SNPs in cytokine genes can have an effect on the transcription levels of the respective genes and resulting in differences in both pro- and anti-inflammatory response activity. A series of polymorphisms in a number of cytokines has been investigated in relation to CRC risk and other cancer types but not for Lynch syndrome [68 - 77]. In addition, genetic variation in pro- and anti-inflammatory cytokine genes has been shown to influence individual response to carcinogen exposure [69], but no association has been identified in the one report focusing on a series of SNPs in cytokine genes and disease expression in Lynch syndrome [28]. Given the complexity of the inflammatory response and the limited number of SNPs utilised in that study, it cannot be ruled out that a relationship between SNPs influencing the immune response and Lynch syndrome exits.

5. Insulin like Growth Factor IGF-1 Gene polymorphisms

The *IGF-1* gene was first reported as a potential modifying gene in Lynch syndrome disease expression in 2006. The CA-repeat polymorphism located near the *IGF-1* promoter region was described as having an association with the age of disease onset in a cohort of 121 Lynch syndrome patients originating from the United States [22]. Certainly this is not the first time that a repeat region has been implicated in disease; with numerous studies reporting a link between DNA repeat regions significantly altering risk of prostate cancer [78 - 80] breast cancer, squamous cell carcinoma, bladder and lung cancers [81 - 84]. DNA microsatellite repeat regions are also strongly associated with Lynch Syndrome by virtue of their instability in tumours which is a consequence of the loss in the fidelity of DNA MMR [8].

IGF-1 is important for cellular proliferation and differentiation however, elevated levels of IGF-1 have been reported to have significant links to diseases such as CRC which is thought to be a result of the mitogenic and anti-apoptotic effects elicited by this protein [22, 85]. Several environmental and physiological reasons have been proposed that influence IGF-1 expression; however there is now evidence to suggest that a genetic role is significant. Rosen *et al.* was the first to report that the length of the CA repeat region in *IGF-1* may be associated with circulating IGF-1 levels [86]. In a similar growth factor related gene, Epidermal Growth Factor Receptor (EGFR), a CA repeat region is located in intron 1. A study of this *EGFR* polymorphic repeat region revealed lower transcriptional activity with increasing numbers of polymorphic CA repeats coinciding with lower levels of gene expression [87]. In 2007, a similar result was reported for the *IGF-1* gene in swine where the length of the CA repeat region was clearly associated with circulating levels of IGF-1 [88]. More recently, additional human data has been published which supports the notion that this polymorphism is linked to serum levels of IGF-1 [89]. From this data a trend is emerging that CA repeat polymorphisms in growth factor related genes, such as *IGF-1*, are related to overall gene expression, which is reflected in the circulating serum levels of the respective proteins. Accumulating evidence suggests that serum IGF-1 levels appear to be linked to disease with recent reports indicating that elevated levels of IGF-1 are observed in breast, prostate and CRC [90 – 93]. There have been estimates that higher circulating levels of IGF-1 result in a 15% increase in the risk of developing disease, insinuating the importance of circulating IGF-1 in disease progression [94].

As CRC involves the accrual of a number of specific molecular alterations [95, 96], consistently high IGF-1 serum levels may increase cellular proliferation, thereby enhancing the rate by which genetic alterations accumulate. Both normal colonic epithelial and transformed cells are IGF-1 responsive; thus, IGF-1 can influence not only the likelihood of disease initiation but also disease progression. This overall process provides some insight into how intracellular serum levels of IGF-1 may have a significant influence in accelerating the accumulation of genetic errors leading to disease, especially in persons who have inherited a predisposition to develop malignancy characterized by a mutator phenotype as observed in Lynch syndrome.

An equally important facet to disease risk as a result of increased levels of IGF-1 is its link with obesity. Obesity and physical inactivity are strong independent determinants of insulin resistance and hyperinsulinaemia [97 – 104] and this is associated with an increased risk of CRC [101, 102]. Increased blood insulin lowers IGF-1 binding protein levels, which often results in an increase of free IGF-1 [105]. As IGF-1 is associated with both percentage body fat and general overall obesity [106], an increased level of IGF-1 expression as a result of shorter CA repeat lengths may have an enhanced effect in persons who are obese where IGF-1 serum levels are already elevated.

In addition to the IGF-1 effect, CRC risk is also increased in obese patients through oxidative stress in adipose tissue. This is caused by increased lipid peroxidation leading to the production of reactive oxygen species. In regards to cancer, reactive oxygen species can damage DNA by several methods including DNA base modification, deletions, frame shifts, strand breaks, DNA-protein cross-links, and chromosomal rearrangements [107]. Both lipid peroxidation and increased DNA damage are likely to promote tumour development by generating reactive oxygen species, increasing hormone production/bioavailability of IGF-1 and providing an energy-rich environment. This combined mechanism is potentially a risk factor for all types of CRC, however in Lynch syndrome this may be of greater significance in a deficient DNA repair environment where enhanced levels of IGF-1 inhibit cell death and encourage cellular proliferation. Together, the relationship between obesity and IGF-1 CA repeat length may be of particular importance in obese Lynch syndrome cases as these may be at greatest risk of developing disease at a younger age.

The role of inherited factors in circulating IGF1 serum levels is likely to be substantial with estimates of the proportion of variance in IGF-1 that is genetically determined varying somewhere between 38% to over 80% [108]. A substantial amount of data has been reported revealing differences in IGF levels across ethnic groups [109 – 111], however this is suggestive of dietary and lifestyle factors having a more modifiable effect on serum levels when combined with genetic ancestry. One such study has shown that the impact of several nutritional factors such as calcium, dairy products and vegetables on IGF1 levels is quite different in racially stratified models as reported between African-American and European American males [112]. This is strongly suggestive of there being population differences that differentially modify the effect of several nutrients on IGF levels. Together this information is suggestive that environmental factors such as calorific intake, lifestyle and demographic factors are probably playing a substantial role in ethnic variation in disease risk in regards to

serum IGF levels. This is intriguing as it may also be contributing to the differences in relative disease risk observed between the Polish and Australian cohorts as reported [22].
The data reported to date [21] indicate a significant interaction between the CA repeat polymorphism length and disease expression in Lynch syndrome which is likely to be linked to circulating levels of IGF-1. The data suggest a significant correlation for earlier onset CRC in participants who carry 17 or less IGF-1 CA repeats in over 400 Lynch syndrome patients. An encouraging aspect of the results of this study is that significance is retained across two different populations where variance in IGF-1 allele size frequencies occur [22]. A limitation however in defining the exact relationship between IGF-1 expression and cancer incidence in Lynch syndrome patients is the genotype–phenotype correlation between the *IGF-1* CA-repeat number and the corresponding serum levels. Assessment of serum IGF-1 concentration, however, has the inherent problem of serum IGF-I measurement, which is typically assessed at only one time point yet for accurate analysis should be performed multiple times from any single patient. Whether it would be feasible to monitor IGF-1 serum levels in families with Lynch syndrome is an area which needs further investigation. Future work should also include additional candidate polymorphisms located within *IGF-1* or *IGFBP-3* that interact with the IGF-1 pathway and may provide further insight into the overall IGF-1 effect. At present, however the IGF-1 pathway remains largely under-investigated, and there is now a requirement for further work to develop a more thorough understanding of the relationship between *IGF-1* genotype, expression and its implication in disease risk.

6. Methylenetetrahydrofolate reductase (MTHFR) gene polymorphisms

There have been tantalizing reports in the literature that polymorphisms in the *MTHFR* gene are associated with altered CRC risk. These polymorphisms occur in relatively high frequency in the general population and the two that promote special attention are both associated with altered enzymatic function. MTHFR is a key folate-metabolizing enzyme involved in both DNA methylation and DNA synthesis. The enzyme catalyses the irreversible conversion of 5,10-methylenetetrahydrofolate (5,10-MTHF), needed for purine and thymidine synthesis, to 5-methyltetrahydrofolate (5-MTHF), which is necessary for methionine production. Insufficient thymidine results in uracil misincorporation into DNA, leading to single-strand and double-strand breaks. This can increase the incidence of DNA damage, thereby increasing the risk of genetic instability. The understanding that folate metabolism can both equally influence DNA synthesis and methylation has made the study of environmental and genetic variants associated with MTHFR particularly attractive as a candidate genetic factor that influences cancer susceptibility. Two common polymorphisms, *C677T* and *A1298C* are located within the MTHFR gene and have been linked to altering the function of the encoded protein. This has lead to these variants being the focus of numerous studies into CRC risk outside the context of an inherited predisposition to disease. Both polymorphisms result in a substitution of an amino acid and have previously been shown to significantly influence MTHFR enzyme activity [113]. *C677T* is located within the coding region for the catalytic domain, resulting in an amino acid substitution from alanine to valine that is associated with a reduction of enzyme activity. The *A1298C* polymorphism, located in the regulatory region of MTHFR, substitutes an amino acid change from glutamine to alanine. Evidence suggests that *A1298C* also reduces MTHFR activity, however it is reported to be less influential than *C677T* [114]. This modifying effect incurred by the presence of one or both polymorphisms in a pivotal folate metabolism pathway and its association with sporadic disease suggests that these polymorphisms are of particular interest with respect to modifying disease risk in Lynch syndrome.

Both *A1298C* and *C677T* are in strong linkage disequilibrium with no evidence of the existence of a *MTHFR* allele that carries both the homozygote (*C1298C/T677T*) variants of these polymorphisms [115 – 117]. Owing to this linkage disequilibrium, no studies have been reported where patients have inherited both homozygote variants. Nevertheless, heterozygote carriers of 1298C and 677T have been reported. The effect of inheriting both alleles in trans (i.e. one allele with the 677T polymorphism and the other with the 1298C polymorphism) effectively reduces overall MTHFR activity, thereby significantly altering the kinetics of folate metabolism. Data reported from an Australian and Polish study on the effects of MTHFR variants and disease expression in Lynch syndrome revealed that heterozygote forms of the *MTHFR* variants were required for a significant protective effect to occur [23]. The Kaplan-Meier survival estimates reported in this study predicted a median age gap of 10 years later for CRC onset in patients carrying the combined heterozygote *MTHFR* genotype which was supported by multi variable regression modelling statistics. The data also suggested this effect was significant in both *hMLH1* and *hMSH2* carriers, where previously only a significant association had been described in *hMLH1* for *C677T* only [118]. The most likely cause for this discrepancy between the Australian/Polish study and those by reported by Pande *et al* (2007) [119] is likely to be due to a type 1 statistical error as the reported association in *hMLH1* carriers were in a considerable smaller sample size, although differences in the ethnicity of Lynch syndrome cohorts cannot be ruled out as a contributing factor.

The mechanism by which *C677T* and *A1298C* appears to influence disease risk can be explained by the functional effects that these polymorphisms have on MTHFR and consequently folate metabolism. Previous reports have demonstrated a reduction of up to 60% in the activity of MTHFR when both *C677T* and *A1298C* heterozygote alleles were present in the gene. The reduction of *MTHFR* activity leads to an increased concentration of its substrate 5,10-MTHF. The increased pool of 5,10-MTHF pushes folate metabolism towards DNA synthesis, in turn reducing the pool of uracil. A reduced quantity of uracil potentially reduces the overall risk of uracil misincorporation as a result of its limited availability. For individuals with a MMR deficiency, the effect of reduced MTHFR enzyme activity may be advantageous since uracil misincorporation could be particularly deleterious in conjunction with an impaired DNA repair pathway. The subsequent lower levels of 5-MTHF may also be beneficial due to a potential reduction in DNA methylation. Hypermethylation of the promoter of tumour suppressor or MMR genes may lead to gene silencing, therefore a reduction in methylation through decreased MTHFR activity could lead to lower probability of this type of gene silencing occurring.

Numerous case control and cohort studies have investigated the relationship between folate intake and CRC risk with the majority reporting a reduction in CRC incidence with higher levels of folate [116]. The outcome of one meta-analysis suggested that CRC risk could be reduced by up to 25% with a high level of dietary folate compared to a low level one [117]. Further studies are required to clarify to what extent total folate has on disease risk; however it is generally accepted that there is an association and that a number of common genetic variants alter either the cellular levels or functioning of folate metabolism enzymes and are likely to have an important role in determining an individual's response to changes in dietary folate. With this in mind further studies into functional polymorphisms in the folate metabolism pathway would benefit significantly by including total folate levels so that a more exact assessment its role could be made. Using this approach a more precise view of the relationship between folate intake and disease risk may become apparent where Lynch syndrome patients could be stratified by *MTHFR* genotype. Accurately estimating dietary folate intake however may prove difficult and therefore the analysis of plasma folate levels may be a more viable alternative. Future studies would benefit by including other dietary factors including alcohol, choline, and methionine intake which are known to effect folate metabolism besides folate and folic acid [119]. An accurate level of plasma folate combined with *MTHFR C677T* and *A1298C* genotypes is an interesting prospect and may provide an indicator of individual risk of developing a Lynch syndrome related CRC.

The identification of *MTHFR* polymorphisms being associated with divergence in disease risk in Lynch syndrome provides the basis for targeted intervention measures that could be used to reduce the risk of disease development. Dietary supplementation of folate/folic acid in Lynch syndrome families may prove to be beneficial in decreasing disease risk or prolonging the time before the diagnosis of malignancy. Dietary supplementation and a change in disease risk however, are more complex than previously thought. Folic acid supplementation has been proven to be beneficial in decreasing neural tube defects (NTD's), [120] and was the catalyst for the United States and Canada introducing the compulsory supplementation of folic acid in flour in 1996 with the aim to reduce the incidence of NTD's. Despite proving successful for this purpose an unexpected trend was observed in both countries as described by Mason et al. (2007) [121] who investigated the relationship between the onset of folic acid fortification and rises in the incidence of CRC. This analysis indicated that in the early part of the 1990's the age-adjusted incidence of CRC had declined gradually in both countries. Between 1995 and 1996 however, the incidence rate in the United States showed a slight increase followed by more marked increases in 1997 and 1998. A similar finding was observed in the Canadian population, which also corresponded to the mandatory supplementation of folic acid. In both populations the increase in CRC incidence was highly significant when compared to pre-existing trends in both men and women. These observations have lead to a hypothesis that mandatory folic acid supplementation was responsible for the spike in CRC rates which after peaking approximately 2-3 years after its introduction have begun to decline once again [121].

The association of increased CRC incidence with folate supplementation has been supported by the results of two large-scale studies which have recently emerged from both the United States and United Kingdom. In both these phase III studies a common trend was observed in participants who supplemented their diets for three years with a daily dose of 1000ug and 500ug folic acid respectively, and an increased risk of developing a colorectal adenoma, with the greater risk in those participants consuming the higher 1000ug dose [122, 123]. Studies in mismatch repair or tumour suppressor gene deficient mice have demonstrated that the timing of folate supplementation is important in the association it may have on disease risk. In the first few months of folate supplementation a threefold decrease in colorectal adenomas has been observed when compared to mice with a moderate folate deficient diet. Dietary folate treatment after the development of carcinomas had the opposite effect however, with folate deficiency significantly decreasing the number of adenomas compared with supplementation [124, 125]. Together, this evidence suggests that as long as an individual is healthy, folate supplementation is protective whereas if a tumour has been initiated folate restriction is more important. This dual modulatory role of folate may be of even greater influence in an impaired DNA mismatch repair pathway as found in Lynch syndrome patients. In this case folate supplementation may be particularly beneficial or deleterious depending upon any early tumour development.

7. Haemochromatosis HFE gene polymorphisms

The role of high body iron levels in modifying the risk of colorectal cancer has been investigated by several groups but remains unclear [126 – 130]. The genetic iron overload disorder hereditary haemochromatosis (HH) is characterised by high iron indices and progressive parenchymal iron overload and occurs due to a problem in restricting iron uptake (reviewed in [131- 133]. While clear associations have been established between haemochromatosis and liver disease, studies investigating the correlation between haemochromatosis and other pathologies have yielded conflicting results [134 – 137].

The primary cause of classical HH has been ascribed to SNPs in the *HFE* gene, in particular the 845G>A SNP which results in the substitution of a tyrosine residue for a cysteine at position 282 (C282Y) and is present in 10-15% of individuals of northern European descent. The more common but less penetrant 163C>G SNP (H63D) is present in 15-30% of individuals [131, 136 – 142]. A longitudinal also study has demonstrated that up to 30% of men and 1% of women homozygous for the C282Y polymorphism develop iron overload that subsequently manifests as a disease phenotype [143]. The risk of developing colorectal cancer increased 3-fold in C282Y homozygotes when compared to matched controls without the mutation [144].

A number of other epidemiological studies have also investigated the impact of *HFE* genotype on colorectal cancer risk, with mixed results [145 -148]. Most studies exploring the link between *HFE* genotype and the risk of developing colorectal cancer have approached the problem by selecting subjects diagnosed with colorectal cancer and comparing the frequency of *HFE* polymorphisms to matched controls.

In regards to Lynch syndrome and the potential influence of disease risk one study has been reported suggesting that homozygosity of the *HFE* H63D mutation may act as a modifier, increasing the risk of developing CRC. In addition, there was evidence for earlier CRC onset age in H63D homozygotes [24]. The results of this study suggest that the median age of disease onset could be as much as 6 years earlier in H63D homozygotes (who represent around 2.5% of the Australian and Polish general populations).

While these findings will require substantiation in other populations, they support a possible relationship between iron dysregulation and colorectal cancer risk. While mechanisms cannot be established by a genetic epidemiological study of this nature, it appears likely that iron is involved, in view of the roles of the HFE gene in iron metabolism, the previously reported effects of H63D homozygosity on iron status [149] and existing evidence that iron status can modify CRC. Since iron levels in haemochromatosis patients can usually be maintained at normal levels through phlebotomy and regulating factors such as diet, this might have the potential to substantially reduce colorectal cancer risks or delay onset by several years in people with HNPCC-associated MMR gene mutations.

However the possibility of other mechanisms not directly reflecting abnormal body iron status cannot be ruled out. Homozygosity of the H63D polymorphism increases the risk of the neurodegenerative brain disease amyotrophic lateral sclerosis in the absence of apparent effects of C282Y polymorphism [150 – 152], suggesting that in some tissues the H63D mutation might have pathological consequences that are not directly related to whole body iron status. It will be important to validate the findings on H63D and also to investigate the effects of C282Y homozygosity in larger HNPCC samples, preferably in conjunction with information on patient iron status, to determine the mechanisms involved and the role of iron.

While this is the first time that the H63D polymorphism has been specifically associated with HNPCC, there is some previous evidence for association of both the H63D and the C282Y polymorphism with colorectal cancer in general [147, 148]. Power has limited past studies, as the homozygous and compound heterozygous mutations that have been associated with the greatest increases in iron loading and potentially the highest disease risks, are relatively rare. For this reason, some studies have analysed all HFE mutation genotypes as a single group, which may dilute observed effects. Although past epidemiological studies of HFE genotype and colorectal cancer risk have had mixed results, an American study of 475 colorectal cancer case patients and 833 control subjects found an odds ratio of 1.4 for participants with any HFE mutation after adjustment for a range of factors including age, gender and total iron intake [148]. The increased risk predominantly occurred in the quartile with greatest dietary iron intakes. In addition, a recent study of a large Australian sample has found that homozygosity for the C282Y SNP is associated with a three-fold increase in the risk of developing colorectal cancer in men [144]. This suggests that the effects of HFE on colorectal cancer may not be limited only to MMR gene mutation carriers, although such effects may be stronger when both types of mutation are present simultaneously.

Heterozygosity for either the H63D or C282Y SNP does not appear to have any modifying effect in either the Australian or Polish samples, although it is possible that small effects may be detectable with very large samples. While heterozygosity for C282Y or H63D has been reported to have a range of effects in other diseases, reviewed in [153], these genotypes are not usually associated with significant changes in iron parameters [26, 154 – 156]. For these reasons, for our final analyses it was considered more appropriate to compare mutant homozygotes to combined heterozygotes and wildtype homozygotes, as is usually done in most studies of HFE gene SNPs. However, while this was effective in revealing the potential modifying effect of H63D homozygosity on HNPCC development, we were not able to do this for the C282Y SNP, due to its relative rarity and the lack of C282Y homozygotes in the samples. Stronger modifying effects may occur in C282Y homozygotes or C282Y/H63D compound heterozygotes, as it is well established that iron indices are increased most in individuals with these genotypes, reviewed in [131, 132, 157].

Gender affects both the onset age and site of first tumour manifestation in HNPCC. In females, the age of onset of colorectal cancer is delayed 5 to 10 years when compared to males [158]. Gender is also a factor in the manifestation of iron loading as a result of HFE genotype, affecting males much earlier in life than females [159]. In a larger sample it is possible that HFE genotype may show a contribution to the earlier onset of CRC in males when compared to females.

8. Candidate polymorphisms not associated with disease risk

Not all polymorphisms which have been associated with hereditary disease have remained consistently significant across cohorts. An example is the delta DNMT3b SNP which was reported to have a significant association in a cohort of participants in the United States [160]. DNMT3B has been identified as a candidate in disease modifying risk due to its role in methylation. DNA methylation is regulated by a family of DNA methyltransferases (DNMTs), of which three active forms (DNMT1, DNMT3A and DNMT3B) have been identified in mammalian cells [161]. It has been reported that an increase in DNA methyltransferase enzyme activity of the DNA methyltransferases DNMT1, and DNMT3A and DNMT3B, is elevated in several types of disease including leukemia, prostate, lung, breast and endometrial cancers [162 -165]. A polymorphism located within *DNMT3b* has been reported to influence enzyme expression through altering promoter activity. It has been suggested that in *in vitro* assays the C>T variant could lead to an increase of promoter activity of up to 30% [161]. Using a study group of over 400 individuals, no association was observed between age of onset and *DNMT3b* genotype in an Australian and Polish Lynch syndrome cohort. The failure to confirm the potential modifying influence of a polymorphism in one population compared to another could be simply due to insufficient numbers of test subjects. If a polymorphism is an effect modifier its response should be similar no matter what population is examined even though it may not reach statistical significance. In the case of the delta *DNMT3b* SNP no such trend was observed. The Australian/Polish study group was approximately three times larger than the participants of a previous study [160] and the most likely explanation for the difference in results is a type 1 error. Notwithstanding, it is worth noting that it does not rule out the possibility that *DNMT3b* expression may be associated with Lynch syndrome disease expression. Different isoforms of DNMT3b exist therefore expression levels of these may vary influencing disease risk. Numerous other polymorphisms have also been reported in the functional domains of DNMT3b which could also alter methylation status and thereby alter disease risk.

Genes involved in DNA repair have also been prime candidates in the search for modifying effects due to their important role in the cell cycle. Polymorphisms located within genes involved in this process have been widely reported to be associated with cancer susceptibility in an extensive range of malignancies that include CRC. For one combined cohort (Australian and Polish Lynch syndrome patients), eight common polymorphisms were selected across several genes involved in the DNA repair pathway including *BRCA2*, *hMSH3*, *Lig4*, *hOGG1* and *XRCC* 1, 2 and 3, which had not previously been assessed for disease risk in Lynch syndrome. When considered separately conflicting data were identified in the two populations. Cox regression modelling indicated a significant protective effect in Polish participants for both polymorphisms *hMSH3* A>G (rs26279) and *XRCC2* G>A (rs1799793). This finding was somewhat contradictory as the homozygote form of both rs26279 and rs1799793 have been previously weakly associated with an increased risk of CRC and bladder cancer respectively [166, 167]. Two points need to be taken into account in interpreting this data. First, since multiple tests were undertaken in evaluating the possible influence of DNA repair gene polymorphisms a correction for multiple testing must be undertaken to ensure that any observed result is not due to a chance association; second, population stratification may adversely affect result outcome but is less likely (Reeves et al. 2011 [168]. Differences in the probabilities of an association with the age of disease onset in relation to DNA repair gene polymorphisms occurring in small study groups is more likely to be a result of a type 1 or 2 statistical error and can be overcome by undertaking an appropriate power calculation to determine the expected power to detect an association. Furthermore, statistical correction (such as Bonferroni) is required especially where multiple testing is undertaken although some types of correction are somewhat conservative and could remove an association where one exists.

9. Summary

There have been a number of studies that demonstrate the role of modifying genes that influence disease risk in Lynch Syndrome. Many studies have been undertaken that have failed to identify a range of candidate modifying genes as a result of studies being too small in size to provide robust statistical results. Nevertheless, there is a growing body of evidence that suggests modifying genes do influence disease risk in Lynch Syndrome and some of these are of particular interest as they suggest potential avenues by which disease risk can be modulated.

The role of genome wide association studies in identifying new agnostic modifier genes is currently generating special interest and at this point two studies have reported intriguing associations that correlate well with disease risk. It remains to be seen if such associations can be verified in larger populations. The use of genome wide data or even target assessment of several thousand potential modifiers is fraught with difficulties not the least of which is the available population size and the number of individual SNPs analysed.

Despite the difficulties encountered in identifying polymorphic modifier genes, their role in improving disease risk assessment is becoming clearer and the search for those that can make for individualised patient care will continue.

10. References

[1] Lengauer, C., et al. Genetic instabilities in human cancers. Nature 1998; 396:643-649.

[2] Boland, C.R. and Goel, A. Clearing the air on smoking and colorectal cancer. J. Natl Cancer Inst. 2010; 102:996-997.

[3] Lynch, H. T. and A. de la Chapelle (1999). Genetic susceptibility to non-polyposis colorectal cancer. Journal of medical genetics 1999; 36:801-818.

[4] Boland, C. R., et al. The biochemical basis of microsatellite instability and abnormal immunohistochemistry and clinical behavior in Lynch syndrome: from bench to bedside." Familial cancer 2008; 7:41-52.

[5] Vasen, H. F.,,, et al. New clinical criteria for hereditary nonpolyposis colorectal cancer (HNPCC, Lynch syndrome) proposed by the International Collaborative group on HNPCC. Gastroenterology 1999;116: 1453-1456.

[6] Lynch H.T., et al. Hereditary factors in cancer. Study of two large Mid-Western kindreds. Arch. Intern. Med. 1996; 117:206-212.

[7] Lindor NM. Familial colorectal cancer type X: the other half of hereditary nonpolyposis colon cancer syndrome. Surg Oncol Clin N Am. 2009;18:637-645.

[8] Peltomaki, P. Deficient DNA mismatch repair: a common etiologic factor for colon cancer. Hum Mol Genet 2001; 10:735-740.

[9] Kunkel, T. A. and D. A. Erie. DNA mismatch repair. Annu Rev Biochem 2001; 74: 681-710.

[10] Jiricny, J. The multifaceted mismatch-repair system. Nat Rev Mol Cell Biol 2006; 7: 335-346.

[11] Bonis, P. A., et al. (2007). Hereditary nonpolyposis colorectal cancer: diagnostic strategies and their implications. Evid Rep Technol Assess 2007; 150: 1-180.

[12] Lynch, H. T., et al. Phenotypic variation in colorectal adenoma/cancer expression in two families. Hereditary flat adenoma syndrome. Cancer 1990; 66: 909-915.

[13] Lynch, H. T., et al. Genetics, natural history, tumor spectrum, and pathology of hereditary nonpolyposis colorectal cancer: an updated review. Gastroenterology 1993; 104:1535-1549.

[14] Scott, R. J., et al. (2001). Hereditary nonpolyposis colorectal cancer in 95 families: differences and similarities between mutation-positive and mutation-negative kindreds. Am J Hum Genet 2001; 68: 118-127.

[15] Rebbeck T.R., et al. Genetic variation and cancer: improving the environment for publication of association studies. Cancer Epidemiol. Biomarkers Prev. 2004; 13:1985-1986.

[16] Pharoah P.D., et al. The reliable identification of disease-gene associations. Cancer Epidemiol. Biomarkers Prev. 2005; 14:1362.

[17] Ross J.A., et al. Genetic variation in the leptin receptor gene and obesity in survivors of childhood acute lymphoblastic leukaemia: a report from the Childhood Cancer Survivor Study. J. Clin. Oncol. 2004; 22:3558-3562.

[18] Terry, K.L., et al. Genetic variation in the progesterone receptor gne and ovarian cancer risk. Am J. Epidemiol. 2005;161:442-451.

[19] Freedman, M.L., et al. Systematic evaluation of genetic variation at the androgen receptor locus and risk of prostate cancer in a multiethnic cohort study. Am. J. Hum. Genet. 2005; 76:82-90.

[20] Eerola, H., et al. Hereditary breast cancer and hanlding of patients risk. Scand J. Surg. 2002; 91:280-287.

[21] Stormorken, A.T., et al. Prevention of colorectal cancer by colonoscopic surveillance in families with hereditary colorectal cancer. Scand. J. Gastroenterol. 2007; 42:611-617.

[22] Zecevic, M., et al. (2006). IGF1 gene polymorphism and risk for hereditary nonpolyposis colorectal cancer. J National Cancer Inst 2006; 98: 139-143.

[23] Reeves, S. G., et al. IGF1 is a modifier of disease risk in hereditary non-polyposis colorectal cancer. International journal of cancer. Journal international du cancer 2008; 123: 1339-1343.

[24] Reeves, S.G., et al., MTHFR 677 C>T and 1298 A>C polymorphisms and the age of onset of colorectal cancer in hereditary nonpolyposis colorectal cancer. Eur J Hum Genet, 2009. 17: 629-635.

[25] Shi, Z., et al. Haemochromatosis HFE gene polymorphisms as potential modifiers of hereditary nonpolyposis colorectal cancer risk and onset age. Int. J. Cancer. 2009; 125: 78-83.

[26] Heinimann, K., et al. N-acetyltransferase 2 influences cancer prevalence in hMLH1/hMSH2 mutation carriers. Cancer research 1999; 59: 3038-3040.

[27] Talseth, B. A., et al. Genetic polymorphisms in xenobiotic clearance genes and their influence on disease expression in hereditary nonpolyposis colorectal cancer patients. Cancer Epidem. Biomarkers & Prevention 2006;15: 2307-2310.

[28] Jones, J. S., et al. ATM polymorphism and hereditary nonpolyposis colorectal cancer (HNPCC) age of onset (United States). Cancer causes & control : 2005; 6: 749-753.

[29] Talseth, B. A., et al. Lack of association between genetic polymorphisms in cytokine genes and disease expression in patients with hereditary non-polyposis colorectal cancer. Scandinavian journal of gastroenterology 2007; 42: 628-632.

[30] Levine, A. J. P53, the cellular gatekeeper for growth and division. Cell 1997; 88(3): 323-331.

[31] Xu, H. and M. R. el-Gewely. P53-responsive genes and the potential for cancer diagnostics and therapeutics development." Biotechnology Ann Rev 2001; 7:131-164.

[32] Jones, J. S., et al. P53 polymorphism and age of onset of hereditary nonpolyposis colorectal cancer in a Caucasian population. Clin. Cancer Res. 2004; 10:5845-5849.

[33] Thomas, M., et al. Two polymorphic variants of wild-type p53 differ biochemically and biologically. Molecular and cellular biology 1999; 19:1092-1100.

[34] Pim, D. and L. Banks. P53 polymorphic variants at codon 72 exert different effects on cell cycle progression." Int. J. Cancer. 2004 108: 196-199.

[35] Storey, A., et al. Role of a p53 polymorphism in the development of human papillomavirus-associated cancer. Nature 1998; 393: 229-234.

[36] Wang, Y. C., et al. (1999). "p53 codon 72 polymorphism in Taiwanese lung cancer patients: association with lung cancer susceptibility and prognosis." Clin. Can Res. 1999; 5:129-134.

[37] Bergamaschi, G., et al. TP53 codon 72 polymorphism in patients with chronic myeloid leukemia. Haematologica 2004; 89:868-869.

[38] Cortezzi, S. S., et al. Analysis of human papillomavirus prevalence and TP53 polymorphism in head and neck squamous cell carcinomas. Cancer Genet and Cytogenet. 2004; 150: 44-49.

[39] Sotamaa, K., et al. P53 codon 72 and MDM2 SNP309 polymorphisms and age of colorectal cancer onset in Lynch syndrome." Clin. Cancer Res 2005; 11: 6840-6844.

[40] Talseth, B. A., et al. Age of diagnosis of colorectal cancer in HNPCC patients is more complex than that predicted by R72P polymorphism in TP53. Int. J. Cancer. 2006; 118:2479-2484.

[41] Bond, G. L., et al. A single nucleotide polymorphism in the MDM2 promoter attenuates the p53 tumor suppressor pathway and accelerates tumor formation in humans. Cell 2004; 119:591-602.

[42] Talseth, B. A., et al. MDM2 SNP309 T>G alone or in combination with the TP53 R72P polymorphism does not appear to influence disease expression and age of diagnosis of colorectal cancer in HNPCC patients. Int. J. Cancer. 2007; 120: 563-565.

[43] Lohmueller, K. E., et al. Variants associated with common disease are not unusually differentiated in frequency across populations. Am J. Hum. Genet. 2006; 78:130-136.

[44] Kong, S., et al. Effects of cyclin D1 polymorphism on age of onset of hereditary nonpolyposis colorectal cancer. Cancer Res. 2000; 60: 249-252.

[45] Chen, J., et al. Association between Aurora-A kinase polymorphisms and age of onset of hereditary nonpolyposis colorectal cancer in a Caucasian population." Mol. Carcinogenesis 2007; 46: 249-256.

[46] Bala, S. and P. Peltomaki. CYCLIN D1 as a genetic modifier in hereditarynonpolyposis colorectal cancer. Cancer Res 2001; 61: 6042-6045.

[47] Kruger, S., et al. Absence of association between cyclin D1 (CCND1) G870A polymorphism and age of onset in hereditary nonpolyposis colorectal cancer. Cancer Letts 2006; 236:191-197.

[48] Talseth, B. A., et al. Aurora-A and Cyclin D1 polymorphisms and the age of onset of colorectal cancer in hereditary nonpolyposis colorectal cancer." Int J. Cancer 2008; 122: 1273-1277.

[49] Ferraz, J. M., et al. Impact of GSTT1, GSTM1, GSTP1 and NAT2 genotypes on KRAS2 and TP53 gene mutations in colorectal cancer. Int. J. Cancer 2004; 110:183-187.

[50] Smith G., et al. Metabolic polymorphisms and cancer susceptibility. Cancer Surv. 1995; 25:27-65.

[51] Campbell, P. T., et al. Cytochrome P450 17A1 and catechol O-methyltransferase polymorphisms and age at Lynch syndrome colon cancer onset in Newfoundland. Clin Cancer Res. 2007; 13:3783-3788.

[52] Esteller, M., et al. Germline polymorphisms in cytochrome-P4501A1 (C4887 CYP1A1) and methylenetetrahydrofolate reductase (MTHFR) genes and endometrial cancer susceptibility. Carcinogenesis 1997; 18:2307-2311.

[53] Felix, R., et al. GSTM1 and GSTT1 polymorphisms as modifiers of age at diagnosis of hereditary nonpolyposis colorectal cancer (HNPCC) in a homogeneous cohort of individuals carrying a single predisposing mutation. Mut. Research 2006; 602:175-181.

[54] Frazier, M. L., et al. Age-associated risk of cancer among individuals with N-acetyltransferase 2 (NAT2) mutations and mutations in DNA mismatch repair genes. Cancer Res. 2001; 61:1269-1271.

[55] He, L.J., et al. Genetic polymorphisms of N-acetyltransferase 2 and colorectal cancer risk. World J Gastroenterol. 2005; 11:4268-4271.

[56] Loktionov, A., et al. Glutathione-S-transferase gene polymorphisms in colorectal cancer patients: interaction between GSTM1 and GSTM3 allele variants as a risk-modulating factor. Carcinogenesis 2001; 22:1053-1060.

[57] Moisio, A. L., et al. Genetic polymorphisms in carcinogen metabolism and their association to hereditary nonpolyposis colon cancer. Gastroenterology 1998; 115: 1387-1394.

[58] Pistorius, S., et al. N-acetyltransferase (NAT) 2 acetylator status and age of onset in patients with hereditary nonpolyposis colorectal cancer (HNPCC). Cancer letters 2006; 241:150-157.

[59] Sivaraman, L., et al. CYP1A1 genetic polymorphisms and in situ colorectal cancer. Cancer Res. 1994; 54:3692-3695

[60] Slattery, M.L., et al. NAT2, GSTM-1, cigarette smoking and risk for colon cancer. Cancer Epidemiol. Biomarkers Prev. 1998; 7:1079-1084.

[61] Ye, Z. and Parry, J.M. Genetic polymorphisms in the cytochrome P4501A1, glutathione S-transferase M1 and T1, and susceptibility to colon cancer. Teratog. Carcinog. Mutagen 2002; 22:385-392.

[62] Brockton, N., et al. N-acetyltransferase polymorphisms and colorectal cancer: A HuGE review. Am. J. Epidemiol. 2000; 151, 846-861.

[63] Shin, J. H., et al. Glutathione S-transferase M1 associated with cancer occurrence in Korean HNPCC families carrying the hMLH1/hMSH2 mutation. Oncology Reports 2003;10: 483-486.

[64] Gyorffy B., Kocsis, I., Vasarhelyi, B. Biallelic genotype distributions in papers publidhed in Gut between 1998 and 2003: altered conclusions after recalculating the Hardy-Weinberg equilibrium. Gut 2004; 53:614-615.

[65] Landi, S., et al. A comprehensive analysis of phase I and phase II metabolism gene polymorphisms and risk of colrectal cancer. Pharmacogenet. Genomics 2005; 15:535-546

[66] Balkwill, F. and Mantovani, A. Inflammation and cancer: back to Virchow? Lancet 2001; 357:539-545

[67] Coussens, L.M. and Webb, Z. Inflammation and cancer. Nature 2002; 420:860-867

[68] Duarte, I., et al. G 308A TNF-alpha polymorphism is associated with an increased risk of invasive cervical cancer. Biochem. Biophys Res Commun. 2005; 334:588-592

[69] El-Omar, E.M., et al Increased risk of noncardia gastric cancaer associated with proinflammatory cytokine gene polymorphisms. Gastroenterology 2003; 124:1193-1201.

[70] Giordani, L., et al. Association of breast cancer and polymorphisms of interleukin-10 and tumor necrosis factor-alpha genes. Clin. Chem. 2003; 49:1664-1667.

[71] Graziano, F. et al. Prognostic role of interleukin-1beta gene and interleukin-1 receptor antagonist gene polymorphisms in patients with advance gastric cancer. J. Clin. Oncol. 2005; 23:2339-2345.

[72] Hefler, L.A., et al. An interleukin-6 gene promotor polymorphism influences the biological phenotype of ovarian cancer. Cancer Res. 2003; 63:3066-3068.

[73] Iacopetta, B., Grieu, F. and Joseph, D. The -174 G/C gene polymorphism in interleukin-6 is associated with an aggressive breast cancer phenotype. Br. J. Cancer 2004; 90: 419-422.

[74] Ikeda, H., Old, L.J., and Schreiber, R.D. The roles of IFN gamma in protection against tumor developmen and cacner immunoediing. Cytokine Growth Factor Res. 2002; 13:95-109.

[75] Landi, S., et al. association of common polymorphisms in inflammatroy genes interleukin (IL)6, IL8, tumor necrosis factor alpha, NFKB1, and peroxisome proliferator-activated recpetor gamma wtih colorectal cancer. Cancer Res. 2003; 3:3560-3566.

[76] Sugaya, K., et al. Molecular analysis of adrenergic receptor genes and interleukin-4/interleukin-4 receptor genes in patients with interstitial cystitis. J. Urol. 2002; 168:26768-2671.

[77] Tsai, F.J., et al. Interleukin-4 gene intron-3 polymorphism is associated with transitional cell carcinoma of the urinary bladder. BJU Int. 2005; 95:432-435

[78] Balic, I., et al., Androgen receptor length polymorphism associated with prostate cancer risk in Hispanic men. J Urol, 2002. 168: 2245-2248.

[79] Beilin, J., et al., A case-control study of the androgen receptor gene CAG repeat polymorphism in Australian prostate carcinoma subjects. Cancer, 2001. 92: 941-949.

[80] Bennett, C.L., et al., Racial variation in CAG repeat lengths within the androgen receptor gene among prostate cancer patients of lower socioeconomic status. J Clin Oncol, 2002. 20: 3599-3604.

[81] Nowacka-Zawisza, M., et al., Dinucleotide repeat polymorphisms of RAD51, BRCA1, BRCA2 gene regions in breast cancer. Pathol Int, 2008. 58: 275-281.

[82] Vashist, Y.K., et al., Microsatellite GTn-repeat polymorphism in the promoter of heme oxygenase-1 gene is an independent predictor of tumor recurrence in male oral squamous cell carcinoma patients. J Oral Pathol Med, 2008. 37: 480-484.

[83] Wang, L., et al., Association of a functional tandem repeats in the downstream of human telomerase gene and lung cancer. Oncogene, 2003. 22: 7123-7129.

[84] Wang, S., et al., A novel variable number of tandem repeats (VNTR) polymorphism containing Sp1 binding elements in the promoter of XRCC5 is a risk factor for human bladder cancer. Mutat Res, 2008. 638: 26-36.

[85] Giovannucci, E., Insulin, insulin-like growth factors and colon cancer: a review of the evidence. J Nutr, 2001. 131(Suppl): 3109S-3120S.

[86] Rosen, C.J., et al., Association between serum insulin growth factor-I (IGF-I) and a simple sequence repeat in IGF-I gene: implications for genetic studies of bone mineral density. J Clin Endocrinol Metab, 1998. 83: 2286-2290.

[87] Gebhardt, F., K.S. Zanker, and B. Brandt, Modulation of epidermal growth factor receptor gene transcription by a polymorphic dinucleotide repeat in intron 1. J Biol Chem, 1999. 274: 13176-13180.

[88] Estany, J., et al., Association of CA repeat polymorphism at intron 1 of insulin-like growth factor (IGF-I) gene with circulating IGF-I concentration, growth, and fatness in swine. Physiol Genomics, 2007. 31: 236-243.

[89] Hoyo, C., et al., Predictors of variation in serum IGF1 and IGFBP3 levels in healthy African American and white men. J Natl Med Assoc, 2009. 101: 711-716.

[90] Chen, W., et al., Phenotypes and genotypes of insulin-like growth factor 1, IGF-binding protein-3 and cancer risk: evidence from 96 studies. Eur J Hum Genet, 2009. 17: 1668-1675.

[91] Espelund, U., et al., Elevated free IGF2 levels in localized, early-stage breast cancer in women. Eur J Endocrinol, 2008. 159: 595-601.

[92] Renehan, A.G., et al., Insulin-like growth factor (IGF)-I, IGF binding protein-3, and cancer risk: systematic review and meta-regression analysis. Lancet, 2004. 363: 1346-1353.

[93] Shi, R., et al., IGF-I and breast cancer: a meta-analysis. Int J Cancer, 2004. 111: 418-423.

[94] Warren, R.S., et al., Induction of vascular endothelial growth factor by insulin-like growth factor 1 in colorectal carcinoma. J Biol Chem, 1996. 271: 29483-29488.

[95] Baserga, R., The insulin-like growth factor I receptor: a key to tumor growth? Cancer Res, 1995. 55: 249-252.

[96] Kaulfuss, S., et al., Dual silencing of insulin-like growth factor-I receptor and epidermal growth factor receptor in colorectal cancer cells is associated with decreased proliferation and enhanced apoptosis. Mol Cancer Ther, 2009. 8: 821-833.

[97] Bjorntorp, P., Metabolic implications of body fat distribution. Diabetes Care, 1991. 14: 1132-1143.

[98] Donahue, R.P. and R.D. Abbott, Central obesity and coronary heart disease in men. Lancet, 1987. 2: 1215.

[99] Kissebah, A.H., et al., Relation of body fat distribution to metabolic complications of obesity. J Clin Endocrinol Metab, 1982. 54: 254-260.

[100] Koivisto, V.A., H. Yki-Jarvinen, and R.A. DeFronzo, Physical training and insulin sensitivity. Diabetes Metab Rev, 1986. 1: 445-481.

[101] Krotkiewski, M., et al., Impact of obesity on metabolism in men and women. Importance of regional adipose tissue distribution. J Clin Invest, 1983. 72: 1150-1162.

[102] Regensteiner, J.G., et al., Relationship between habitual physical activity and insulin levels among nondiabetic men and women. San Luis Valley Diabetes Study. Diabetes Care, 1991. 14: 1066-1074.

[103] Potter, J.D., et al., Colon cancer: a review of the epidemiology. Epidemiol Rev, 1993. 15: 499-545.

[104] Riccardi, G. and A.A. Rivellese, Effects of dietary fiber and carbohydrate on glucose and lipoprotein metabolism in diabetic patients. Diabetes Care, 1991. 14: 1115-1125.

[105] Powell, D.R., et al., Insulin inhibits transcription of the human gene for insulin-like growth factor-binding protein-1. J Biol Chem, 1991. 266: 18868-18876.

[106] Kajantie, E., et al., Serum insulin-like growth factor (IGF)-I and IGF-binding protein-1 in elderly people: relationships with cardiovascular risk factors, body composition, size at birth, and childhood growth. J Clin Endocrinol Metab, 2003. 88: 1059-1065.

[107] Valko, M., et al., Role of oxygen radicals in DNA damage and cancer incidence. Mol Cell Biochem, 2004. 266: 37-56.

[108] Palles, C., et al., Identification of genetic variants that influence circulating IGF1 levels: a targeted search strategy. Hum Mol Genet, 2008. 17: 1457-1464.

[109] Colangelo, L.A., et al., IGF-1, IGFBP-3, and nutritional factors in young black and white men: the CARDIA Male Hormone Study. Nutr Cancer, 2005. 53: 57-64.

[110] Cruickshank, J.K., et al., Epidemiology of the insulin-like growth factor system in three ethnic groups. Am J Epidemiol, 2001. 154: 504-513.

[111] Platz, E.A., et al., Racial variation in insulin-like growth factor-1 and binding protein-3 concentrations in middle-aged men. Cancer Epidemiol Biomarkers Prev, 1999. 8: 1107-1110.

[112] McGreevy, K.M., et al., Impact of nutrients on insulin-like growth factor-I, insulin-like growth factor binding protein-3 and their ratio in African American and white males. Public Health Nutr, 2007. 10: 97-105.

[113] Weisberg, I., et al., A second genetic polymorphism in methylenetetrahydrofolate reductase (MTHFR) associated with decreased enzyme activity. Mol Genet Metab, 1998. 64: 169-172.

[114] Chen, J., et al., Linkage disequilibrium between the 677C>T and 1298A>C polymorphisms in human methylenetetrahydrofolate reductase gene and their contributions to risk of colorectal cancer. Pharmacogenetics, 2002. 12: 339-342.

[115] Yin, G., et al., Methylenetetrahydrofolate reductase C677T and A1298C polymorphisms and colorectal cancer: the Fukuoka Colorectal Cancer Study. Cancer Sci, 2004. 95: 908-913.

[116] Sharp, L. and J. Little, Polymorphisms in genes involved in folate metabolism and colorectal neoplasia: a HuGE review. Am J Epidemiol, 2004. 159: 423-443.

[117] Giovannucci, E., Epidemiologic studies of folate and colorectal neoplasia: a review. J Nutr, 2002. 132(Suppl): 2350S-2355S.

[118] Pande, M., et al., Influence of methylenetetrahydrofolate reductase gene polymorphisms C677T and A1298C on age-associated risk for colorectal cancer in a caucasian lynch syndrome population. Cancer Epidemiol Biomarkers Prev, 2007. 16: 1753-1759.

[119] Sanjoaquin, M.A., et al., Folate intake and colorectal cancer risk: a meta-analytical approach. Int J Cancer, 2005. 113: 825-828.

[120] Hubner, R.A. and R.S. Houlston, Folate and colorectal cancer prevention. Br J Cancer, 2009. 100: 233-239.

[121] Mason, J.B., et al., A temporal association between folic acid fortification and an increase in colorectal cancer rates may be illuminating important biological principles: a hypothesis. Cancer Epidemiol Biomarkers Prev, 2007. 16: 1325-1329.

[122] Cole, B.F., et al., Folic acid for the prevention of colorectal adenomas: a andomized clinical trial. Jama, 2007. 297: 2351-2359.

[123] Logan, R.F., et al., Aspirin and folic acid for the prevention of recurrent colorectal adenomas. Gastroenterology, 2008. 134: 29-38.

[124] Song, J., et al., Effects of dietary folate on intestinal tumorigenesis in the apcMin mouse. Cancer Res, 2000. 60: 5434-5440.

[125] Song, J., et al., Chemopreventive effects of dietary folate on intestinal polyps in Apc+/- Msh2-/- mice. Cancer Res, 2000. 60: 3191-3199.

[126] Kabat GC, et al. A cohort study of dietary iron and heme iron intake and risk of colorectal cancer in women. *British journal of cancer* 2007;97:118-22.

[127] Kato I, et al. Iron intake, body iron stores and colorectal cancer risk in women: a nested case-control study. *International journal of cancer* 1999;80:693-8.

[128] Larsson SC, et al. Red meat consumption and risk of cancers of the proximal colon, distal colon and rectum: the Swedish Mammography Cohort. *International journal of cancer* 2005;113:829-34.

[129] Nelson RL. Iron and colorectal cancer risk: human studies. *Nutrition reviews* 2001;59:140-8.

[130] Norat T, Riboli E. Meat consumption and colorectal cancer: a review of epidemiologic evidence. *Nutrition reviews* 2001;59:37-47.

[131] Beutler E. Hemochromatosis: genetics and pathophysiology. *Annu Rev Med* 2006;57:331-347.

[132] Camaschella C. Understanding iron homeostasis through genetic analysis of hemochromatosis and related disorders. *Blood* 2005;106:3710-7.

[133] Pietrangelo A. Hereditary hemochromatosis. *Annual review of nutrition* 2006;26;251-270.

[134] Adams PC, et al. Hemochromatosis and iron-overload screening in a racially diverse population. *The New England journal of medicine* 2005;352:1769 78.

[135] Ellervik C, et al. Hemochromatosis genotypes and risk of 31 disease endpoints: meta analyses including 66,000 cases and 226,000 controls. *Hepatology (Baltimore, Md* 2007;46:1071-80.

[136] Olynyk JK, et al. A population-based study of the clinical expression of the hemochromatosis gene. *The New England journal of medicine* 1999;341:718-24.

[137] Whitlock EP, et al. Screening for hereditary hemochromatosis: a systematic review for the U.S. Preventive Services Task Force. *Annals of internal medicine* 2006;145:209-23.

[138] Chua AC, et al. The regulation of cellular iron metabolism. *Critical reviews in clinical laboratory sciences* 2007;44:413-59.

[139] Gochee PA, et al.. A population-based study of the biochemical and clinical expression of the H63D hemochromatosis mutation. *Gastroenterology* 2002;122:646-51.

[140] Jackson HA, et al.. HFE mutations, iron deficiency and overload in 10,500 blood donors. *Brit J Haematol* 2001;114:474-484.

[141] Milman N, et al. Frequency of the C282Y and H63D mutations of the hemochromatosis gene (HFE) in 2501 ethnic Danes. *Annals of hematology* 2004;83:654-7.

[142] Steinberg KK, et al. Prevalence of C282Y and H63D mutations in the hemochromatosis (HFE) gene in the United States. *Jama* 2001;285:2216-22.

[143] Allen KJ, et al. Iron-overload-related disease in HFE hereditary hemochromatosis. *The New England journal of medicine* 2008;358:221-30.

[144] Osborne NJ, et al. Homozygosity for the C282Y mutation in the HFE gene is associated with increased risk of colorectal and breast cancer in Australian population. *Am J Hematol.* 2007;82:575.

[145] Chan AT, et al. Hemochromatosis gene mutations, body iron stores, dietary iron, and risk of colorectal adenoma in women. *Journal of the National Cancer Institute* 2005;97:917-926.

[146] Macdonald GA, et al. No evidence of increased risk of colorectal cancer in individuals heterozygous for the Cys282Tyr haemochromatosis mutation. *Journal of gastroenterology and hepatology* 1999;14:1188-1191.

[147] Robinson JP, et al. Evidence for an association between compound heterozygosity for germ line mutations in the hemochromatosis (HFE) gene and increased risk of colorectal cancer. *Cancer Epidemiol Biomarkers Prev* 2005,14.1460-1463.

[148] Shaheen NJ, et al. Association between hemochromatosis (HFE) gene mutation carrier status and the risk of colon cancer. *Journal of the National Cancer Institute* 2003;95:154-159.

[149] Barton JC, et al. Initial screening transferrin saturation values, serum ferritin concentrations, and HFE genotypes in Native Americans and whites in the Hemochromatosis and Iron Overload Screening Study. *Clinical genetics* 2006;69(1):48-57.

[150] Goodall EF, et al. Association of the H63D polymorphism in the hemochromatosis gene with sporadic ALS. *Neurology* 2005;65:934-7.

[151] Sutedja NA, et al. The association between H63D mutations in HFE and amyotrophic lateral sclerosis in a Dutch population. *Archives of neurology* 2007;64:63-7.

[152] Wang XS, et al. Increased incidence of the Hfe mutation in amyotrophic lateral sclerosis and related cellular consequences. *Journal of the neurological sciences* 2004;227:27-33.

[153] Weinberg ED. Do some carriers of hemochromatosis gene mutations have higher than normal rates of disease and death? *Biometals* 2002;15:347-50.

[154] Beutler E, et al.. Penetrance of 845G--> A (C282Y) HFE hereditary haemochromatosis mutation in the USA. *Lancet* 2002;359:211-8.

[155] Hunt JR, Zeng H. Iron absorption by heterozygous carriers of the HFE C282Y mutation associated with hemochromatosis. *The American journal of clinical nutrition* 2004;80:924-31.

[156] Singh M, et al. Risk of iron overload in carriers of genetic mutations associated with hereditary haemochromatosis: UK Food Standards Agency workshop. *The British journal of nutrition* 2006;96:770-3.

[157] Pietrangelo A. Hereditary hemochromatosis. *Biochim Biophys Acta* 2006;1763:700-10.

[158] Parc Y, et al.. Cancer risk in 348 French MSH2 or MLH1 gene carriers. *Journal of medical genetics* 2003;40:208-13.

[159] Ayonrinde OT, et al. Clinical perspectives on hereditary hemochomatosis. *Critical reviews in clinical laboratory sciences* 2008; 45; 451-458.

[160] Jones, J.S., et al., DNMT3b polymorphism and hereditary nonpolyposis colorectal cancer age of onset. Cancer Epidemiol Biomarkers Prev, 2006. 15: 886-891.

[161] Shen, H., et al., A novel polymorphism in human cytosine DNA-methyltransferase-3B promoter is associated with an increased risk of lung cancer. Cancer Res, 2002. 62: 4992-4995.

[162] Jin, F., et al., Up-regulation of DNA methyltransferase 3B expression in endometrial cancers. Gynecol Oncol, 2005. 96: 531-538.

[163] Mizuno, S., et al., Expression of DNA methyltransferases DNMT1, 3A, and 3B in normal hematopoiesis and in acute and chronic myelogenous leukemia. Blood, 2001. 97: 1172-1179.

[164] Montgomery, K.G., et al., The DNMT3B C-->T promoter polymorphism and risk of breast cancer in a British population: a case-control study. Breast Cancer Res, 2004. 6: 390-394.

[165] Patra, S.K., et al., DNA methyltransferase and demethylase in human prostate cancer. Mol Carcinog, 2002. 33: 163-171.

[166] Chang, C.H., et al., Significant association of XPD codon 312 single nucleotide polymorphism with bladder cancer susceptibility in Taiwan. Anticancer Res, 2009. 29: 3903-3907.

[167] Koessler, T., et al., Common variants in mismatch repair genes and risk of colorectal cancer. Gut, 2008. 57: 1097-1101.

[168] Reeves S.G. et al. DNA repair gene polymorphisms and risk of early onset colorectal cancer in Lynch syndrome. 2011. doi:10.1016/j.canep.2011.09.003

Part 3

Tumor Microenvironment

5

Modulation of Tumor Angiogenesis by a Host Anti-Tumor Response in Colorectal Cancer

N. Britzen-Laurent[1], V.S. Schellerer[2], R.S. Croner[2],
M. Stürzl[1] and E. Naschberger[1]
*[1]Division of Molecular and Experimental Surgery, Department of Surgery,
University Medical Center Erlangen, Erlangen,
[2]Department of Surgery, University Medical Center Erlangen, Erlangen,
Germany*

1. Introduction

Colorectal carcinoma (CRC) is the second most frequently occurring cancer in industrialized countries, in both men and women. The cumulative lifetime risk of developing colorectal carcinoma is about 6%, and the cancer-related five year survival rate is 62% (Smith et al., 2002). Malignant transformation of CRC occurs in a multistep process via three different pathways: the chromosomal instability pathway, the microsatellite instability pathway (Vogelstein et al., 1988) and the methylation pathway (Jass, 2002). Moreover, putative tumor-initiating cells with increased malignancy were isolated from CRC (O'Brien et al., 2007; Ricci-Vitiani et al., 2007). These cells exhibited stem cell-like characteristics; however, their role in CRC pathogenesis is still controversial (Shmelkov et al., 2008). Tumor development and metastasis require the presence of a newly formed vasculature. Tumor cells can directly promote angiogenesis but the tumor microenvironment plays also a crucial role in this process. The tumor microenvironment consists of a variety of conjunctive tissue components and cells, as well as infiltrating immune cells. It is inflammatory and undergoes constant remodelling. Immune cells are not only recruited in order to eliminate the tumor, they can also be attracted by tumor cells in order to support a tumor-promoting inflammation. In CRC, the type of immune cells infiltrating the tumor has been shown to influence tumor growth and patient survival (Galon et al., 2007; Tosolini et al., 2011). In addition, immune cells have been shown to exert antagonistic effects on tumor angiogenesis. In this chapter, we focus on the modulation of tumor angiogenesis by tumor infiltrating immune cells and on its implications in terms of diagnosis and prognosis in CRC.

2. Tumor angiogenesis and tumor vessels

Tumor growth beyond two to three millimeters in diameter and metastasis requires angiogenesis, the formation of new blood vessels. Angiogenesis plays a crucial role in the development and progression of CRC, and this has been convincingly documented in the literature. It has been shown that microvessel density is increased in primary tumors compared to normal mucosa or adenoma tissues (Bossi et al., 1995), and this is a strong independent predictor of poor outcome (Takebayashi et al., 1996). A high microvessel density is associated with a more than threefold increased relative risk of cancer-related death from CRC (Choi et al., 1998). Moreover, the expression of vascular endothelial growth factor (VEGF), a potent angiogenesis-promoting factor, is significantly increased in all stages of colorectal carcinoma (Kumar et al., 1998). The major sources of VEGF are either the tumor cells themselves or monocytes/macrophages recruited into the tumor tissue through paracrine signalling. Intratumor expression of VEGF was also found to increase the relative risk of cancer-related death from CRC by twofold (Kang et al., 1997; Ishigami et al., 1998; Kahlenberg et al., 2003).

The recruitment and growth of tumor vessels is a critical adaption step that has to be achieved during the development of clinically relevant solid tumors such as the CRC. This process has been termed "angiogenic switch" (Folkman, 1995) and the "induction of angiogenesis" has been included in the eight hallmarks of cancer defined by Hanahan and Weinberg (Hanahan & Weinberg, 2000; Hanahan & Weinberg, 2011). New vessels may arise through different ways in the organism under physiological and/or pathological conditions. During embryonic development angioblasts differentiate into endothelial cells in a process called vasculogenesis whereas new vessels in adults are generated through angiogenesis (Risau, 1997). The major driving molecules for angiogenic processes are VEGF, VEGF-C, angiopoietin-2, fibroblast growth factors and chemokines (Carmeliet & Jain, 2011). Active angiogenesis is achieved either by vessel sprouting, non-sprouting intussusception (splitting of existing vessels), vessel co-option (tumor cells hijack vasculature), vascular mimicry (tumor cells line vessels), luminal incorporation of bone marrow-derived endothelial progenitor cells or a recently described non-VEGF-dependent biomechanical mechanism (Risau, 1997; Kilarski et al., 2009; Carmeliet & Jain, 2011).

The role of so called "tumor stem cells" in tumor angiogenesis is currently heavily discussed. Cancer stem cells might not only have an impact on the growth and assembly of the CRC tumor cells themselves (O'Brien et al., 2007; Ricci-Vitiani et al., 2007) but also on the formation of tumor vessels (Ricci-Vitiani et al., 2010; Wang et al., 2010). The two latter studies described for the first time the differentiation of putative cancer stem cells not only into functional tumor cells but also into tumor endothelial cells. However, these findings were demonstrated for the brain tumor glioblastoma. Of note, normal neuronal stem cells are able to differentiate into endothelial cells under physiological conditions, which questions whether these findings can be also applied to non-brain tumors such as colorectal carcinoma.

Tumor vessels are structurally and functionally abnormal compared to vessels in healthy tissues (Carmeliet & Jain, 2000; Hida et al., 2008). In contrast to normal vessels, they show a deficient support provided by only few perivascular cells with loose connections to the endothelium and the vessels maintain an immature structure. The tumor vasculature is commonly disorganized and heterogenous, with excessive branching and shunts, reduced interendothelial cell contacts, reduced barrier function and uneven vessel lumen. This disturbs the blood flow in the tumors, leads to hypoxia and acidification as well as high fluid pressure concomitant with increased resistance to the application of systemic drugs [reviewed in (Carmeliet & Jain, 2000; Hida et al., 2008; Carmeliet & Jain, 2011)]. Tumor cells attempt to overcome this issue by the expression of more pro-angiogenic factors such as VEGF resulting in amplified formation of abnormal vessels. However, tumor hypoxia cannot be rescued by the formation of abnormal vessels (Leite de Oliveira et al., 2011).

When anti-angiogenic treatment was initially developed, tumor endothelial cells (TECs) were thought to be similar in all tumor types and, in contrast to tumor cells, genetically stable. However, subsequent studies showed that TECs are different in tumors from different organs and are actually genetically instable. It has been suggested that this is due to the involvement of endothelial cells (ECs) from different vascular beds. In addition, tumor cells and TECs interact strongly with each other and with additional cells present in the stroma via paracrine and possibly also juxtacrine pathways. Importantly, these interactions might induce microenvironment-dependent abnormalities in TECs that could differentiate them from normal endothelial cells. Recently, studies in mice and humans showed that abnormalities observed in TECs are maintained over long periods in cell culture, and include chromosomal abnormalities (Streubel et al., 2004; Hida & Klagsbrun, 2005; Akino et al., 2009), resistance to apoptosis (Bussolati et al., 2003), increased adhesiveness for tumor cells (Bussolati et al., 2003), drug resistance (Xiong et al., 2009), abnormal angiogenic capability (Ghosh et al., 2008; Xiong et al., 2009), and pronounced growth in the absence of serum (Bussolati et al., 2003).

TECs have been isolated from numerous animal models and from a limited number of human tumors mentioned above (Bussolati et al., 2003; Streubel et al., 2004; Buckanovich et al., 2007; Xiong et al., 2009). Until recently, no viable, pure TEC cultures from human colorectal carcinomas were available, and the biological phenotype of these cells was not characterized at the functional level. We have developed the first protocol for the routine isolation of both CRC TECs and the corresponding ECs from normal colon tissue (NECs) by collagenase II-digestion followed by multiple CD31-MACS selections (Schellerer et al., 2007). It was demonstrated that the cells were of endothelial blood cell origin (CD31-, CD105-, VE-cadherin-positive; E-selectin-, VCAM-1-, ICAM-1-positive after stimulation with inflammatory cytokines; capability to form capillaries in matrigel, take up acetylated LDL and bind *ulex europaeus*; CD45-, CD68-, CK-20-, podoplanin-negative). Moreover, the isolated TECs maintained differences from NECs during long-term culture for example by decreased von Willebrand factor (vWF) levels in the isolated tumor endothelial cells as well as in the original cancer tissue biopsies compared to the corresponding normal endothelial cells and normal colon biopsy (Schellerer et al., 2007). Meanwhile, we could show that the TEC isolated from CRC differ from each other also at the transcriptome and genome level (data unpublished).

TEC-specific markers were isolated from CRC by serial analysis of gene expression after laser-microdissection of tumor vessels (St Croix et al., 2000). The identified genes were designated as tumor endothelial markers (TEMs) (St Croix et al., 2000; Nanda et al., 2004). However, out of the nine different TEMs initially described, five were not pursued in future studies and two were shown to be expressed by other cells rather than tumor endothelial cells (Lee et al., 2006; Christian et al., 2008). These results indicated that the initial samples were most likely contaminated with non-endothelial cells such as pericytes that cover the mature vessel. Up to now, no widely accepted specific marker for tumor vessel endothelial cells in the CRC or other human tumors has been identified. Accordingly, a superior approach would be to specifically isolate pure, viable TEC cultures from CRC and then use these cells to identify TEC-specific markers.

In summary, the described results indicate that the induction and maintenance of tumor angiogenesis is an important feature in CRC growth and progression and that the interaction of TECs with tumor cells and other stromal cells changes the TEC phenotype.

Furthermore, pure viable TEC cultures isolated from CRC might be a valuable tool, allowing functional analysis of the TEC phenotype in CRC and the identification of TEC-specific markers. Pure CRC-derived TEC cultures will shed light on the manifold interactions between tumor and endothelial cells and their impact on the pathogenesis and prognosis of this tumor. This understanding will lead to improved anti-angiogenic treatment strategies in the CRC.

3. Host anti-tumor response and angiogenesis in colorectal cancer

3.1 Tumor infiltrating immune cells and angiogenesis in CRC

In CRC, tumor progression is tightly associated with and partly promoted by the tumor microenvironment. The tumor microenvironment consists of extracellular matrix, the vasculature and tumor-infiltrating cells. Infiltrating cells are recruited through inflammation and chemoattractants produced by the tumor cells or by cells of the stroma. Tumor infiltrating cells comprise cancer-associated fibroblasts (CAFs), endothelial cells, platelets, mesenchymal stem cells and various types of immune cells. Initial studies addressing the prognostic role of intratumoral immune cells infiltrates in colorectal cancer were partly contradictory. Some studies supported a protective role of inflammatory infiltrates (Jass, 1986; Harrison et al., 1994; Ropponen et al., 1997; Naito et al., 1998; Leo et al., 2000; Guidoboni et al., 2001; Galon et al., 2006) but other reports did not (Roncucci et al., 1996; Nielsen et al., 1999).

It is now clear that the type, the subtype and the localization of the infiltrating immune cells determine their effects on the tumor cells and the tumor microenvironment. Both the innate and the adaptive immune responses are involved in this process. For instance, the infiltration of cytotoxic T cells and type I helper T cells (Th1 cells) in CRC correlates with a prolonged disease-free survival, whereas the presence of infiltrating Th17 cells is of poor prognosis (Galon et al., 2006). In the same way, polarization of tumor-associated macrophages towards either M1 or M2 subpopulation results in anti-tumorigenic (M1) or pro-tumorigenic (M2) effects (Mantovani & Sica, 2010). Some forms of inflammatory infiltrates participate to the anti-tumor immune response while other immune cells are actively recruited by the tumor to exploit their pro-angiogenic and pro-metastatic effects (Balkwill & Mantovani, 2001; Coussens & Werb, 2001).

In addition, there is a growing body of evidence that tumor infiltrating immune cells can modulate tumor angiogenesis in cancer and particularly in CRC as summarized in table 1 and discussed in more detail below.

Pro-angiogenic	Anti-angiogenic
Tumor-associated macrophages (M2)	Lymphocytes (Th1)
TIE-2 expressing monocytes	NK cells
Mast cells	NKT cells
Neutrophils	Dendritic cells
MDSCs	
Immature DCs	
Th17 lymphocytes	
Immature dendritic cells	

Table 1. Pro-angiogenic or anti-angiogenic features of tumor infiltrating immune cells.

3.1.1 Tumor-associated macrophages

The recruitment of tumor-associated macrophages (TAMs) is mediated by various factors such as colony-stimulating factor-1 (CSF-1), which is produced by colon carcinoma cells, or the chemokines CCL2, CCL3, CCL4 and CCL5 (Sica et al., 2008a; Sica et al., 2008b). Tumors are predominantly infiltrated by TAMs with M2 polarization and high TAM infiltration in CRC is associated with a poor prognosis (Bacman et al., 2007). TAMs express pro-angiogenic factors including VEGF, basic fibroblast growth factor (bFGF), TNF-α, IL-8, IL-1β or platelet derived growth factor-β (PDGF-β) (Figure 1) (Barbera-Guillem et al., 2002; Sica et al., 2008a; Sica et al., 2008b). In addition, TAMs secrete matrix metalloproteases (MMP-7, MMP12) which participate in tumor angiogenesis by remodelling the extracellular matrix (Peddareddigari et al., 2010).

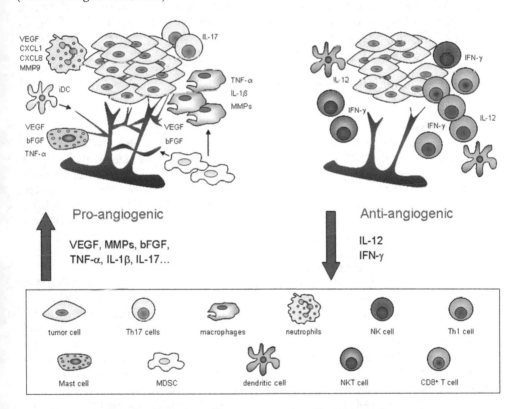

Fig. 1. Tumor-infiltrating immune cells exert opposite effects on angiogenesis.

3.1.2 TIE-2 expressing monocytes

TIE-2 expressing monocytes (TEMs) represent a subset of monocytes differing from the classical inflammatory monocytes (De Palma et al., 2005). The number of TEMs is increased in the blood of cancer patients and the tumor stroma of various types of cancers including CRC (De Palma et al., 2007; Venneri et al., 2007). TIE-2 is an angiopoietin receptor which is normally found at the surface of endothelial cells or haematopoietic stem cells. TEM recruitment in tumors is mediated by the chemokines CCL3, CCL5 and CCL8, and the expression of angiopoietin-2 by tumor cells or tumor endothelial cells (De Palma & Naldini, 2009; De Palma & Naldini, 2011). TEMs have been shown to promote tumor angiogenesis and tumor growth in tumor mouse models (De Palma & Naldini, 2011).

3.1.3 Mast cells

Mast cells are myeloid-derived cells which contain numerous granules rich in histamine and heparin. They are resident in tissues and represent key effectors of allergic reactions. Mast cells can also infiltrate tumors where they localize in the vicinity of blood vessels (Maltby et al., 2009). A high mast cell infiltration is usually associated with increased tumor growth, invasion and vascularisation. It has been shown that low mast cell numbers in CRC samples correlate with a better patient survival and hypovascularization (Gulubova & Vlaykova, 2009). Mast cells are able to produce numerous pro-angiogenic factors such as VEGF, bFGF, angiopoietin-1, TNF-α, heparin, histamine or various proteases (Maltby et al., 2009). It has been suggested that mast cell infiltration triggers the "angiogenic switch" during tumor growth: mast cells might be involved in angiogenesis at early stages of tumor growth, while at late stages the tumor cells control growth and angiogenesis in a mast cell-independent manner (Coussens et al., 1999).

3.1.4 Neutrophils

Infiltrates of neutrophils have been observed in various cancers including CRC (Roncucci et al., 2008; Tazzyman et al., 2009). In addition, neutrophils are involved in the pathogenesis of inflammatory bowel disease (Roessner et al., 2008). The recruitment of neutrophils is mediated by the chemokines CXCL1 and CXCL8 (Eck et al., 2003). Neutrophils stimulate tumor angiogenesis by releasing proteins including VEGF, CXCL1, CXCL8 or MMP9. The latter induces the release of VEGF from the extracellular matrix by cleavage of heparan sulfates (Hawinkels et al., 2008; Tazzyman et al., 2009).

3.1.5 Tumor infiltrating lymphocytes

Recent studies have highlighted the prognostic importance of tumor infiltrating lymphocytes (TILs) in colorectal carcinoma (Galon et al., 2006; Katz et al., 2009). The type, density and localization of T-cells in colorectal tumors have been found to be a better predictor of patient survival than the classical histopathological staging (Galon et al., 2006). T-cells can be divided in different subtypes. Naïve CD4+ T-cells differentiate in T helper (Th) cells of type 1 (Th1) in the presence of IL-12 or of type 2 (Th2) in the presence of IL-4 (Zhou et al., 2009). Th1 and Th2 cells inhibit each other. The presence of a Th1 adaptive immune response in CRC correlates with a better survival and an anti-angiogenic phenotype (Galon et al., 2006; Naschberger et al., 2008). Th1 cells facilitate the recruitment and the action of CD8+ cytotoxic T cells (Zhang et al., 2009). In CRC, CD8+ infiltrating T cells are the cell type most strongly associated with an improved survival (Galon et al., 2006). Th1 cells and CD8+ T-cells produce IL-12 and IFN-γ, both anti-angiogenic cytokines (Figure 1) (Zhu & Paul, 2010; Briesemeister et al., 2011). IL-12 promotes the production of IFN-γ by CD8+ T-cells and reduces the production of pro-angiogenic proteases such as MMP-9 by endothelial cells (Tartour et al., 2011). IFN-γ induces the production of angiostatic chemokines (CXCL9 and CXCL10) by endothelial cells and blocks the production of both VEGF and bFGF (Tartour et al., 2011).

Besides Th1 and Th2 cells, two other populations of T-cells have been shown to be involved in cancer, namely the regulatory T-cells (Treg) and the Th17 cells. In CRC, the infiltration of Treg, as well as of Th2 cells, seems to have no influence on patient survival (Tosolini et al., 2011). However, a direct association was found between the presence of a Th17 response and a worse prognosis (Tosolini et al., 2011). Th17 cells differentiate from naïve CD4+ T-cells upon exposure to IL-6 or TGF-β, and produce IL-17, IL-17F and IL-22 (Zhou et al., 2009). IL-17 promotes angiogenesis by inducing the production of angiogenic growth factors and chemokines by tumor cells and fibroblasts (Figure 1). Furthermore, IL-17 exerts a direct effect on endothelial cells, increasing migration and tube formation. Finally, IL-17 can indirectly promote angiogenesis by recruiting neutrophils to the tumor site (Tartour et al., 2011).

3.1.6 Myeloid-derived suppressor cells

Myeloid-derived suppressor cells (MDSCs) are immature myeloid cells including progenitors of macrophages, granulocytes and DCs. The number of MDSCs has been shown to be increased in the blood of CRC patients (Mandruzzato et al., 2009). MDSCs are immunosuppressive and in particular inhibit T-cells (Condamine & Gabrilovich, 2011). In addition, they modulate the action of NK cells and induce Treg cells. MDSCs exert their functions through up-regulation of NO, arginase or ROS (Gabrilovich & Nagaraj, 2009). In mouse models, MDSCs have been shown to promote angiogenesis, tumor cell invasion and metastasis (Youn & Gabrilovich, 2010). MDSCs are very heterogenic but one can distinguish two different subtypes: the granulocytic (G)-MDSCs and the monocytic (M)-MDSCs (Youn & Gabrilovich, 2010). G-MDSCs are found in the spleen or in peripheral lymphoid organs, use primarily ROS for immune suppression, require cell-cell contact with T cells and are dependent on antigen-specific interactions (Youn & Gabrilovich, 2010). M-MDSCs are found in tumors, use primarily iNOS, arginase and cytokines for immune suppression, their action does not require direct cell-cell contact. M-MDSCs exert a non-specific suppression and are more potent (Youn & Gabrilovich, 2010). M-MDSCs are able to differentiate towards TAMs under hypoxic conditions (Corzo et al., 2010). Some MDSCs express endothelial markers such as CD31 or VEGFR2 and are able to incorporate into the tumor endothelium (Figure 1) (Yang et al., 2004).

3.1.7 Dendritic cells

Dendritic cells (DCs) are bone-marrow derived cells and represent the most important antigen-presenting cells (Salama & Platell, 2008). In CRC, DCs localize at the invasive margin of the tumor and in lymph nodes (Ambe et al., 1989; Suzuki et al., 2002). The presence of a high number of DCs in CRC correlates with a better prognosis, in particular when DCs infiltrate the intra-epithelial compartment of the tumor (Dadabayev et al., 2004; Sandel et al., 2005). Mature DCs are able to produce IL-12 which induces the polarization of immune cells towards the Th1 anti-tumorigenic and anti-angiogenic phenotype. Tumors are in addition able to recruit immature DCs (iDCs) which have been shown in ovarian cancer to secrete pro-angiogenic factors and to be capable of incorporating in newly formed vessels (Figure 1) (Curiel et al., 2004).

3.1.8 NK and NKT cells

NK cells are lymphocytes from the innate immune system which are able to recognize tumor cells as target. The immune infiltration of NK cells represents a positive prognostic marker in various solid tumors including CRC (Coca et al., 1997). They represent together with CD8+ T cells the most likely effectors of the anti-tumor immunity. NK cells exert their anti-tumorigenic effects notably through the production of IFN-γ and participate therefore in the anti-angiogenic immune response (Levy et al., 2011).

NKT cell are a small population of T cells which also exhibit NK cells markers. They have the property to modulate immune responses and to link the innate and the adaptive immune responses. NKT cells are able to recognize lipid antigens that are not recognized by other T cell subsets (Terabe & Berzofsky, 2008). Two subtypes of NKT cells have been described. The most frequent type of NKT cells, called type I, has a very restricted T-cell receptor (TCR) repertoire and expresses the invariant Vα24Jα18 TCR. On the contrary, the type II NKT cells express different TCRs (Terabe & Berzofsky, 2008). NKT type I cells exert anti-tumor effects through IFN-γ but independently of perforin (van der Vliet et al., 2008). In addition, they activate DCs to produce IL-12. In colorectal carcinoma, a high infiltration of type I NKT cells, which are Vα24 positive, correlates with a better overall and disease-free survival (Tachibana et al., 2005). Through their production of IFN-γ and their activation of DCs, type I NKT cells participate in the Th1 anti-angiogenic immune response in CRC (Figure 1). While type I NKT cells enhance anti-tumor immunity, mouse models showed that type II NKT cells repress it (Terabe & Berzofsky, 2008).

Tumor angiogenesis is promoted by the production of VEGF from the tumor cells but also from mast cells, M2 macrophages and neutrophils. In addition, macrophages and mast cells produce IL-1β and TNF-α, which can promote a local pro-angiogenic inflammation through the further recruitment of macrophages *in vivo*, even if their direct action on endothelial cells *in vitro* is anti-angiogenic. Neutrophils and macrophages produce MMPs, inducing a matrix remodeling necessary for angiogenesis. Th17 cells directly promote angiogenesis through the secretion of IL-17, which enhances the recruitment of neutrophils. Immature MDSCs can differentiate towards M2 macrophages or, like immature dendritic cells, can be incorporated into newly formed vessels. On the contrary, a Th1 dominated immune response exerts anti-angiogenic effects, mainly through the production of IFN-γ by Th1 cells, CD8+ T cells, NK or NKT cells. Th1 cells are activated by IL-12, notably produced by some DCs.

3.2 Markers for the interplay of angiogenesis and a host anti-tumor response in CRC

The impact of angiogenesis on colorectal tumor growth and progression described in the previous paragraphs was convincingly supported by a clinical phase III study in which an anti-VEGF antibody (bevacizumab) was added to fluorouracil-based combination chemotherapy. The combination therapy led to a statistically significant and clinically meaningful improvement in overall survival (20.3 months vs. 15.6 months for the control group) and progression-free survival among patients with metastatic CRC (Hurwitz et al., 2004). Based on these results bevacizumab was approved as the first solely anti-angiogenic drug used as anti-cancer agent by the FDA in 2004. Moreover, two additional anti-angiogenic drugs for the same molecular target have been approved for the clinics meanwhile: sunitinib and sorafenib. These drugs are both broad-spectrum receptor tyrosine kinase (RTK) inhibitors that target VEGFR1, VEGFR2, VEGFR3 or PDGFR-α/β among other RTKs (Escudier et al., 2007; Motzer et al., 2007).

However, in all of the clinical studies employing anti-angiogenic treatment for human tumors including CRC, only a fraction of the treated patients responded completely or partially to the therapy (10-49.3% maximum partial response rates) (Hurwitz et al., 2004;

Demetri et al., 2006; Escudier et al., 2007; Motzer et al., 2007; Sobrero et al., 2009). Additionally, in some cases, severe side effects such as cardiovascular damage, perforation of the colon or venous thromboembolic events have been observed (Hurwitz et al., 2004; Sobrero et al., 2009). Furthermore, anti-angiogenic treatment is very expensive and puts a significant cost burden on the health system. This raises important questions: (1) which subset of patients will benefit most from these therapies? (2) How can these patients be preselected? (3) Can the side effects be decreased by patient preselection?

From these questions it becomes obvious that valid biomarkers able to indicate different angiogenic or angiostatic tumor microenvironments, and in consequence patients who will benefit most from anti-angiogenic therapy, are urgently required. Numerous efforts have been undertaken to identify predictive and/or prognostic biomarkers and this research field is rapidly expanding. By definition a predictive biomarker is able to foretell the response of the patient to a certain treatment whereas a prognostic biomarker predicts the potential outcome of the disease independently of the applied therapy. Promising results have been reported in the last few years, however, none of the proposed markers has been accepted widely (Asghar et al., 2010; Gerger et al., 2011).

Different kinds of potential biomarkers for anti-angiogenic treatment have been reported in the literature in the past few years: serum, tissue and genetic markers. Initially, for obvious reasons, VEGF tissue and serum levels were heavily investigated but surprisingly did not make it into the clinics due to the inability to predict response at the tissue level (Jubb et al., 2006) and contradictory results at the serum level (Loupakis et al., 2007; Willett et al., 2009). Efforts have also been undertaken to investigate the impact of genetic polymorphisms of VEGF and VEGFR-2 as potential biomarkers (Schneider et al., 2008). Many other potential biomarkers were reported in the last few years in the literature to be measured either at the tissue or serum/plasma level. Examples for these markers are tissue CD31 and PDGFR-β expression in breast cancer (Yang et al., 2008), soluble angiopoietin-2 (Goede et al., 2010), circulating endothelial cells (Ronzoni et al., 2010), TNF-α, MMP-9 (Perez-Gracia et al., 2009), soluble KIT (Deprimo et al., 2009) as well as IL-8 (Kopetz et al., 2010). However, all of these potential markers require confirmation in larger cohorts and unfortunately lack either prognostic or predictive value.

From these results it becomes clear that very likely different biomarkers will be required for the different kinds of anti-angiogenic treatments and the different kinds of cancers. In addition, as discussed in the section 3 of this review, a broad range of immune cells can infiltrate tumors and have been detected in CRC samples. These cells interact with tumor endothelial cells during their extravasation and some of them are able to modulate tumor angiogenesis (Figure 1). While tumor infiltrating macrophages, mast cells, Th17 lymphocytes and neutrophils are recognized to exert pro-angiogenic effects in CRC, Th1 lymphocytes are associated with an anti-angiogenic microenvironment. On the other end, tumor vessels can be more or less permissive for the infiltration of immune cells. Therefore, the interplay between immune cells and tumor endothelial cells represents an important issue with implications for the anti-tumor host response and angiogenesis.

3.2.1 GBP-1 as a marker for the anti-angiogenic Th1 immune response in CRC

As mentioned above, the presence of a Th1 microenvironment is associated with a significantly improved prognosis in CRC (Galon et al., 2006). A Th-1 microenvironment is characterized by increased IFN-γ expression, often combined with the increased expression of pro-inflammatory cytokines IL-1β and TNF-α (Dayer, 2002b; Dayer, 2002a; Cui et al., 2007). The guanylate-binding protein 1 (GBP-1) has been identified as a marker of the Th1 microenvironment in CRC (Naschberger et al., 2008). GBP-1 expression is induced upon stimulation by IFN-γ but also by other pro-inflammatory cytokines such as IL-1β and/or TNF-α (Guenzi et al., 2001; Lubeseder-Martellato et al., 2002). In CRC, GBP-1 is strongly expressed in infiltrating cells and in the vasculature. Its expression correlates with expression of IFN-γ-induced genes, chemokines and immune reaction-associated genes (Naschberger et al., 2008). Among them, three anti-angiogenic chemokines known to play a role in tumors (CXCL9, CXCL10, CXCL11) could also be detected (Romagnani et al., 2004). GBP-1 expression in CRC stroma is associated with an increase of the cancer-related five-year survival rate and GBP-1 represents an independent prognostic factor indicating a reduction of the relative risk of cancer-related death by the half (Naschberger et al., 2008). In tumor-associated endothelial cells the presence of GBP-1 is associated with a decreased angiogenic activity (Naschberger et al., 2008; Guenzi et al., 2001; Guenzi et al., 2003). GBP-1 is presently the only marker available to specifically indicate whether endothelial cells in tissues are exposed to an angiostatic Th-1-like tumor microenvironment.

3.2.2 Modulation of lymphocytes infiltration by endothelial cells

The relationship between tumor angiogenesis and immunity is actually bidirectional. As described above, infiltrating immune cells can positively or negatively regulate angiogenesis in tumors. On the other hand, tumor endothelial cells are able to regulate extravasation of immune cells, notably through the expression of surface molecules. Among the potential molecular effectors identified, endothelin, endothelin receptor and CD137 seem to play a prominent role.

The endothelin-endothelin receptor axis

The endothelin (ET) family comprises four members designated ET-1 to -4 (Kandalaft et al., 2009). ETs derive from precursor proteins after cleavage by membrane-bound metalloproteinases. ET-1 is the most potent ligand and the most widely expressed in endothelial cells (Kandalaft et al., 2009). In addition, ET-1 is overexpressed in many tumor cell lines and many tumors, including CRC (Kusuhara et al., 1990; Arun et al., 2004; Bagnato & Rosano, 2008). Two endothelin receptors have been identified: the endothelin A and the endothelin B receptor, respectively ET_AR and ET_BR (Kandalaft et al., 2009). In normal tissues, ET_AR and ET_BR regulate vasoconstriction and are also involved in inflammation. Both receptors exert opposite effects. In particular, ET_AR promote T-cell adhesion to endothelial cells, whereas ET_BR inhibits it. In tumor cells, concomitant up-regulation of ET-1 and ET_AR inhibits apoptosis and promotes cell proliferation, invasion and metastasis (Kedzierski & Yanagisawa, 2001; Kandalaft et al., 2009). In a study comparing the expression profiles of tumor associated endothelial cells (TECs) in ovarian cancer with or without TILs, ET_BR has been associated with the absence of TILs and short patient survival time (Buckanovich et al., 2008). Of note, in this study, GBP-1 expression in TECs correlated with the presence of TILs. The inhibition of T cells homing in tumor by ET_BR is mediated by an increase of NO synthase and NO release and by a decrease in the expression of the adhesion molecule ICAM-1. In CRC, ET-1 and ET_AR are expressed by the tumor cells, generating a stimulatory loop, while ET_BR expression in TECs is reduced as compared to normal colon blood vessels (Ali et al., 2000a; Ali et al., 2000b; Asham et al., 2001; Hoosein et al., 2007).

Investigation of the expression of ET_BR in TECs in relation to TILs infiltration might provide further insights into the molecular regulation of immune cells extravasation by endothelial cells in CRC.

CD137 (TNFRSF9)

CD137 is a surface glycoprotein of the TNF-α receptor family involved in T-cell co-stimulation (Shao & Schwarz, 2011). CD137 is expressed on the surface of activated T cells, NK cells, DCs, macrophages or B cells, while its ligand, CD137L is expressed by APCs (Shao & Schwarz, 2011). CD137 is induced under hypoxia and by TNF-α, LPS or IL-1β. CD137 is however also expressed in human tumor capillaries, notably in CRC (Broll et al., 2001; Wang et al., 2008). In tumors, CD137 is expressed on the vessel walls whereas CD137L is expressed on tumor cells (Salih et al., 2000; Broll et al., 2001). The effects of CD137 are mediated by the up-regulation of V-CAM, I-CAM and E-selectin, inducing thereby the recruitment of T lymphocytes (Palazon et al., 2011). In addition, it has been shown that the ligation of CD137L on lung squamous carcinoma cells with CD137 on T cells induced IFN-γ production by T cells (Salih et al., 2000). Therefore, expression of CD137 by TECs might promote the recruitment of T cells in CRC and their polarization towards the anti-tumorigenic and anti-angiogenic Th1 subtype.

4. Conclusions

In this review we tried to shed light on the current understanding of tumor angiogenesis and its modulation by a potential host anti-tumor response with a specific focus on colorectal carcinoma. Our major aim was to point out the connection of these two processes. A host anti-tumor response does not only have a direct effect on the tumor cells but also a major impact on the development and function of the tumor vasculature. Different tumor microenvironments, which can either inhibit or foster angiogenesis, are established during a specific immune response. These various microenvironments are achieved by different means: (1) immune cells such as Th1-T-cells are attracted into the tumor tissue within the context of a specific host anti-tumor response that secrete soluble mediators (e.g. IFN-γ) directly acting on tumor endothelial cells in an anti-angiogenic manner. (2) The tumor cells themselves also attract immune cells such as M2 macrophages or Th17-T-cells that might release mediators which modulate the microenvironment in a pro-angiogenic manner. (3) Endothelial cells can also modulate the stromal composition of infiltrating leukocytes which alters the soluble mediator profile to which the tumor and its vasculature are exposed. Therefore, biomarkers are required in order to characterize the specific angiogenic phenotype of each CRC patient. Moreover, these biomarkers should have prognostic and/or predictive potential for anti-angiogenic treatment and at best also give information about the presence of a host anti-tumor immune response. A potential candidate for such a biomarker might be the guanylate binding protein-1 (GBP-1).

5. References

Akino, T.; Hida, K.; Hida, Y.; Tsuchiya, K.; Freedman, D.; Muraki, C.; Ohga, N.; Matsuda, K.; Akiyama, K.; Harabayashi, T.; Shinohara, N.; Nonomura, K.; Klagsbrun, M. & Shindoh, M. (2009). Cytogenetic abnormalities of tumor-associated endothelial cells in human malignant tumors. *Am J Pathol*, Vol.175, No.6, (Dec 2009), pp. 2657-2667

Ali, H.; Dashwood, M.; Dawas, K.; Loizidou, M.; Savage, F. & Taylor, I. (2000a). Endothelin
    receptor expression in colorectal cancer. *J Cardiovasc Pharmacol*, Vol.36, No.5 Suppl
    1, (Nov 2000a), pp. S69-71
Ali, H.; Loizidou, M.; Dashwood, M.; Savage, F.; Sheard, C. & Taylor, I. (2000b). Stimulation
    of colorectal cancer cell line growth by ET-1 and its inhibition by ET(A) antagonists.
    Gut, Vol.47, No.5, (Nov 2000b), pp. 685-688
Ambe, K.; Mori, M. & Enjoji, M. (1989). S-100 protein-positive dendritic cells in colorectal
    adenocarcinomas. Distribution and relation to the clinical prognosis. *Cancer*, Vol.63,
    No.3, (Feb 1 1989), pp. 496-503
Arun, C.; London, N. J. & Hemingway, D. M. (2004). Prognostic significance of elevated
    endothelin-1 levels in patients with colorectal cancer. *Int J Biol Markers*, Vol.19,
    No.1, (Jan-Mar 2004), pp. 32-37
Asghar, U.; Hawkes, E. & Cunningham, D. (2010). Predictive and prognostic biomarkers for
    targeted therapy in metastatic colorectal cancer. *Clin Colorectal Cancer*, Vol.9, No.5,
    (Dec 2010), pp. 274-281
Asham, E.; Shankar, A.; Loizidou, M.; Fredericks, S.; Miller, K.; Boulos, P. B.; Burnstock, G.
    & Taylor, I. (2001). Increased endothelin-1 in colorectal cancer and reduction of
    tumour growth by ET(A) receptor antagonism. *Br J Cancer*, Vol.85, No.11, (Nov 30
    2001), pp. 1759-1763
Bacman, D.; Merkel, S.; Papadopoulos, T.; Croner, R. S.; Brueckl, W. M. & Dimmler, A.
    (2007). TGF-beta receptor 2 downregulation in tumour-associated stroma worsens
    prognosis and high-grade tumours show more tumour-associated macrophages
    and lower TGF-beta1 expression in colon carcinoma: a retrospective study. *BMC
    Cancer*, Vol.7, No.1, (Aug 10 2007), pp. 156
Bagnato, A. & Rosano, L. (2008). The endothelin axis in cancer. *Int J Biochem Cell Biol*, Vol.40,
    No.8, 2008), pp. 1443-1451
Balkwill, F. & Mantovani, A. (2001). Inflammation and cancer: back to Virchow? *Lancet*,
    Vol.357, No.9255, (Feb 17 2001), pp. 539-545
Barbera-Guillem, E.; Nyhus, J. K.; Wolford, C. C.; Friece, C. R. & Sampsel, J. W. (2002).
    Vascular endothelial growth factor secretion by tumor-infiltrating macrophages
    essentially supports tumor angiogenesis, and IgG immune complexes potentiate
    the process. *Cancer Res*, Vol.62, No.23, (Dec 1 2002), pp. 7042-7049
Bossi, P.; Viale, G.; Lee, A. K.; Alfano, R.; Coggi, G. & Bosari, S. (1995). Angiogenesis in
    colorectal tumors: microvessel quantitation in adenomas and carcinomas with
    clinicopathological correlations. *Cancer Res*, Vol.55, No.21, (Nov 1 1995), pp. 5049-
    5053
Briesemeister, D.; Sommermeyer, D.; Loddenkemper, C.; Loew, R.; Uckert, W.; Blankenstein,
    T. & Kammertoens, T. (2011). Tumor rejection by local interferon gamma induction
    in established tumors is associated with blood vessel destruction and necrosis. *Int J
    Cancer*, Vol.128, No.2, (Jan 15 2011), pp. 371-378
Broll, K.; Richter, G.; Pauly, S.; Hofstaedter, F. & Schwarz, H. (2001). CD137 expression in
    tumor vessel walls. High correlation with malignant tumors. *Am J Clin Pathol*,
    Vol.115, No.4, (Apr 2001), pp. 543-549
Buckanovich, R. J.; Facciabene, A.; Kim, S.; Benencia, F.; Sasaroli, D.; Balint, K.; Katsaros, D.;
    O'Brien-Jenkins, A.; Gimotty, P. A. & Coukos, G. (2008). Endothelin B receptor

mediates the endothelial barrier to T cell homing to tumors and disables immune therapy. *Nat Med*, Vol.14, No.1, (Jan 2008), pp. 28-36

Buckanovich, R. J.; Sasaroli, D.; O'Brien-Jenkins, A.; Botbyl, J.; Hammond, R.; Katsaros, D.; Sandaltzopoulos, R.; Liotta, L. A.; Gimotty, P. A. & Coukos, G. (2007). Tumor vascular proteins as biomarkers in ovarian cancer. *J Clin Oncol*, Vol.25, No.7, (Mar 1 2007), pp. 852-861

Bussolati, B.; Deambrosis, I.; Russo, S.; Deregibus, M. C. & Camussi, G. (2003). Altered angiogenesis and survival in human tumor-derived endothelial cells. *FASEB J*, Vol.17, No.9, (Jun 2003), pp. 1159-1161

Carmeliet, P. & Jain, R. K. (2000). Angiogenesis in cancer and other diseases. *Nature*, Vol.407, No.6801, (Sep 14 2000), pp. 249-257

Carmeliet, P. & Jain, R. K. (2011). Molecular mechanisms and clinical applications of angiogenesis. *Nature*, Vol.473, No.7347, (May 19 2011), pp. 298-307

Choi, H. J.; Hyun, M. S.; Jung, G. J.; Kim, S. S. & Hong, S. H. (1998). Tumor angiogenesis as a prognostic predictor in colorectal carcinoma with special reference to mode of metastasis and recurrence. *Oncology*, Vol.55, No.6, (Nov-Dec 1998), pp. 575-581

Christian, S.; Winkler, R.; Helfrich, I.; Boos, A. M.; Resemfelder, E.; Schadendort, D. & Augustin, H. G. (2008). Endosialin (Tem1) is a marker of tumor-associated myofibroblasts and tumor vessel-associated mural cells. *Am J Pathol*, Vol.172, No.2, (Feb 2008), pp. 486-494

Coca, S.; Perez-Piqueras, J.; Martinez, D.; Colmenarejo, A.; Saez, M. A.; Vallejo, C.; Martos, J. A. & Moreno, M. (1997). The prognostic significance of intratumoral natural killer cells in patients with colorectal carcinoma. *Cancer*, Vol.79, No.12, (Jun 15 1997), pp. 2320-2328

Condamine, T. & Gabrilovich, D. I. (2011). Molecular mechanisms regulating myeloid-derived suppressor cell differentiation and function. *Trends Immunol*, Vol.32, No.1, (Jan 2011), pp. 19-25

Corzo, C. A.; Condamine, T.; Lu, L.; Cotter, M. J.; Youn, J. I.; Cheng, P.; Cho, H. I.; Celis, E.; Quiceno, D. G.; Padhya, T.; McCaffrey, T. V.; McCaffrey, J. C. & Gabrilovich, D. I. (2010). HIF-1alpha regulates function and differentiation of myeloid-derived suppressor cells in the tumor microenvironment. *J Exp Med*, Vol.207, No.11, (Oct 25 2010), pp. 2439-2453

Coussens, L. M.; Raymond, W. W.; Bergers, G.; Laig-Webster, M.; Behrendtsen, O.; Werb, Z.; Caughey, G. H. & Hanahan, D. (1999). Inflammatory mast cells up-regulate angiogenesis during squamous epithelial carcinogenesis. *Genes Dev*, Vol.13, No.11, (Jun 1 1999), pp. 1382-1397

Coussens, L. M. & Werb, Z. (2001). Inflammatory cells and cancer: think different! *J Exp Med*, Vol.193, No.6, (Mar 19 2001), pp. F23-26

Cui, G.; Goll, R.; Olsen, T.; Steigen, S. E.; Husebekk, A.; Vonen, B. & Florholmen, J. (2007). Reduced expression of microenvironmental Th1 cytokines accompanies adenomas-carcinomas sequence of colorectum. *Cancer Immunol Immunother*, Vol.56, No.7, (Jul 2007), pp. 985-995

Curiel, T. J.; Cheng, P.; Mottram, P.; Alvarez, X.; Moons, L.; Evdemon Hogan, M.; Wei, S.; Zou, L.; Kryczek, I.; Hoyle, G.; Lackner, A.; Carmeliet, P. & Zou, W. (2004). Dendritic cell subsets differentially regulate angiogenesis in human ovarian cancer. *Cancer Res*, Vol.64, No.16, (Aug 15 2004), pp. 5535-5538

Dadabayev, A. R.; Sandel, M. H.; Menon, A. G.; Morreau, H.; Melief, C. J.; Offringa, R.; van der Burg, S. H.; Janssen-van Rhijn, C.; Ensink, N. G.; Tollenaar, R. A.; van de Velde, C. J. & Kuppen, P. J. (2004). Dendritic cells in colorectal cancer correlate with other tumor-infiltrating immune cells. *Cancer Immunol Immunother*, Vol.53, No.11, (Nov 2004), pp. 978-986

Dayer, J. M. (2002a). Evidence for the biological modulation of IL-1 activity: the role of IL-1Ra. *Clin Exp Rheumatol*, Vol.20, No.5 Suppl 27, (Sep-Oct 2002a), pp. S14-20

Dayer, J. M. (2002b). Interleukin 1 or tumor necrosis factor-alpha: which is the real target in rheumatoid arthritis? *J Rheumatol Suppl*, Vol.65, (Sep 2002b), pp. 10-15

De Palma, M.; Murdoch, C.; Venneri, M. A.; Naldini, L. & Lewis, C. E. (2007). Tie2-expressing monocytes: regulation of tumor angiogenesis and therapeutic implications. *Trends Immunol*, Vol.28, No.12, (Dec 2007), pp. 519-524

De Palma, M. & Naldini, L. (2009). Tie2-expressing monocytes (TEMs): Novel targets and vehicles of anticancer therapy? *Biochim Biophys Acta*, (Apr 10 2009),

De Palma, M. & Naldini, L. (2011). Angiopoietin-2 TIEs Up Macrophages in Tumor Angiogenesis. *Clin Cancer Res*, (May 16 2011),

De Palma, M.; Venneri, M. A.; Galli, R.; Sergi Sergi, L.; Politi, L. S.; Sampaolesi, M. & Naldini, L. (2005). Tie2 identifies a hematopoietic lineage of proangiogenic monocytes required for tumor vessel formation and a mesenchymal population of pericyte progenitors. *Cancer Cell*, Vol.8, No.3, (Sep 2005), pp. 211-226

Demetri, G. D.; van Oosterom, A. T.; Garrett, C. R.; Blackstein, M. E.; Shah, M. H.; Verweij, J.; McArthur, G.; Judson, I. R.; Heinrich, M. C.; Morgan, J. A.; Desai, J.; Fletcher, C. D.; George, S.; Bello, C. L.; Huang, X.; Baum, C. M. & Casali, P. G. (2006). Efficacy and safety of sunitinib in patients with advanced gastrointestinal stromal tumour after failure of imatinib: a randomised controlled trial. *Lancet*, Vol.368, No.9544, (Oct 14 2006), pp. 1329-1338

Deprimo, S. E.; Huang, X.; Blackstein, M. E.; Garrett, C. R.; Harmon, C. S.; Schoffski, P.; Shah, M. H.; Verweij, J.; Baum, C. M. & Demetri, G. D. (2009). Circulating levels of soluble KIT serve as a biomarker for clinical outcome in gastrointestinal stromal tumor patients receiving sunitinib following imatinib failure. *Clin Cancer Res*, Vol.15, No.18, (Sep 15 2009), pp. 5869-5877

Eck, M.; Schmausser, B.; Scheller, K.; Brandlein, S. & Muller-Hermelink, H. K. (2003). Pleiotropic effects of CXC chemokines in gastric carcinoma: differences in CXCL8 and CXCL1 expression between diffuse and intestinal types of gastric carcinoma. *Clin Exp Immunol*, Vol.134, No.3, (Dec 2003), pp. 508-515

Escudier, B.; Eisen, T.; Stadler, W. M.; Szczylik, C.; Oudard, S.; Siebels, M.; Negrier, S.; Chevreau, C.; Solska, E.; Desai, A. A.; Rolland, F.; Demkow, T.; Hutson, T. E.; Gore, M.; Freeman, S.; Schwartz, B.; Shan, M.; Simantov, R. & Bukowski, R. M. (2007). Sorafenib in advanced clear-cell renal-cell carcinoma. *N Engl J Med*, Vol.356, No.2, (Jan 11 2007), pp. 125-134

Folkman, J. (1995). Angiogenesis in cancer, vascular, rheumatoid and other disease. *Nat Med*, Vol.1, No.1, (Jan 1995), pp. 27-31

Gabrilovich, D. I. & Nagaraj, S. (2009). Myeloid-derived suppressor cells as regulators of the immune system. *Nat Rev Immunol*, Vol.9, No.3, (Mar 2009), pp. 162-174

Galon, J.; Costes, A.; Sanchez-Cabo, F.; Kirilovsky, A.; Mlecnik, B.; Lagorce-Pages, C.; Tosolini, M.; Camus, M.; Berger, A.; Wind, P.; Zinzindohoue, F.; Bruneval, P.;

Cugnenc, P. H.; Trajanoski, Z.; Fridman, W. H. & Pages, F. (2006). Type, density, and location of immune cells within human colorectal tumors predict clinical outcome. *Science*, Vol.313, No.5795, (Sep 29 2006), pp. 1960-1964

Galon, J.; Fridman, W. H. & Pages, F. (2007). The adaptive immunologic microenvironment in colorectal cancer: a novel perspective. *Cancer Res*, Vol.67, No.5, (Mar 1 2007), pp. 1883-1886

Gerger, A.; LaBonte, M. & Lenz, H. J. (2011). Molecular predictors of response to antiangiogenesis therapies. *Cancer J*, Vol.17, No.2, (Mar-Apr 2011), pp. 134-141

Ghosh, K.; Thodeti, C. K.; Dudley, A. C.; Mammoto, A.; Klagsbrun, M. & Ingber, D. E. (2008). Tumor-derived endothelial cells exhibit aberrant Rho-mediated mechanosensing and abnormal angiogenesis in vitro. *Proc Natl Acad Sci U S A*, Vol.105, No.32, (Aug 12 2008), pp. 11305-11310

Goede, V.; Coutelle, O.; Neuneier, J.; Reinacher-Schick, A.; Schnell, R.; Koslowsky, T. C.; Weihrauch, M. R.; Cremer, B.; Kashkar, H.; Odenthal, M.; Augustin, H. G.; Schmiegel, W.; Hallek, M. & Hacker, U. T. (2010). Identification of serum angiopoietin-2 as a biomarker for clinical outcome of colorectal cancer patients treated with bevacizumab-containing therapy. *Br J Cancer*, Vol.103, No.9, (Oct 26 2010), pp. 1407-1414

Guenzi, E.; Töpolt, K.; Cornali, E.; Lubeseder-Martellato, C.; Jörg, A.; Matzen, K.; Zietz, C.; Kremmer, E.; Nappi, F.; Schwemmle, M.; Hohenadl, C.; Barillari, G.; Tschachler, E.; Monini, P.; Ensoli, B. & Stürzl, M. (2001). The helical domain of GBP-1 mediates the inhibition of endothelial cell proliferation by inflammatory cytokines. *Embo J*, Vol.20, No.20, 2001), pp. 5568-5577.

Guenzi, E.; Töpolt, K.; Lubeseder-Martellato, C.; Jörg, A.; Naschberger, E.; Benelli, R.; Albini, A. & Stürzl, M. (2003). The guanylate binding protein-1 GTPase controls the invasive and angiogenic capability of endothelial cells through inhibition of MMP-1 expression. *Embo J*, Vol.22, No.15, (Aug 1 2003), pp. 3772-3782

Guidoboni, M.; Gafa, R.; Viel, A.; Doglioni, C.; Russo, A.; Santini, A.; Del Tin, L.; Macri, E.; Lanza, G.; Boiocchi, M. & Dolcetti, R. (2001). Microsatellite instability and high content of activated cytotoxic lymphocytes identify colon cancer patients with a favorable prognosis. *Am J Pathol*, Vol.159, No.1, (Jul 2001), pp. 297-304

Gulubova, M. & Vlaykova, T. (2009). Prognostic significance of mast cell number and microvascular density for the survival of patients with primary colorectal cancer. *J Gastroenterol Hepatol*, Vol.24, No.7, (Jul 2009), pp. 1265-1275

Hanahan, D. & Weinberg, R. A. (2000). The hallmarks of cancer. *Cell*, Vol.100, No.1, (Jan 7 2000), pp. 57-70

Hanahan, D. & Weinberg, R. A. (2011). Hallmarks of cancer: the next generation. *Cell*, Vol.144, No.5, (Mar 4 2011), pp. 646-674

Harrison, J. C.; Dean, P. J.; el-Zeky, F. & Vander Zwaag, R. (1994). From Dukes through Jass: pathological prognostic indicators in rectal cancer. *Hum Pathol*, Vol.25, No.5, (May 1994), pp. 498-505

Hawinkels, L. J.; Zuidwijk, K.; Verspaget, H. W.; de Jonge-Muller, E. S.; van Duijn, W.; Ferreira, V.; Fontijn, R. D.; David, G.; Hommes, D. W.; Lamers, C. D. & Sier, C. F. (2008). VEGF release by MMP-9 mediated heparan sulphate cleavage induces colorectal cancer angiogenesis. *Eur J Cancer*, Vol.44, No.13, (Sep 2008), pp. 1904-1913

Hida, K.; Hida, Y. & Shindoh, M. (2008). Understanding tumor endothelial cell abnormalities to develop ideal anti-angiogenic therapies. *Cancer Sci*, Vol.99, No.3, (Mar 2008), pp. 459-466

Hida, K. & Klagsbrun, M. (2005). A new perspective on tumor endothelial cells: unexpected chromosome and centrosome abnormalities. *Cancer Res*, Vol.65, No.7, (Apr 1 2005), pp. 2507-2510

Hoosein, M. M.; Dashwood, M. R.; Dawas, K.; Ali, H. M.; Grant, K.; Savage, F.; Taylor, I. & Loizidou, M. (2007). Altered endothelin receptor subtypes in colorectal cancer. *Eur J Gastroenterol Hepatol*, Vol.19, No.9, (Sep 2007), pp. 775-782

Hurwitz, H.; Fehrenbacher, L.; Novotny, W.; Cartwright, T.; Hainsworth, J.; Heim, W.; Berlin, J.; Baron, A.; Griffing, S.; Holmgren, E.; Ferrara, N.; Fyfe, G.; Rogers, B.; Ross, R. & Kabbinavar, F. (2004). Bevacizumab plus irinotecan, fluorouracil, and leucovorin for metastatic colorectal cancer. *N Engl J Med*, Vol.350, No.23, (Jun 3 2004), pp. 2335-2342

Ishigami, S. I.; Arii, S.; Furutani, M.; Niwano, M.; Harada, T.; Mizumoto, M.; Mori, A.; Onodera, H. & Imamura, M. (1998). Predictive value of vascular endothelial growth factor (VEGF) in metastasis and prognosis of human colorectal cancer. *Br J Cancer*, Vol.78, No.10, (Nov 1998), pp. 1379-1384

Jass, J. R. (1986). Lymphocytic infiltration and survival in rectal cancer. *J Clin Pathol*, Vol.39, No.6, (Jun 1986), pp. 585-589

Jass, J. R. (2002). Pathogenesis of colorectal cancer. *Surg Clin North Am*, Vol.82, No.5, (Oct 2002), pp. 891-904

Jubb, A. M.; Hurwitz, H. I.; Bai, W.; Holmgren, E. B.; Tobin, P.; Guerrero, A. S.; Kabbinavar, F.; Holden, S. N.; Novotny, W. F.; Frantz, G. D.; Hillan, K. J. & Koeppen, H. (2006). Impact of vascular endothelial growth factor-A expression, thrombospondin-2 expression, and microvessel density on the treatment effect of bevacizumab in metastatic colorectal cancer. *J Clin Oncol*, Vol.24, No.2, (Jan 10 2006), pp. 217-227

Kahlenberg, M. S.; Sullivan, J. M.; Witmer, D. D. & Petrelli, N. J. (2003). Molecular prognostics in colorectal cancer. *Surg Oncol*, Vol.12, No.3, (Nov 2003), pp. 173-186

Kandalaft, L. E.; Facciabene, A.; Buckanovich, R. J. & Coukos, G. (2009). Endothelin B receptor, a new target in cancer immune therapy. *Clin Cancer Res*, Vol.15, No.14, (Jul 15 2009), pp. 4521-4528

Kang, S. M.; Maeda, K.; Onoda, N.; Chung, Y. S.; Nakata, B.; Nishiguchi, Y. & Sowa, M. (1997). Combined analysis of p53 and vascular endothelial growth factor expression in colorectal carcinoma for determination of tumor vascularity and liver metastasis. *Int J Cancer*, Vol.74, No.5, (Oct 21 1997), pp. 502-507

Katz, S. C.; Pillarisetty, V.; Bamboat, Z. M.; Shia, J.; Hedvat, C.; Gonen, M.; Jarnagin, W.; Fong, Y.; Blumgart, L.; D'Angelica, M. & DeMatteo, R. P. (2009). T cell infiltrate predicts long-term survival following resection of colorectal cancer liver metastases. *Ann Surg Oncol*, Vol.16, No.9, (Sep 2009), pp. 2524-2530

Kedzierski, R. M. & Yanagisawa, M. (2001). Endothelin system: the double-edged sword in health and disease. *Annu Rev Pharmacol Toxicol*, Vol.41, 2001), pp. 851-876

Kilarski, W. W.; Samolov, B.; Petersson, L.; Kvanta, A. & Gerwins, P. (2009). Biomechanical regulation of blood vessel growth during tissue vascularization. *Nat Med*, Vol.15, No.6, (Jun 2009), pp. 657-664

Kopetz, S.; Hoff, P. M.; Morris, J. S.; Wolff, R. A.; Eng, C.; Glover, K. Y.; Adinin, R.; Overman, M. J.; Valero, V.; Wen, S.; Lieu, C.; Yan, S.; Tran, H. T.; Ellis, L. M.; Abbruzzese, J. L. & Heymach, J. V. (2010). Phase II trial of infusional fluorouracil, irinotecan, and bevacizumab for metastatic colorectal cancer: efficacy and circulating angiogenic biomarkers associated with therapeutic resistance. *J Clin Oncol*, Vol.28, No.3, (Jan 20 2010), pp. 453-459

Kumar, H.; Heer, K.; Lee, P. W.; Duthie, G. S.; MacDonald, A. W.; Greenman, J.; Kerin, M. J. & Monson, J. R. (1998). Preoperative serum vascular endothelial growth factor can predict stage in colorectal cancer. *Clin Cancer Res*, Vol.4, No.5, (May 1998), pp. 1279-1285

Kusuhara, M.; Yamaguchi, K.; Nagasaki, K.; Hayashi, C.; Suzaki, A.; Hori, S.; Handa, S.; Nakamura, Y. & Abe, K. (1990). Production of endothelin in human cancer cell lines. *Cancer Res*, Vol.50, No.11, (Jun 1 1990), pp. 3257-3261

Lee, H. K.; Kang, D. S.; Seo, I. A.; Choi, E. J.; Park, H. T. & Park, J. I. (2006). Expression of tumor endothelial marker 7 mRNA and protein in the dorsal root ganglion neurons of the rat. *Neurosci Lett*, Vol.402, No.1-2, (Jul 10 2006), pp. 71-75

Leite de Oliveira, R.; Hamm, A. & Mazzone, M. (2011). Growing tumor vessels: More than one way to skin a cat - Implications for angiogenesis targeted cancer therapies. *Mol Aspects Med*, Vol.32, No.2, (Apr 2011), pp. 71-87

Leo, E.; Belli, F.; Andreola, S.; Gallino, G.; Bonfanti, G.; Ferro, F.; Zingaro, E.; Sirizzotti, G.; Civelli, E.; Valvo, F.; Gios, M. & Brunelli, C. (2000). Total rectal resection and complete mesorectum excision followed by coloendoanal anastomosis as the optimal treatment for low rectal cancer: the experience of the National Cancer Institute of Milano. *Ann Surg Oncol*, Vol.7, No.2, (Mar 2000), pp. 125-132

Levy, E. M.; Roberti, M. P. & Mordoh, J. (2011). Natural killer cells in human cancer: from biological functions to clinical applications. *J Biomed Biotechnol*, Vol.2011, 2011), pp. 676198

Loupakis, F.; Falcone, A.; Masi, G.; Fioravanti, A.; Kerbel, R. S.; Del Tacca, M. & Bocci, G. (2007). Vascular endothelial growth factor levels in immunodepleted plasma of cancer patients as a possible pharmacodynamic marker for bevacizumab activity. *J Clin Oncol*, Vol.25, No.13, (May 1 2007), pp. 1816-1818

Lubeseder-Martellato, C.; Guenzi, E.; Jörg, A.; Töpolt, K.; Naschberger, E.; Kremmer, E.; Zietz, C.; Tschachler, E.; Hutzler, P.; Schwemmle, M.; Matzen, K.; Grimm, T.; Ensoli, B. & Stürzl, M. (2002). Guanylate-Binding Protein-1 Expression Is Selectively Induced by Inflammatory Cytokines and Is an Activation Marker of Endothelial Cells during Inflammatory Diseases. *Am J Pathol*, Vol.161, No.5, (Nov 2002), pp. 1749-1759

Maltby, S.; Khazaie, K. & McNagny, K. M. (2009). Mast cells in tumor growth: angiogenesis, tissue remodelling and immune-modulation. *Biochim Biophys Acta*, Vol.1796, No.1, (Aug 2009), pp. 19-26

Mandruzzato, S.; Solito, S.; Falisi, E.; Francescato, S.; Chiarion-Sileni, V.; Mocellin, S.; Zanon, A.; Rossi, C. R.; Nitti, D.; Bronte, V. & Zanovello, P. (2009). IL4Ralpha+ myeloid-derived suppressor cell expansion in cancer patients. *J Immunol*, Vol.182, No.10, (May 15 2009), pp. 6562-6568

Mantovani, A. & Sica, A. (2010). Macrophages, innate immunity and cancer: balance, tolerance, and diversity. *Curr Opin Immunol*, Vol.22, No.2, (Apr 2010), pp. 231-237

Motzer, R. J.; Hutson, T. E.; Tomczak, P.; Michaelson, M. D.; Bukowski, R. M.; Rixe, O.; Oudard, S.; Negrier, S.; Szczylik, C.; Kim, S. T.; Chen, I.; Bycott, P. W.; Baum, C. M. & Figlin, R. A. (2007). Sunitinib versus interferon alfa in metastatic renal-cell carcinoma. *N Engl J Med*, Vol.356, No.2, (Jan 11 2007), pp. 115-124

Naito, Y.; Saito, K.; Shiiba, K.; Ohuchi, A.; Saigenji, K.; Nagura, H. & Ohtani, H. (1998). CD8+ T cells infiltrated within cancer cell nests as a prognostic factor in human colorectal cancer. *Cancer Res*, Vol.58, No.16, (Aug 15 1998), pp. 3491-3494

Nanda, A.; Buckhaults, P.; Seaman, S.; Agrawal, N.; Boutin, P.; Shankara, S.; Nacht, M.; Teicher, B.; Stampfl, J.; Singh, S.; Vogelstein, B.; Kinzler, K. W. & St Croix, B. (2004). Identification of a binding partner for the endothelial cell surface proteins TEM7 and TEM7R. *Cancer Res*, Vol.64, No.23, (Dec 1 2004), pp. 8507-8511

Naschberger, E.; Croner, R. S.; Merkel, S.; Dimmler, A.; Tripal, P.; Amann, K. U.; Kremmer, E.; Brueckl, W. M.; Papadopoulos, T.; Hohenadl, C.; Hohenberger, W. & Stürzl, M. (2008). Angiostatic immune reaction in colorectal carcinoma: Impact on survival and perspectives for antiangiogenic therapy. *Int J Cancer*, Vol.123, No.9, (Nov 1 2008), pp. 2120-2129

Nielsen, H. J.; Hansen, U.; Christensen, I. J.; Reimert, C. M.; Brunner, N. & Moesgaard, F. (1999). Independent prognostic value of eosinophil and mast cell infiltration in colorectal cancer tissue. *J Pathol*, Vol.189, No.4, (Dec 1999), pp. 487-495

O'Brien, C. A.; Pollett, A.; Gallinger, S. & Dick, J. E. (2007). A human colon cancer cell capable of initiating tumour growth in immunodeficient mice. *Nature*, Vol.445, No.7123, (Jan 4 2007), pp. 106-110

Palazon, A.; Teijeira, A.; Martinez-Forero, I.; Hervas-Stubbs, S.; Roncal, C.; Penuelas, I.; Dubrot, J.; Morales-Kastresana, A.; Perez-Gracia, J. L.; Ochoa, M. C.; Ochoa-Callejero, L.; Martinez, A.; Luque, A.; Dinchuk, J.; Rouzaut, A.; Jure-Kunkel, M. & Melero, I. (2011). Agonist anti-CD137 mAb act on tumor endothelial cells to enhance recruitment of activated T lymphocytes. *Cancer Res*, Vol.71, No.3, (Feb 1 2011), pp. 801-811

Peddareddigari, V. G.; Wang, D. & Dubois, R. N. (2010). The tumor microenvironment in colorectal carcinogenesis. *Cancer Microenviron*, Vol.3, No.1, 2010), pp. 149-166

Perez-Gracia, J. L.; Prior, C.; Guillen-Grima, F.; Segura, V.; Gonzalez, A.; Panizo, A.; Melero, I.; Grande-Pulido, E.; Gurpide, A.; Gil-Bazo, I. & Calvo, A. (2009). Identification of TNF-alpha and MMP-9 as potential baseline predictive serum markers of sunitinib activity in patients with renal cell carcinoma using a human cytokine array. *Br J Cancer*, Vol.101, No.11, (Dec 1 2009), pp. 1876-1883

Ricci-Vitiani, L.; Lombardi, D. G.; Pilozzi, E.; Biffoni, M.; Todaro, M.; Peschle, C. & De Maria, R. (2007). Identification and expansion of human colon-cancer-initiating cells. *Nature*, Vol.445, No.7123, (Jan 4 2007), pp. 111-115

Ricci-Vitiani, L.; Pallini, R.; Biffoni, M.; Todaro, M.; Invernici, G.; Cenci, T.; Maira, G.; Parati, E. A.; Stassi, G.; Larocca, L. M. & De Maria, R. (2010). Tumour vascularization via endothelial differentiation of glioblastoma stem-like cells. *Nature*, Vol.468, No.7325, (Dec 9 2010), pp. 824-828

Risau, W. (1997). Mechanisms of angiogenesis. *Nature*, Vol.386, No.6626, (Apr 17 1997), pp. 671-674

Roessner, A.; Kuester, D.; Malfertheiner, P. & Schneider-Stock, R. (2008). Oxidative stress in ulcerative colitis-associated carcinogenesis. *Pathol Res Pract*, Vol.204, No.7, 2008), pp. 511-524

Romagnani, P.; Lasagni, L.; Annunziato, F.; Serio, M. & Romagnani, S. (2004). CXC chemokines: the regulatory link between inflammation and angiogenesis. *Trends Immunol*, Vol.25, No.4, (Apr 2004), pp. 201-209

Roncucci, L.; Fante, R.; Losi, L.; Di Gregorio, C.; Micheli, A.; Benatti, P.; Madenis, N.; Ganazzi, D.; Cassinadri, M. T.; Lauriola, P. & Ponz de Leon, M. (1996). Survival for colon and rectal cancer in a population-based cancer registry. *Eur J Cancer*, Vol.32A, No.2, (Feb 1996), pp. 295-302

Roncucci, L.; Mora, E.; Mariani, F.; Bursi, S.; Pezzi, A.; Rossi, G.; Pedroni, M.; Luppi, D.; Santoro, L.; Monni, S.; Manenti, A.; Bertani, A.; Merighi, A.; Benatti, P.; Di Gregorio, C. & de Leon, P. M. (2008). Myeloperoxidase-positive cell infiltration in colorectal carcinogenesis as indicator of colorectal cancer risk. *Cancer Epidemiol Biomarkers Prev*, Vol.17, No.9, (Sep 2008), pp. 2291-2297

Ronzoni, M.; Manzoni, M.; Mariucci, S.; Loupakis, F.; Brugnatelli, S.; Bencardino, K.; Rovati, B.; Tinelli, C.; Falcone, A.; Villa, E. & Danova, M. (2010). Circulating endothelial cells and endothelial progenitors as predictive markers of clinical response to bevacizumab-based first-line treatment in advanced colorectal cancer patients. *Ann Oncol*, Vol.21, No.12, (Dec 2010), pp. 2382-2389

Ropponen, K. M.; Eskelinen, M. J.; Lipponen, P. K.; Alhava, E. & Kosma, V. M. (1997). Prognostic value of tumour-infiltrating lymphocytes (TILs) in colorectal cancer. *J Pathol*, Vol.182, No.3, (Jul 1997), pp. 318-324

Salama, P. & Platell, C. (2008). Host response to colorectal cancer. *ANZ J Surg*, Vol.78, No.9, (Sep 2008), pp. 745-753

Salih, H. R.; Kosowski, S. G.; Haluska, V. F.; Starling, G. C.; Loo, D. T.; Lee, F.; Aruffo, A. A.; Trail, P. A. & Kiener, P. A. (2000). Constitutive expression of functional 4-1BB (CD137) ligand on carcinoma cells. *J Immunol*, Vol.165, No.5, (Sep 1 2000), pp. 2903-2910

Sandel, M. H.; Dadabayev, A. R.; Menon, A. G.; Morreau, H.; Melief, C. J.; Offringa, R.; van der Burg, S. H.; Janssen-van Rhijn, C. M.; Ensink, N. G.; Tollenaar, R. A.; van de Velde, C. J. & Kuppen, P. J. (2005). Prognostic value of tumor-infiltrating dendritic cells in colorectal cancer: role of maturation status and intratumoral localization. *Clin Cancer Res*, Vol.11, No.7, (Apr 1 2005), pp. 2576-2582

Schellerer, V. S.; Croner, R. S.; Weinländer, K.; Hohenberger, W.; Stürzl, M. & Naschberger, E. (2007). Endothelial cells of human colorectal cancer and healthy colon reveal phenotypic differences in culture. *Lab Invest*, Vol.87, No.11, (Nov 2007), pp. 1159-1170

Schneider, B. P.; Wang, M.; Radovich, M.; Sledge, G. W.; Badve, S.; Thor, A.; Flockhart, D. A.; Hancock, B.; Davidson, N.; Gralow, J.; Dickler, M.; Perez, E. A.; Cobleigh, M.; Shenkier, T.; Edgerton, S. & Miller, K. D. (2008). Association of vascular endothelial growth factor and vascular endothelial growth factor receptor-2 genetic polymorphisms with outcome in a trial of paclitaxel compared with paclitaxel plus bevacizumab in advanced breast cancer: ECOG 2100. *J Clin Oncol*, Vol.26, No.28, (Oct 1 2008), pp. 4672-4678

Shao, Z. & Schwarz, H. (2011). CD137 ligand, a member of the tumor necrosis factor family, regulates immune responses via reverse signal transduction. *J Leukoc Biol*, Vol.89, No.1, (Jan 2011), pp. 21-29

Shmelkov, S. V.; Butler, J. M.; Hooper, A. T.; Hormigo, A.; Kushner, J.; Milde, T.; St Clair, R.; Baljevic, M.; White, I.; Jin, D. K.; Chadburn, A.; Murphy, A. J.; Valenzuela, D. M.; Gale, N. W.; Thurston, G.; Yancopoulos, G. D.; D'Angelica, M.; Kemeny, N.; Lyden, D. & Rafii, S. (2008). CD133 expression is not restricted to stem cells, and both CD133+ and CD133- metastatic colon cancer cells initiate tumors. *J Clin Invest*, Vol.118, No.6, (Jun 2008), pp. 2111-2120

Sica, A.; Allavena, P. & Mantovani, A. (2008a). Cancer related inflammation: the macrophage connection. *Cancer Lett*, Vol.267, No.2, (Aug 28 2008a), pp. 204-215

Sica, A.; Larghi, P.; Mancino, A.; Rubino, L.; Porta, C.; Totaro, M. G.; Rimoldi, M.; Biswas, S. K.; Allavena, P. & Mantovani, A. (2008b). Macrophage polarization in tumour progression. *Semin Cancer Biol*, Vol.18, No.5, (Oct 2008b), pp. 349-355

Smith, R. A.; Cokkinides, V.; von Eschenbach, A. C.; Levin, B.; Cohen, C.; Runowicz, C. D.; Sener, S.; Saslow, D. & Eyre, H. J. (2002). American Cancer Society guidelines for the early detection of cancer. *CA Cancer J Clin*, Vol.52, No.1, (Jan-Feb 2002), pp. 8-22

Sobrero, A.; Ackland, S.; Clarke, S.; Perez-Carrion, R.; Chiara, S.; Gapski, J.; Mainwaring, P.; Langer, B. & Young, S. (2009). Phase IV study of bevacizumab in combination with infusional fluorouracil, leucovorin and irinotecan (FOLFIRI) in first-line metastatic colorectal cancer. *Oncology*, Vol.77, No.2, 2009), pp. 113-119

St Croix, B.; Rago, C.; Velculescu, V.; Traverso, G.; Romans, K. E.; Montgomery, E.; Lal, A.; Riggins, G. J.; Lengauer, C.; Vogelstein, B. & Kinzler, K. W. (2000). Genes expressed in human tumor endothelium. *Science*, Vol.289, No.5482, (Aug 18 2000), pp. 1197-1202

Streubel, B.; Chott, A.; Huber, D.; Exner, M.; Jager, U.; Wagner, O. & Schwarzinger, I. (2004). Lymphoma-specific genetic aberrations in microvascular endothelial cells in B-cell lymphomas. *N Engl J Med*, Vol.351, No.3, (Jul 15 2004), pp. 250-259

Suzuki, A.; Masuda, A.; Nagata, H.; Kameoka, S.; Kikawada, Y.; Yamakawa, M. & Kasajima, T. (2002). Mature dendritic cells make clusters with T cells in the invasive margin of colorectal carcinoma. *J Pathol*, Vol.196, No.1, (Jan 2002), pp. 37-43

Tachibana, T.; Onodera, H.; Tsuruyama, T.; Mori, A.; Nagayama, S.; Hiai, H. & Imamura, M. (2005). Increased intratumor Valpha24-positive natural killer T cells: a prognostic factor for primary colorectal carcinomas. *Clin Cancer Res*, Vol.11, No.20, (Oct 15 2005), pp. 7322-7327

Takebayashi, Y.; Aklyama, S.; Yamada, K.; Akiba, S. & Aikou, T. (1996). Angiogenesis as an unfavorable prognostic factor in human colorectal carcinoma. *Cancer*, Vol.78, No.2, (Jul 15 1996), pp. 226-231

Tartour, E.; Pere, H.; Maillere, B.; Terme, M.; Merillon, N.; Taieb, J.; Sandoval, F.; Quintin-Colonna, F.; Lacerda, K.; Karadimou, A.; Badoual, C.; Tedgui, A.; Fridman, W. H. & Oudard, S. (2011). Angiogenesis and immunity: a bidirectional link potentially relevant for the monitoring of antiangiogenic therapy and the development of novel therapeutic combination with immunotherapy. *Cancer Metastasis Rev*, Vol.30, No.1, (Mar 2011), pp. 83-95

Tazzyman, S.; Lewis, C. E. & Murdoch, C. (2009). Neutrophils: key mediators of tumour angiogenesis. *Int J Exp Pathol*, Vol.90, No.3, (Jun 2009), pp. 222-231

Terabe, M. & Berzofsky, J. A. (2008). The role of NKT cells in tumor immunity. *Adv Cancer Res*, Vol.101, 2008), pp. 277-348

Tosolini, M.; Kirilovsky, A.; Mlecnik, B.; Fredriksen, T.; Mauger, S.; Bindea, G.; Berger, A.; Bruneval, P.; Fridman, W. H.; Pages, F. & Galon, J. (2011). Clinical impact of different classes of infiltrating T cytotoxic and helper cells (Th1, th2, treg, th17) in patients with colorectal cancer. *Cancer Res*, Vol.71, No.4, (Feb 15 2011), pp. 1263-1271

van der Vliet, H. J.; Wang, R.; Yue, S. C.; Koon, H. B.; Balk, S. P. & Exley, M. A. (2008). Circulating myeloid dendritic cells of advanced cancer patients result in reduced activation and a biased cytokine profile in invariant NKT cells. *J Immunol*, Vol.180, No.11, (Jun 1 2008), pp. 7287-7293

Venneri, M. A.; De Palma, M.; Ponzoni, M.; Pucci, F.; Scielzo, C.; Zonari, E.; Mazzieri, R.; Doglioni, C. & Naldini, L. (2007). Identification of proangiogenic TIE2-expressing monocytes (TEMs) in human peripheral blood and cancer. *Blood*, Vol.109, No.12, (Jun 15 2007), pp. 5276-5285

Vogelstein, B.; Fearon, E. R.; Hamilton, S. R.; Kern, S. E.; Preisinger, A. C.; Leppert, M.; Nakamura, Y.; White, R.; Smits, A. M. & Bos, J. L. (1988). Genetic alterations during colorectal-tumor development. *N Engl J Med*, Vol.319, No.9, (Sep 1 1988), pp. 525-532

Wang, Q.; Zhang, P.; Zhang, Q.; Wang, X.; Li, J.; Ma, C.; Sun, W. & Zhang, L. (2008). Analysis of CD137 and CD137L expression in human primary tumor tissues. *Croat Med J*, Vol.49, No.2, (Apr 2008), pp. 192-200

Wang, R.; Chadalavada, K.; Wilshire, J.; Kowalik, U.; Hovinga, K. E.; Geber, A.; Fligelman, B.; Leversha, M.; Brennan, C. & Tabar, V. (2010). Glioblastoma stem-like cells give rise to tumour endothelium. *Nature*, Vol.468, No.7325, (Dec 9 2010), pp. 829-833

Willett, C. G.; Duda, D. G.; di Tomaso, E.; Boucher, Y.; Ancukiewicz, M.; Sahani, D. V.; Lahdenranta, J.; Chung, D. C.; Fischman, A. J.; Lauwers, G. Y.; Shellito, P.; Czito, B. G.; Wong, T. Z.; Paulson, E.; Poleski, M.; Vujaskovic, Z.; Bentley, R.; Chen, H. X.; Clark, J. W. & Jain, R. K. (2009). Efficacy, safety, and biomarkers of neoadjuvant bevacizumab, radiation therapy, and fluorouracil in rectal cancer: a multidisciplinary phase II study. *J Clin Oncol*, Vol.27, No.18, (Jun 20 2009), pp. 3020-3026

Xiong, Y. Q.; Sun, H. C.; Zhang, W.; Zhu, X. D.; Zhuang, P. Y.; Zhang, J. B.; Wang, L.; Wu, W. Z.; Qin, L. X. & Tang, Z. Y. (2009). Human hepatocellular carcinoma tumor-derived endothelial cells manifest increased angiogenesis capability and drug resistance compared with normal endothelial cells. *Clin Cancer Res*, Vol.15, No.15, (Aug 1 2009), pp. 4838-4846

Yang, L.; DeBusk, L. M.; Fukuda, K.; Fingleton, B.; Green-Jarvis, B.; Shyr, Y.; Matrisian, L. M.; Carbone, D. P. & Lin, P. C. (2004). Expansion of myeloid immune suppressor Gr+CD11b+ cells in tumor-bearing host directly promotes tumor angiogenesis. *Cancer Cell*, Vol.6, No.4, (Oct 2004), pp. 409-421

Yang, S. X.; Steinberg, S. M.; Nguyen, D.; Wu, T. D.; Modrusan, Z. & Swain, S. M. (2008). Gene expression profile and angiogenic marker correlates with response to neoadjuvant bevacizumab followed by bevacizumab plus chemotherapy in breast cancer. *Clin Cancer Res*, Vol.14, No.18, (Sep 15 2008), pp. 5893-5899

Youn, J. I. & Gabrilovich, D. I. (2010). The biology of myeloid-derived suppressor cells: the blessing and the curse of morphological and functional heterogeneity. *Eur J Immunol*, Vol.40, No.11, (Nov 2010), pp. 2969-2975

Zhang, S.; Zhang, H. & Zhao, J. (2009). The role of CD4 T cell help for CD8 CTL activation. *Biochem Biophys Res Commun*, Vol.384, No.4, (Jul 10 2009), pp. 405-408

Zhou, L.; Chong, M. M. & Littman, D. R. (2009). Plasticity of CD4+ T cell lineage differentiation. *Immunity*, Vol.30, No.5, (May 2009), pp. 646-655

Zhu, J. & Paul, W. E. (2010). Heterogeneity and plasticity of T helper cells. *Cell Res*, Vol.20, No.1, (Jan 2010), pp. 4-12

6

The Role of Infectious Agents
in Colorectal Carcinogenesis

Hytham K. S. Hamid[1] and Yassin M. Mustafa[2]
[1]Department of Surgery, Waterford Regional Hospital, Waterford,
[2] Department of Internal Medicine,
Howard University Hospital, Washington D. C.,
[1]Ireland
[2]USA

1. Introduction

Infectious agents have been increasingly recognized as bona fide etiologic factors of human malignancies, particularly gastrointestinal cancers. The estimated total of infection-attributed malignancies per year is 1.9 million cases, accounting for 17.8% of the global cancer burden (Parkin, 2006). Given that colorectal cancer (CRC) is the third most common incident cancer worldwide (World health organization, 2003), it seems prudent to explore the role of microbial pathogens in colorectal carcinogenesis. By elucidating the probable mechanisms by which infectious agents contribute to colorectal oncogenesis, the management of CRC may one day parallel what is already in place for cancers such as gastric lymphoma and cervical cancer. Antimicrobial therapy and vaccination against some of these infections may herald a future with a curtailed role for traditional therapies of surgery and chemo-radiotherapy.

Unlike gastric cancer, which is chiefly linked to a single infectious agent, multiple organisms may contribute to the genesis of CRC. Epidemiological and experimental evidence strongly implicate several bacterial and parasitic agents in promotion of colorectal carcinogenesis. Most of these agents incite continual inflammation, which generates a procarcinogenic microenvironment (Parsonnet, 1995; Vennervald & Polman, 2009). Viruses have not attained the same status as other microorganisms as probable causative agents, though merit attention because of their inherent oncogenic properties and the increasing strength of their association with other malignancies (McLaughlin-Drubin & Munger, 2008). Yet, putative viral agents seemingly display an immense geographic variation that has led to much debate regarding the relative importance of one organism versus another. The present review summarizes the data available on the possible relationship of certain micro-organisms and CRC. These include but not limited to *Helicobacter pylori, Streptococcus bovis, Bacteroides fragilis*, JC virus (JCV), and human papillomavirus (HPV), and intestinal schistosomes. The consistency and nature of these associations are discussed, as are the mechanisms whereby each pathogen participates in the malignant transformation of the colonic mucosa.

2. Bacteria

2.1 *Helicobacter pylori*

H. pylori is a gastric microbiome that colonizes approximately 50% of the population worldwide (EUROGAST study group, 1993). Gastric infection with *H. pylori* fosters chronic inflammation and significantly increases the risk of developing peptic ulcer disease and gastric cancer. Indeed, the bacterium has been designated by the International Agency for Research in Cancer (IARC, 1994), as a class I carcinogen in human causing gastric cancer. Recently, promotion of tumour development by *H. pylori* infection in extragastric target organs, such as the colorectum, has been reported, though causal relationship is presently controversial.

Cancer in human

Numerous comparative and case-control studies have examined the relationship between *H. pylori* IgG seropositivity and colorectal neoplasia risk, but the results have been inconsistent. While some studies demonstrated positive correlations between colorectal neoplastic lesions, especially adenomas, and *H. pylori* seroprevalence (Aydin et al., 1999; Hartwich et al., 2001b; Meucci et al., 1997; Mizuno et al., 2005; Zumkeller et al., 2007), others showed null or inverse associations (Moss et al., 1995; Penman et al., 1994; Fireman et al., 2000; Shmuely et al., 2001; Siddheshwar et al., 2001; Machida-Montani et al., 2007; D'Onghia et al., 2007). Most of these studies were, however, confounded by uncontrolled extraneous variables. Breuer-Katschinski et al. (1999) compared *H. pylori* serostatus between 98 colorectal adenoma patients and age/sex-matched hospitalized and populations-based control groups. The results clearly demonstrated an increase in the risk of colorectal adenoma in association with *H. pylori* infection following adjustment for dietary and lifestyle factors. Importantly, two case-control studies nested in large population-based cohorts failed to establish any association between *H. pylori* seroprevalence and incident CRC, irrespective of adjustment for potential confounders (Thorburn et al., 1998; Limburg et al., 2002). In each study, the presence of *H. pylori* was determined in subjects who developed CRC years after serum donation. The inconclusive findings in these studies have been partially attributed to small sample size, lack of control heterogeneity, and incomplete colonoscopic evaluation (Takeda & Asaka, 2005). Besides, serologic methods may not always reflect real-time *H. pylori* infection and likely yield positive results for infections caused by *Helicobacter* species other than *H. pylori*, which commonly colonize the human colonic mucosa (Keenan et al., 2010).

Other studies have utilized more reliable diagnostic tools for detection of *H. pylori* infection. Lin et al. (2010) conducted a cross-sectional study using biopsy urease test, and demonstrated a significantly increased risk of colorectal adenoma among *H. pylori* infected-patients, particularly those with concomitant metabolic syndrome. Conversely, two case control studies, using 13C-Urea breath test (UBT), did not substantiate any significant associations of *H. pylori* infection with colorectal tumours (Penman et al., 1994; Liou et al., 2006). Fujimori et al. (2005) evaluated 699 patients for *H. pylori* infection using combination of three tests; UBT, rapid urease test, and gastric biopsy histology. Their analysis revealed a significantly higher prevalence of colorectal adenoma and adenocarcinoma among *H. pylori*-positive female patients compared to their *H. pylori*-free counterparts.

Of note, in a metanalysis of 11 case-control studies, the summary odd ratio for the association of *H. pylori* infection with the risk for colorectal carcinoma or adenoma was found to be 1.4 (95% CI, 1.1–1.8). Different testing methods were, nevertheless, combined to assess the *H. pylori* infection status in these studies (Zumkeller et al., 2006). More recently, a meta-analysis comprising 13 studies and 1709 patients with colorectal neoplasms, arrived at summary odd ration of 1.49 (95% CI 1.17–1.91). Further analysis of studies using serologic response as the sole indicator of infection revealed a higher summary odd ratio of 1.56 (95% CI, 1.14–2.14) (Y. S. Zhao et al., 2008).

Recently, Soylu et al. (2008) have investigated the presence of *H. pylori* in colorectal neoplasms using immunohistochemical methods, which allowed more accurate detection of the non-spiral forms of the bacterium. The prevalence of *H. pylori* was higher in villous type polyps than in tubular type polyps and adenocarcinomas. Contrary to this finding, Jones et al. (2007) demonstrated that villous adenoma had the lowest rate of *H. pylori* positivity compared to other premalignant and malignant colonic lesions. Their results also showed significant associations of *H. pylori* positivity with tubular and tubulovillous adenomas, and adenocarcinomas, but not with villous adenomas.

Likewise, studies employing PCR analysis for detection of *H. pylori* genomic material in the cancerous tissue have yielded conflicting results. A Swedish group detected *H. pylori* DNA in 27% of CRC specimens (Bulajic et al., 2007). In contrast, Grahn et al. (2005) identified *H. pylori* DNA in 1.2% of the malignant tissues and, unexpectedly, in 6% of normal mucosal samples among patients with CRC. Additionally, there was no statistical correlation between *H. pylori* PCR positivity and CRC. This finding was further confirmed in a later study on a separate population (Keenan et al., 2010).

Cancer in experimental animals

Studies have shown that amidated gastrins have no stimulatory effect on colon mucosal growth or progression of colon cancer in different experimental models (Hakanson et al., 1986, 1988). Others demonstrated that non-amidated gastrins, including progastrin and Gly-gastrin, have a mitogenic effect on the colonic mucosa in transgenic mice (T.C. Wang., 1996; Koh et al., 1999). Singh et al. (2000a, 2000b) reported that transgenic mice with elevated plasma progastrin, but not amidated gastrins, exhibit increased aberrant crypt foci, adenomas, and adenocarcinomas after treatment with azoxymethane, whilst no tumours developed in mice exposed to either progastrin or azoxymethane only. These results suggest that non-amidated gastrin is not a carcinogen on its own, but rather promotes oncogenic progression.

Mechanisms/Mechanistic studies

Various pathogenetic mechanisms have been suggested by which *H. pylori* exerts its oncogenic potential. First, persistent *H. pylori* exposure induces hypergastrinemia, which is a putative trophic factor for the human colorectal mucosa, thereby increasing the mutation susceptibility (Renga et al., 1997). Moreover, studies showed that most human colon cancers secrete gastrin, primarily non-amidated gastrins, which likely function in autocrine fashion (Baldwin et al., 1998). Non-amidated gastrin induces proliferation and invasiveness of human tumour cells *in vitro* (Kermorgant & Lehy, 2001). In conjunction with these findings, the overexpression of cyclooxygenase-2 (COX-2) was shown to stimulate the cancer cells to release excessive amount of prostaglandin E_2 (PGE$_2$), leading to further proliferation (Hartwich et al., 2001b).

Although some reports, including a well-controlled prospective study, provided statistical evidence that high fasting plasma gastrin level is associated with increased risk of colorectal adenoma and carcinoma (Hartwich et al., 2001b; Thorburn et al., 1998; Georgopoulos et al.,

2006), others showed no associations (Penman et al., 1994; Fireman et al., 2000; Machida-Montani et al., 2007; Robertson et al., 2009). In a majority of these studies only amidated gastrin was measured, which may have contributed to the discrepancy in results (Dickinson, 1995). In a recent study, circulating forms of both amidated and non-amidated gastrins were measured. Non-amidated gastrins were significantly higher in patients with colorectal carcinomas, compared with levels in control patients (Ciccotosto et al., 1995).

Second, *H. pylori*-related chronic gastritis might contribute to colorectal carcinogenesis by reducing gastric acid secretion with consequent alteration in the normal gastrointestinal flora (Kanno et al., 2009). Another possibility is that CagA protein (Fig 1.), which is produced by virulent strain of *H. pylori*, may contribute to colorectal carcinogenesis by inducing an enhanced inflammatory response and potentiating gastrin secretion (Peek et al., 1995; J.H. Kim et al., 1999). As for the correlation between colorectal neoplasia and CagA+ *H. pylori* serostatus, three studies indicated positive correlations between CagA+ *H. pylori* seropositivity and colorectal tumours (Hartwich et al., 2001b; Shmuely et al., 2001; Georgopoulos et al., 2006), while two other studies found no such correlation (Zumkeller et al., 2007; Limburg et al., 2002).

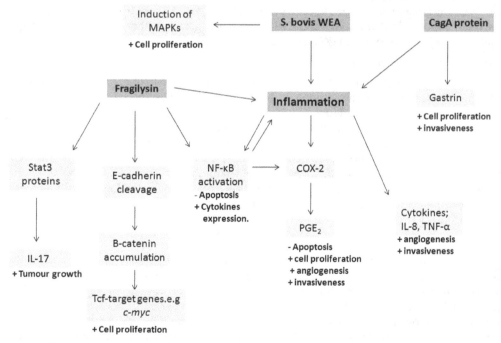

Fig. 1. Illustration of the possible mechanisms of bacterial-toxin-induced carcinogenesis.

2.2 Streptococcus bovis

S. bovis, a nonenterococcal lancefield group D *streptococcus*, is a transient colonic commensal with fecal carriage rate of 5 - 13 % in healthy adults (Potter et al., 1998; Dubrow et al., 1991), and accounts for 11-12% of infective endocarditis (Ballet et al., 1995; Kupferwasser et al., 1998). Traditionally, *S. bovis* has been classified into three distinct biotypes; I, II/1, and II/2, based on phenotypical and genetic characteristics (Coykendall & Gustafson, 1985). Further studies using phylogenetic analysis allowed clear and unambiguous differentiation of human clinical isolates and indicated that all strains of *S. bovis* I and II/2 be identified as *S. gallolyticus* (Schlegel et al., 2003). The latter accounts for most of the human strains isolated from blood or faeces, and is often responsible for endocarditis cases associated with colonic cancer (Schlegel et al., 2003).

Cancer in humans

The association between *S. bovis* endocarditis and colorectal carcinoma was first brought to light by Keusck (1974). Subsequent case studies showed a wide range of prevalence of colorectal neoplasms in patients with *S. bovis* bacteraemia (6 - 67%), depending on the diligence with which the diagnosis was sought (Pigrau et al., 1988; Klein et al, 1979; H.W. Murray & Roberts, 1978; Friedrich et al., 1982a; Reynolds et al., 1983; Zarkin et al., 1990; Gold et al, 2004; Alazmi et al, 2006; Beeching et al., 1985). Additionally, some patients developed new colonic tumours 2 to 4 years following the incidence of *S. bovis* endocarditis, pointing to a possible temporal relationship between the two events (Zarkin et al., 1990; Robbins & Klein, 1983; Muhlemann et al., 1999; Friedrich et al., 1982b). Other studies reported that patients with *S. bovis* endocarditis had significantly higher rates of colorectal neoplasms than those with endocarditis due to other pathogens or non-endocarditis patients (Pergola et al., 2001; Hoen et al., 1994). More particularly, Ruoff et al. (1989) showed that *S. bovis* I bacteraemia was highly correlated with malignant and premalignant colonic lesions, compared to bacteraemia due to other *S. bovis* biotypes. This conclusion was affirmed by several recent analyses, in which the incidence of colonic tumours in patients with *S. bovis* I infection ranged between 27 - 94% (Herrero et al., 2002; Tripodi et al., 2004; Corredoira et al., 2008; Vaska & Faoagali, 2009; Ruoff et al, 1999).

Several investigators have studied the association between the fecal carriage rate of *S. bovis* and both malignant and premalignant colorectal lesions, with the results being contradictory (Klein et al., 1977; Potter et al., 1998; Norfleet & Mitchell, 1993; Burns et al., 1985). Comparing the growth of *S. bovis* from tissue biopsy of adenomas or carcinomas did not show increased frequency compared to normal mucosa from the same patients or non-cancer-patients group (Potter et al., 1998; Norfleet & Mitchell, 1993). In contrast, Abdulamir et al. (2010), using bacteriological studies and molecular techniques to detect *S. gallolyticus* in tissue or faeces, revealed a significantly higher frequency of *S. gallolyticus* isolation from tumorous and non-tumorous tissue in CRC patients than from normal mucosa in control subjects. In parallel, the faecal carriage rate of *S. gallolyticus* was similar in cancer and control groups.

In another aspect, Darjee and Gibb (1993) used immunoblotting and enzyme-linked immunosorbent assay (ELISA) to compare anti-*S. bovis* IgG levels in sera of 16 colonic cancer patients and 16 age-matched controls. Immunoblot assay showed no significant difference in the serologic parameters between patients and controls, whilst ELISA demonstrated higher median *S. bovis* IgG antibody titres in patients with colonic cancer, compared to controls. Using immunocapture mass spectrometry, Tjalsma et al. (2006) showed a higher frequency of anti-*S. bovis* seropositivity in patients with colonic polyps and cancer than age-matched controls. Importantly, recent studies reported that CRC and adenoma were associated with higher levels of serum anti-*S. gallolyticus* IgG antibody in comparison with healthy and tumour-free control subjects (Abdulamir et al., 2009).

It is clear that a strong association does exist between symptomatic *S. bovis* infection and colorectal neoplasia, which has important clinical implications. Patients who have *S. bovis* bacteraemia, with or without endocarditis, require extensive endoscopic evaluation for occult premalignant and malignant colonic cancer (Konda & Duffy, 2008). Further, recent evidence indicates that serum antibodies to *S. bovis* represent a promising potential for early diagnosis and prevention of CRC (Tjalsma et al., 2006).

Cancer in experimental animals

Studies have shown that administration of *S. bovis* or *S. bovis* wall extracted antigens (WEA) to azoxymethane- treated rats resulted in almost two-fold increase in the number of aberrant colonic crypts, compared to azoxymethane-only treated control rats. Fifty percent of the rats receiving WEA developed colonic adenomas, whereas no tumour was detected in the other groups. It is noteworthy to mention that normal rats did not develop hyperplastic colonic crypts upon treatment with *S. bovis* suspension, implying that *S. bovis* proteins are involved in promoting rather than initiating oncogenesis (Ellmerich et al., 2000b). Similar results were obtained by Biarc et al., (2004) who also reported that a purified form of S. bovis WEA (S300 fraction) is even more potent inducer of neoplastic progression than WEA or the intact bacteria.

Mechanisms/Mechanistic studies

Although Klein et al. (1977) originally theorized that *S. bovis* may play a role in producing carcinogens in the large bowel, recent data showed that *S. bovis* wall proteins (Fig. 1.) have proinflammatory potential and procarcinogenic properties (Nguyen et al., 2006). *In vitro* studies indicated that activation of human colonic epithelial cell line Caco-2 by *S. bovis* cell wall proteins, especially S300 fraction, resulted in significant increase in IL-8 production, COX-2 expression, and PGE_2 release (Biarc et al., 2004), whereas binding of *S. bovis* activated human leucocytes cell line to release TNF-α (Ellmerich et al., 2000a). These results are in agreement with those obtained in *in vivo* experiments showing that *S. bovis* as well as cell wall antigens from this bacterium are able to increase the production of IL-8 and PGE_2 in the colonic mucosa of rats (Ellmerich et al., 2000b; Biarc et al., 2004). More recently, human studies have provided evidence for a strong association between *S. gallolyticus* IgG seropositivity and nuclear factor kappa B (NF-κB) and IL-8 expression in tumorous sections of both colorectal adenomas and carcinomas (Abdulamir et al., 2009). Using quantitative PCR analysis to measure bacterial count in cancerous tissue, the same group observed a positive correlation between the levels of expression of IL-1, COX-2, and IL-8 and the *S. gallolyticus* load in tumorous colorectal tissue (Abdulamir et al., 2010). Apart from its inflammatory potential, *S. bovis* cell wall proteins may activate mitogen-activated protein kinases (MAPKs), stimulating a proliferative response in the host cells and increasing the likelihood of cell transformation (Biarc et al., 2004).

Notably, the chemokine 1L-8 is potent angiogenic factor and neutrophil chemoattractant (Li et al., 2001), which as well as other cytokine such as TNF-α, IL-1β, and IL-6, trigger a chronic inflammation with resultant production of highly mutagenic reactive oxygen and nitrogen species (Ohshima & Bartsch., 1994). COX-2, through production of excessive amounts of prostaglandins, inhibits apoptosis, and promotes tumour cell proliferation, angiogenesis, and tumour invasiveness (Hartwich et al., 2001a). In addition, activation of NF-κB pathway induces the expression of downstream mediators such as COX-2, TNF-α, and IL-6, all contributing to inflammation-related tumorigenesis (S. Wang et al., 2009).

2.3 *Bacteroides fragilis*

B. fragilis is a gram-positive, anaerobic colonic microflora in most mammals, and is the leading cause of anaerobic bacteraemia and intraabdominal suppurative infection in human adults (Wexler et al., 2007). The pathogenicity of this bacterium is attributed to several virulence determinants, including a recently identified metalloprotease toxin, called fragilysin. Fragilysin-producing *B. fragilis*, termed enterotoxigenic *B. fragilis* (ETBF), causes acute inflammatory diarrheal disease and asymptomatically colonizes up to 20 -35 % of adults (Sears et al., 2008). As well, it has been recently linked to flare-ups of inflammatory bowel disease (Basset et al., 2004; Prindiville et al., 2000).

Cancer in human

The epidemiological evidence on the association *B. fragilis* infection and colorectal neoplasia is limited. Early studies by Legakis et al. (1981) indicated that the incidence of fecal *B. fragilis* in CRC patients was significantly higher than in healthy subjects, suggesting a possible role for *B. fragilis* in colon carcinogenesis. Moore et al. (1995), however, did not find any significant difference in the frequency of fecal carriage of *B. fragilis* between colorectal adenoma patients and low-risk healthy controls. Similarly, a seroepidemiological study showed lack of associations between *B. fragilis* IgG serostatus and colorectal adenoma and carcinoma (Abdulamir et al., 2009). Using PCR methods, Toprak et al. (2006) recently compared the prevalence of ETBF in stool specimens from 73 patients with CRC with 59 age-matched controls. The frequency of isolation of the organism was significantly higher in the CRC patients (38%) than in the control group (12%). These findings, however, have not been replicated in another population.

Cancer in experimental animals

Studies of murine models have demonstrated that ETBF induced persistent subclinical colonic inflammation and hyperplasia in specific pathogen-free C57BL/6 mice (Rhee et al., 2009). The same group used the adenomatous polyposis coli multiple intestinal neoplasia ($Apc^{Min/+}$) mice to model human CRC. ETBF-colonized $Apc^{Min/+}$ mice developed inflammatory colitis and unusually early onset microadenomas. In addition, *de novo* colon tumours appeared as early as 4 weeks and distributed predominantly in the distal colon, similar to those found in humans (Wu et al., 2009).

Mechanisms/Mechanistic studies

The current experimental evidence suggests a potential role of fragilysin in the oncogenic transformation of the colonic mucosa (Fig. 1.). *In vitro* studies have shown that fragilysin induces IL-8 expression and NF-κB activation in human colonic epithelial cell lines HT29 and Caco-2 (Sanfiloppo et al., 2000; J.M. Kim et al., 2001). IL-8 is a potent neutrophil chemokine, whereas NF-κB is an essential transcription factor that regulates neutrophils migration and the host epithelial cell chemokine response (J.M. Kim et al., 2002). Additionally, it was demonstrated that fragilysin binds to human colonic epithelial cell line HT29/C1 and stimulates cleavage of the tumour suppressor protein, E-cadherin. The resultant nuclear translocation of the adhesion molecule β-catenin causes increased expression of T-cell factor-target genes, including *c-myc*, with consequent persistent cellular proliferation (Wu et al., 1998, 2003).

Recent showed that all ETBF-induced tumours in $Apc^{Min/+}$ mice exhibited intense Stat3 protein activation, which in turn induces dominant colonic IL-17-producing CD4+ T-cells infiltrate. Tumour formation was significantly inhibited by administration of blocking antibodies to IL-17 (Wu et al., 2009). The latter is known to promote tumour growth *in vitro* and *in vivo* through induction of IL-6 synthesis (L. Wang et al., 2009). These results emphasized the contribution of endogenous T cell immune response in ETBF infection-derived colorectal carcinogenesis.

In addition, *B. fragilis* may indirectly promote colon carcinogenesis through production of cytotoxic metabolites such as deoxycholic acid and fecapentaenes. Studies have shown that deoxycholic acid induce proliferation of colonic cells in vitro and promote colonic tumour progression in experimental animals (Peiffer et al., 1997; T. Hori et al., 1998). Several epidemiological studies found a positive association between high faecal deoxycholic acid concentration and colorectal adenoma and carcinoma risk (Little et al., 2002; Reddy & Wynder, 1977), including a prospective study assessing faecal deoxycholic acid levels before the diagnosis of colorectal tumours (Kawano et al., 2010). Fecapentaenes are other fecal mutagens synthesized by *Bacteroides* species, which were shown to be highly genotoxic in both mammalian and bacterial *in vitro* assays (Plummer et al., 1986; Curren et al., 1987). Clinical studies, however, indicated that fecal fecapentaenes levels are not associated with colorectal adenomas and inversely associated with carcinomas (de Kok et al., 1993; Schiffman et al., 1989). It was concluded that if fecapentaenes form a relevant factor in colorectal carcinogenesis, their role is more likely to be related to the transformation of late adenomas into malignant tumors.

2.4 Other bacterial species

There are very few reports on the role of enteric bacterial flora other than *B. fragilis* in colorectal tumorigenesis. Severe distal colitis, rectal dysplasia, and adenocarcinoma were observed in IL-10 knockout mice colonized with *Enterococcus faecalis* (Balish & Warner, 2002; S.C. Kim et al., 2005). *E. faecalis* has been shown to produce reactive oxygen species and induce DNA damage, aneuploidy and tetraploidy in colonic epithelial cells both *in vivo* and *in vitro* (Huycke et al., 2002; X. Wang et al., 2008). Furthermore, it was demonstrated that *E. faecalis* promotes chromosomal instability in mammalian cells, possibly through COX-2 dependent mechanism (X. Wang & Huycke, 2007). Epidemiological studies, however, could not establish any association between colonic colonization of *E. faecalis* and development of CRC (Winters et al., 1998).

Studies showed that mucosa-associated and intramucosal *Escherichia coli* were significantly associated with Crohn's disease, and colorectal adenomas and carcinomas (Swidsinski et al., 1998; Martin et al., 2004). *E. coli* stimulates IL-8 release from the I407 and HT29 cell lines (Martin, 2004), and acts synergistically with *E. faecalis* to induce aggressive pancolitis with reactive atypia in IL-10 deficient mice (S.C. Kim et al., 2007). Recently, Maddocks et al. (2009) reported that enteropathogenic *E. coli* downregulates DNA mismatch repair proteins which increases the susceptibility of colonic epithelial cells to mutations and therefore promotes colonic tumorigenesis.

3. Viruses

3.1 Human papilloma virus

Human papilloma virus is a double stranded DNA virus that is transmitted through direct contact with infected skin or mucous membrane, and causes the most common sexually transmitted disease among sexually active individuals (Koutsky, 1997). While it is well established that HPV is a necessary cause of cervical cancer, studies suggest HPV may be involved in the malignant transformation of the oropharynx and the anogenital tract (D'Souza et al., 2007; Steenbergen et al., 2005). There are more than 100 subtypes of HPV; some of these subtypes, particularly HPV-16 and HPV-18, are referred to as high risk oncogenic infections (Wiley & Masongsong, 2006; Munoz et al., 2003).

Cancer in human

Early case studies have failed to show any association between HPV infection and colorectal carcinoma in relatively small samples of colorectal carcinoma tissue (Boguszakova et al., 1988; Koulos et al., 1991; Shah et al., 1992; Shroyer et al., 1992). Subsequent studies have employed more stringent methods for HPV detection, including PCR and immunohistochemistry. Despite the variation in the control specimen, all studies confirmed an association between HPV detection rates, specifically subtypes 16 and 18, and CRC with odd ratio ranging between 2.7 (95% CI, 1.1–6.2) and 9.1 (95% CI, 3.7–22.3). (Cheng et al., 1995; Kirgan et al., 1990). Moreover, the strength of association was related to the degree of tumour dysplasia. On the contrary, two of three large prospective cohort studies, with sample sizes ranging between 21,222 and 104,760 cases of cervical cancer, reported no increased risk of subsequent CRC in patients with cervical cancer (Weinberg et al., 1999; Rex, 2000). The other study has shown increased risk of anorectal cancer among patients with cervical cancer, though with lack of clarity over whether it was due to HPV infection or radiation (Chaturvedi et al., 2007).

Mechanism/ mechanistic studies

The oncogenic property of the virus is related to early genes which encode the regulatory proteins E6 an E7. It was hypothesized that these proteins interact and inactivate suppressor genes p53 and pRb, and thus inhibiting apoptosis (Steenbergen et al., 2005). Although about 50% of all colorectal cancer has mutated *p53* (Slattery et al., 2002), Buyru et al. (2003) reported that only 3.6% of HPV-positive colorectal cancers contained mutations in *p53*, suggesting that HPV may have direct oncogenic effects independent of any *p53* mutations.

3.2 John Cunningham virus

JC virus is a widespread neurotropic polyoma virus, with seroprevalence rates of 39-90% among healthy adult population (Kean et al., 2009; Shah, 1996). Primary JCV infection typically occurs during early childhood, probably via fecal-oral route, followed by latency of the virus in the kidney and gastrointestinal tract (Khalili et al., 2003, Ricciardiello et al., 2000). The virus may be reactivated in the presence of severe immunosuppression, and replicates in the central nervous system causing a fatal demyelinating disease, progressive multifocal leukoencephalopathy. Furthermore, there is mounting evidence suggesting that JCV infection may be associated with several human malignancies including brain tumours and upper gastrointestinal cancers (Caldarelli-Stefano et al., 2000; Del Valle et al., 2001, 2005; Shin et al., 2006).

Cancer in human

The potential association between JCV infection and colorectal neoplasia has been examined using nested PCR, Southern blotting and *in situ* hybridization techniques. Ten studies, with sample sizes ranging from 18 to 186, detected JCV genomic sequences in 9-89% of colorectal carcinomas and 5-82% of adenomatous tissue (Laghi et al., 1999; Theodoropoulos et al., 2005;

R. Hori et al., 2005; Casini et al., 2005; Enam et al., 2002; Goel et al., 2006; P. Y. Lin et al., 2008, Niv et al., 2010a; Karpinski et al., 2011; Jung et al., 2008). Comparing neoplastic tissues with normal mucosa, three of these studies showed consistently higher detection rates for JCV in colorectal cancerous tissues and adenomas than in normal tissue (Theodoropoulos et al., 2005; R. Hori et al., 2005; Enam et al., 2002). As well, significantly higher viral copy numbers were observed in colorectal carcinomas and adenomas compared to adjacent normal mucosa (Laghi et al., 1999; Theodoropoulos et al., 2005). Of note, a sequence of the Mad-1 variant of JCV, which lacks 98 nucleotides repeats, has been found preferentially in colon cancers, raising the possibility that certain strains may be selectively activated in colonic epithelial cells (Ricciardello et al., 2001). Other studies have employed real-time PCR, a less sensitive molecular technique, to detect JCV genetic material in colorectal carcinomas, adenomas, normal mucosa, and urine samples from CRC patients and controls. While JCV carrier frequencies in urine were comparable to previously published reports (Agostini et al., 1999), none of the neoplastic tissues and less than 1% of the normal tissues tested positive for JCV DNA (Newcomb et al., 2004; Campello et al., 2010; Militello et al., 2009). The discordant results in previous investigations may be explained by the small sample sizes, variable prevalence of viral infection among the studied populations, inherent lack of uniformity in the sensitivity of the assay used, and possible laboratory contamination particularly in studies where Mad 1 viral sequence was used as a positive template control (Newcomb et al., 2004).

The expression pattern of JCV T-antigen has also been studied in both colorectal neoplastic and normal mucosa. About 35%-94% of CRC tissues and 5-50% of colorectal adenomas were found to host JCV T-antigen, which is often concentrated in the nucleus (Enam et al., 2002; P. Y. Lin et al., 2008; Goel et al., 2006; Link et al., 2009; Nosho et al., 2008, 2009; Ogino et al., 2009; Selgrad et al., 2008; Jung et al., 2008). The expression of JCV T-antigen was significantly higher in colorectal adenomas from liver transplant recipients compared to adenomas in normal controls, pointing to a possible etiologic role for immunosuppression (Selgrad et al., 2008). Interestingly, viral DNA has always been detected more frequently than Tag expression in both colonic adenomas and carcinomas. This suggests that either in some samples, the viral copy number is too low to determine expression of the early gene or, alternatively, that the growing tumour tends to lose viral sequences (Ricciardello et al., 2003). In another aspect, two prospective nested case-control investigated the association between JC seroprevalence and colorectal neoplasms in large groups of patients from whom blood samples were collected months or years before colorectal cancer diagnosis (Rollison et al., 2009; Lundstig et al., 2007). Although there was no association between JC seropositivity and colorectal cancer, one study showed a significantly increased risk of adenomas among seropositive male subjects (Rollison et al., 2009). More recently, Niv et al. (2010b) observed positive correlation between the presence of neoplastic colonic lesion and the titre of JCV antibody in the serum, pointing to JCV infection as an early event for the formation of colorectal adenoma.

Mechanism/ mechanistic studies

The JCV T-antigen is a potent oncogenic protein capable of transforming mammalian cells and is likely involved the early stages of colorectal carcinogenesis though "hit and run" mechanisms. These include disruption of the Wnt signalling pathway and inactivation of tumour suppressor genes such as *pRb* and *p53* (Ludlow, 1993). Both in vitro and in vivo studies have shown that coexpression of *p53* and JCV T-antigen in CRC cells (Enam et al., 2002; Nosho et al., 2009; Ricciardello et al., 2003). Similarly, colocalization of T-antigen and B-catenin was observed in the nuclei of neoplastic columnar cells (Enam et al., 2002; nosho et al., 2009). Cooperativity between B-catenin and JCV T-antigen increased in vitro transcription of *c-myc*, leading to chromosomal instability (Enam et al., 2002). Ricciardiello et al. (2003) demonstrated that JCV can induce chromosomal instability in vitro using the diploid CRC cell line, which defines loss of heterozygosity (LOH). Subsequent studies reported a significant association between JCV T-antigen expression and CRC with LOH (Nosho et al., 2009; Goel et al., 2006; Ogino et al., 2009). This deletional event probably provides the second hit at the tumour suppressor genes, and eventually leads to clonal expansion. The role of DNA hypermethylation has recently been explored in both colorectal carcinoma and adenoma, nevertheless the results were contradictory (Nosho et al., 2008, 2009; Goel et al., 2006).

3.3 Other viruses
Epstein-Barr virus (EBV) is a DNA virus with strong association with several lymphoreticular malignancies, especially Burkett's lymphoma, as well as certain epithelial tumours such as the nasopharyngeal carcinoma (Parkin, 2006). Additionally, EBV has also been reported with gastric cancer (Koriyama et al., 2001; Takada, 2000), breast (Labrecque et al., 1995; Bonnet et al., 1999; Fina et al., 2001) and lung cancer (Castro et al., 2001; Han et al., 2001; M.P. Wong et al., 1995). For colorectal cancer, although early studies have detected high rates of EBV infection in colorectal carcinoma tissue, using PCR, immunohistochemisrty and fluorescence in situ hybridization (Song et al., 2006; Liu et al., 2002, 2003), only one study reported significant difference in EBV detection rates between colorectal carcinoma tissue and adjacent normal mucosa (Song et al., 2006). Follow-up studies failed to show any evidence that EBV was detected at a significantly higher rate in colorectal carcinoma (Grinstein et al., 2002; Yuen et al., 1994), even in higher risk populations such as patients with ulcerative colitis (N.A. Wong et al., 2003).

In the case of Cytomegalovirus (CMV), early limited studies have detected CMV genome in the colon carcinoma tissue, whereas controls from normal colons and cases of Crohn disease were negative (Huang & Roche, 1978; Hashiro et al., 1979). Further studies then showed that CMV was not detected at a significantly higher rate in carcinoma tissue than normal tissue by multiple detection methods, such as FISH, immunohistochemistry, or DNA hybridization (Hart et al., 1982; Ruger & Fleckenstein, 1985). It was found that patients with colorectal cancer who were treated with chemotherapy had significantly increased CMV IgG titre (Avni et al., 1981). However, this finding appeared to be related to CMV infection or reactivation secondary to immunosuppression by chemotherapy rather than primary infection causing colorectal cancer.

4. Helminths

4.1 *Schistosoma japonicum*
The epidemiologic parallel between schistosomiasis japonica endemicity and the distribution of large bowel cancer has been noted in the eastern provinces of China in the 1970s (E. S. Zhao, 1981). Subsequently, ecological studies in the same endemic areas showed

a strong geographical correlation between the prevalence of schistosomiasis japonica and CRC incidence and mortality (Xu & Su, 1984). Likewise, significant association was observed between the mortality from CRC and from schistosomiasis japonica in rural China, even after adjustment for dietary factors (Chen et al., 1990; Guo et al., 1993). The authors attributed the continuing high incidence of colorectal cancer in endemic regions to persistent large populations of chronically infected individuals. This conclusion was further bolstered by a retrospective cohort study conducted in an endemic area in Japan, where the standardized mortality ratio for colonic cancer was significantly high in females who lived in the area for 50 years or more (Inaba, 1984).

More importantly, a case-control study carried out in the endemic area of Jiangsu Province, China, showed that the risk of rectal cancer was increased among subjects with a previous diagnosis of S. japonicum infection with odds ratios of 4.5 and 8.3 (depending on the type of controls used), but the risk of colon cancer was not significantly increased in the same patients group (Xu & Su, 1984). A similar investigation in the same endemic area has confirmed strong associations between colon cancer and early and late-stage S. japonicum infection, regardless of the type of control used for comparison. When the results were adjusted to smoking and family history of colon cancer, statistically significant associations were still noted. In addition, the estimated relative risk increased with the duration of exposure to S. japonicum infection (Mayer & Fried, 2007). Of interest also is a recent matched case-control study which reported that patients with chronic schistosomiasis japonica have more than three times risk to develop colon cancer than those with no previous exposure to schistosomal infection. Moreover, the authors attributed 24% of colon cancer cases to long-standing schistosomal infestation (Qiu et al., 2005).

The consensus of available pathological data strongly implicates an association between S. japonicum infestation and induction of CRC. In a review of the literature between 1898 and 1974, 276 cases of schistosomiasis japonica associated with cancer of the large intestine were analysed. The results showed significant differences between carcinoma with schistosomiasis and ordinary carcinoma in symptoms, age range, sex ratio, and histopathologic findings, indicating that schistosomiasis may induce carcinoma (Shindo, 1976). Ming-Chai et al. (1965) reported similar findings in their study of 90 cases of simultaneous CRC and schistosomiasis, and proposed that S. japonicum colitis, in its late phases, is a premalignant condition not infrequently leading to cancer. Supporting their previous results and giving better insight into the pathogenesis of schistosomal colorectal carcinoma, the same group has examined the mucosal changes in the immediate vicinity of the tumours of patients with schistosomiasis, and referred to the close similarity between certain schistosome-induced lesions and those associated with long-standing ulcerative colitis. Pointing to mimicry of cancer evolution in these two clinical entities, they described presence of pseudopolyps, multiple ulcers, and hyperplastic ectopic submucosal glands, with evidence of oviposition and precancerous and cancerous transformation in these lesions (Ming-Chai et al., 1980). It was also demonstrated that the closer to the tumour the area is the more ova tend to be detected (Matsuda et al., 1999). In a following study, Ming-Chai et al. (1981) observed variable degree of colonic epithelial dysplasia in 60% of cases with S. japonicum colitis and regarded these changes as the transition on the way towards cancer development in schistosomal colonic disease. A similar conclusion was drawn by Yu et al. (1991) from their studies on different types of schistosomal egg polyps.

Of note, distinct clinico-pathologic characteristics of S. japonicum-related colorectal cancer seem emerge from the existing literature. Bearing in mind the early environmental exposure to schistosomal infection in childhood, schistosomal colorectal cancer was notably shown to occur in younger age group with a maximum age incidence 6 to 16 years earlier than ordinary colorectal cancer (Shindo, 1976; Ming-Chai et al., 1965, 1980). Furthermore, the gender ratio of male to female in schistosomal colorectal cancer is consistently higher than in nonschistosomal cancer (Shindo, 1976; Ming-Chai et al., 1980). This can be attributed to the fact that men are more prone to schistosomal infection through contact with cercariae-infested waters during agricultural activities.

4.2 Schistosoma mansoni

The epidemiological evidence associating S. mansoni infection with CRC is lacking, of poor quality, or conflicting. Supporting the absence of such a causal association, Parkin et al. (1986) pointed out that although there is a great disparity in the geographical distribution of S. mansoni, CRC occurs in the African continent with clear uniformity. In a recent hospital-based study in Uganda and Zimbabwe, Waku et al. (2005) compared 950 cases of infective gastrointestinal disease, particularly schistosomiasis and amebiasis, with 249 patient controls admitted for various diseases other than GI disease. The cases were thoroughly investigated and further stratified into three groups on the basis of the stage of the disease; cured, acute, and chronic patients group. Colorectal cancer was found in 34 patients; nearly all of them had chronic schistosomiasis or amebiasis, whereas no CRC was detected in the other patients or control groups. It was concluded that large bowel cancer is strongly associated with chronic infectious gastrointestinal diseases. This study, though, was limited by the inability to adjust for potential confounders such as age and gender. Furthermore, the issue of correspondence between the population giving rise to the cases and that sampled for the controls was not addressed. To date, there have been no epidemiological studies conducted at the population level to verify the link between S. mansoni infestation and large bowel cancer.

The pathological evidence supporting an association between S. mansoni infestation and colorectal carcinoma is rather weak. In 1956, Dimmette et al. (1956) failed to demonstrate any specific pathological changes in patients with simultaneous CRC and S. mansoni infestation, and considered the two conditions unrelated. Contrasting to these results, a recent study by Madbouly et al. (2007) has shown that S. mansoni-associated colorectal cancer has distinctive pathological features often similar to those of colitis-induced carcinoma (Fig. 2a,b). These include high percentage of multicentric tumours and mucinous adenocarcinoma, and the tendency of the tumour to present at an advanced stage with high risk of malignant lymph node invasion. Although direct causal inference is limited, this study indicates that S. mansoni infestation may exercise some influence on the prognosis of patients with CRC. Other studies have examined the pathological changes in endoscopic biopsies and cadaveric specimens from the colon of patients with S. mansoni colitis (Mohamed et al., 1990; Cheever et al., 1987). The gross pathological lesions were akin to those observed in patients with S. japonicum colitis. However, histological analysis of the specimens showed no evidence of atypism or carcinomatous changes. This discrepancy in pathologic findings may be explained by the larger number of eggs deposited by S. japonicum than S. mansoni worms, thus causing more pathological problems (Ishii et al., 1994).

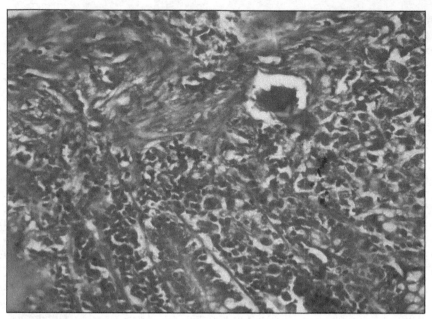

Fig. 2a. Photomicrograph showing S. mansoni egg shell in a background of mucinous adenocarcinoma. H&E × 40

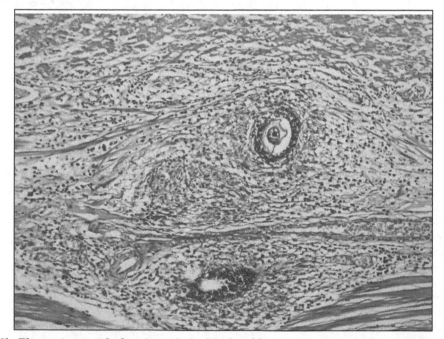

Fig. 2b. Photomicrograph showing calcified and viable S. mansoni ova with granuloma formation in the muscularis propria of the sigmoid colon. H&E × 20

4.3 Mechanisms of tumorigenesis

The exact etiopathogenesis of schistosomal colorectal cancer is enigmatic. Several explanations have been advanced for the possible role of schistosomiasis in colorectal tumorigenesis: the presence of endogenously produced carcinogens (Rosin et al., 1994), chronic immunomodulation resulting in impairment of immunological surveillance (van Riet et al., 2007), symbiotic action of other infective agents (Shindo, 1976), and the presence of schistosomal toxins (Long et al., 2004). While these factors may interact to induce carcinogenesis, chronic inflammation appears to play a central role. In support of this view are data showing that CRC tends to occur mainly in patients who had history of schistosomiasis for 10 years or more and in whom the large bowel is wholly involved (Shindo, 1976; Ming-Chai et al., 1980). Moreover, there is significantly higher rate of synchronous tumours in patients with schistosomal colorectal cancer than in patients with spontaneous colorectal cancer (Ming-Chai et al., 1980; Madbouly et al., 2007). This can be ascribed to the field effect caused by chronic schistosomal inflammation throughout the colon, a phenomenon analogous to that described in the context of colitis-associated cancer.

It has been suggested that chronic inflammatory reaction provoked by schistosome antigens provides the proliferative stimulus necessary to promote cancer growth from potentially malignant foci produced by other carcinogens (Ming-Chai et al., 1980). However, whereas increased epithelial cell proliferation likely contributes to carcinogenesis, it is insufficient to cause cancer. Rather, inflammatory cells generate potentially genotoxic mediators during the course of schistosomal infection such as reactive oxygen and nitrogen species and proinflammatory cytokines, which cause genomic instability and dysregulation of oncogenes and oncosuppresor genes (Herrera et al., 2005; Trakatelli et al., 2005). The accumulation of these molecular disturbances, in turn, drives the progression toward dysplasia and carcinoma. Another factor that may play a major role in colorectal carcinogenesis of schistosomiasis patients is the presence of concomitant enterobacterial infections. In both clinical and experimental studies, various strains of enterobacteriaceae have been described in association with schistosome infection which confers a survival advantage to bacteria by inducing immunosuppression (Chieffi, 1992; Tuazon et al., 1985). Some of these organisms are thought to promote colorectal carcinogenesis through multiple pathways such as production of reactive oxygen intermediates, dysregulation in the T cell response, and alterations in host epithelial carbohydrate expression (Hope et al., 2005).

A further explanation for the carcinogenic process of schistosomal CRC is a possible direct mutagenic effect of the schistosome soluble antigens. Evidence against this hypothesis has come from a study by Ishii et al. (1989), who evaluated the mutagenicity of S. japonicum extracts using the Ames Salmonella/E. coli test in the presence and absence of rat liver S9 mixture. They did not identify any mutagenic activity for the soluble extracts of both eggs and adult worms. Nevertheless, a weak but significant tumour-promoting activity was noted for the S. japonicum soluble egg antigen when tested using cultured viral genome-carrying human lymphoblastoid cells. Osada et al. (2005) tested the adult worm and egg extracts of S. mansoni using more reliable genetic toxicology assays, the Salmonella Umu test and the hypoxanthine guanine phosphoribosyltransferase (HGPRT) gene mutation assay. They could not demonstrate any mutagenic potential in either parasite extracts of S. mansoni before and after addition of S9 mixture.

Recent studies have thrown some light on the molecular events associated with schistosomal colorectal cancer, taking the latter as a separate clinical entity. Zhang et al. (1998) investigated the mutation pattern in the *p53* gene in S. japonicum-associated rectal carcinomas. They observed a higher proportion of base-pair substitutions at CpG dinucleotides and arginine missense mutations among schistosomal rectal cancer patients than in patients with ordinary CRC, albeit the differences were of marginal significance. Their results also indicated that the majority of mutations in *p53* gene were in exon 7 in schistosomal group compared to exon 5 in non-schistosomal group. Barrowing from the ulcerative colitis example, nitric oxide, an endogenously produced genotoxic agent, is capable of inducing similar transition mutations and activation of *p53* gene in the inflamed colonic mucosa (Goodman et al., 2004). Conceivably therefore, it seems plausible that chronic colonic inflammation induced by schistosomal infection may follow a similar pathway.

For *S. mansoni*-associated colorectal carcinomas, it was demonstrated that parasitism is strongly associated with microsatellite instability, which is a sign of defective DNA repair (Soliman et al., 2001). This genomic instability results in DNA replication errors that preferentially affect target genes such as transforming growth factor (*TGH*)*βRII* and insulin-like growth factor (IGF)2R, and render them incapable of normal colonocytes homeostasis resulting in malignant growth (Itzkowitz & Yio, 2004). In another aspect, Madbouly et al. (2007) evaluated the expression of *p53* in patients with *S. mansoni*-related colorectal cancer, and found that mutant *p53* overexpression was significantly more frequent in schistosomal than in non-schistosomal colorectal cancer. Moreover, *p53* overexpression in schistosomal CRC correlated well with mucinous carcinoma, nodal metastasis, and tumour multicentricity. Zalata et al. (2005) developed a more comprehensive study of the expression pattern of *p53*, *Bcl-2*, and *c-myc* in seventy five CRC cases, 24 of these had pathological evidence of *S. mansoni* infection. Although they did not find a significant association between parasitism and *p53* and *c-myc* expression, their results showed that S. mansoni-associated colorectal tumours characterized by *Bcl-2* overexpression and less apoptotic activity than ordinary colorectal tumours. This supports the contention that evasion of apoptosis through change in the expression of *Bcl-2* may be an alternative molecular pathway through which genotoxic agents can induce carcinogenesis in intestinal schistosomiasis.

5. Concluding remarks

It is clearly evident that a wide array of microbial agents is associated with colorectal cancer. Nonetheless, establishing a causal link between a certain organism and colorectal cancer is a complicated process, considering the long latency of infection during which numerous endogenous and exogenous factors interact to obscure causality. For most of these putative agents, the association has been inconsistent, and may either define subsets of the tumour, or may act to modify phenotype of an established tumour, possibly contributing to some phase of oncogenesis.

Despite the fact that *H. pylori* and *S. bovis* were discovered in colorectal tumours and linked to the malignancy by seroepidemiologic studies and molecular analyses, these pathogens are considered to be at most contributing cofactors. The two reasons for this loss of etiological status were the inconsistency in the epidemiological data regarding *H. pylori* and *S. bovis* infections and risk of colorectal cancer (Gold et al, 2004; Y. S. Zhao et al., 2008), whereas none of these agents produced *de novo* colorectal cancer in animal models (Singh et al., 2000a; Biarc et al., 2004). The relation between gut mictobiota such as *B. fragilis* and *E.*

faecalis and colorectal cancer is far less convincing. Although the oncogenic potential of *B. fragilis* and *E. faecalis* is not disputed, the scarcity of epidemiological evidence renders any association hypothetical.

In case of viral agents, while HPV and JCV have oncogenic properties both in cell culture and experimental animals (Butel, 2000), the detection of viral genomes in tumour tissues is inconsistent, which can be attributed to the fact that PCR technique, used for detection of viral DNA in most studies, is subject to contamination. At this point, this precludes a causative role for these viruses in colorectal cancer, and obtaining more credible results mandates employment of combination of in situ methods for detection of viral genome and its products such as *in situ* cytohybridization and immunohistochemistry (Panago et al., 2004).

In case of *S. japonicum*, the growing epidemiological evidence and the unique clinic-pathological features of schistosome-related colorectal cancer point to a reasonably consistent association. However, *S. japonicum* has been classified by IARC as possible and not as definite carcinogen in human leading to colorectal cancer (IARC, 1994). This perhaps reflects the confounding uncertainties presented by epidemiological studies and the lack of experimental evidence. For *S. mansoni* species, it is still a matter of controversy as to whether or not *S. mansoni* infection is an association factor in colorectal cancer development and progression.

Infection-related colorectal carcinogenesis is a complex multistage process that utilizes several mechanisms. For most bacterial species and helminths associated with colorectal cancer, chronic inflammatory response and immunomodulation induced by secretory or structural proteins are the principal mechanisms of carcinogenesis. These involve release of protumorigenic mediators and dysregulation of multiple cellular transcriptional pathways including NF-κB and β–catenin. Others such as *H. pylori* primarily induce production of growth factor resulting disruption of proliferation-antiproliferation pathways. DNA tumour viruses, such as HPV and JCV, primarily target cellular tumour suppressor proteins, thus modulating cell cycle progression (Butel, 2000).

Together, our observations underpin the necessity of epidemiological studies focusing on specific strains such as CagA+ H. pylori, *S. gallolyticus*, ETBF, and Mad-1 JCV. In addition, the interaction between various infectious agents in relation to carcinogenesis, as illustrated in the additive effect of *B. fragilis* and *E. faecalis* needs further evaluation. Finally it is likely that more agents, both known and unidentified, have yet to be implicated in human colorectal cancer. In the meantime, study of tumorigenic infectious agents will continue to illuminate molecular oncogenic processes.

6. Acknowledgement

Acknowledgement to Dr. Salwa O. Mekki, Director of Pathology Department, Soba University Hospital, to Ms. Abeer Musa, Lab Technician for preparing the slides, and to the patients who gave us the permission to add their pictures in our chapter.

7. References

Abdulamir, A. S., Hafidh, R. R. & Abu Bakar, F. (2010). Molecular detection, quantification, and isolation of *Streptococcus gallolyticus* bacteria colonizing colorectal tumors:

inflammation-driven potential of carcinogenesis via IL-1, COX-2, and IL-8. *J Exp Clin Cancer Res*, 9, 249.

Abdulamir, A. S., Hafidh, R. R., Mahdi, L. K., Al-jeboori, T. & Abubaker F. (2009) Investigation into the controversial association of *Streptococcus gallolyticus* with colorectal cancer and adenoma. *BMC Cancer*, 9, 403.

Agostini, H. T., Jobes, D. V., Chima, S. C., Ryschkewitsch, C. F. & Stoner, G. L. (1999). Natural and pathogenic variation in the JC virus genome. *Recent Res Dev Virol*, 1, 683–701.

Alazmi, W., Bustamante, M., O'Loughlin, C., Gonzalez, J. & Raskin, J. B. (2006). The association of *Streptococcus bovis* bacteremia and gastrointestinal diseases: a retrospective analysis. *Dig Dis Sci*, 51, 732 – 736.

Avni, A., Haikin, H., Feuchtwanger, M. M., Sacks, M., Naggan, L., Sarov, B. & Sarov, I. (1981). Antibody pattern to human cytomegalovirus in patients with adenocarcinoma of the colon. *Intervirology*, 16, 4, 244–249.

Aydin, A., Karasu, Z., Zeytinoglu, A., Kumanlioglu, K. & Ozacar, T. (1999). Colorectal adenomateous polyps and Helicobacter pylori infection. *Am J Gastroenterol*, 94, 4, 1121–1122.

Baldwin, G. S. & Shulkes, A. (1998). Gastrin, gastrin receptors and colorectal carcinoma. *Gut*, 42, 4, 581–584.

Balish, E. & Warner, T. (2002). *Enterococcus faecalis* induces inflammatory bowel disease in interleukin-10 knockout mice. *Am J Pathol*, 160, 6, 2253–2257.

Ballet, M., Gevigney, G., Gare, J. P., Delahaye, F., Etienne, J. & Delahaye J. P. (1995). Infective endocarditis due to *Streptococcus bovis*. A report of 53 cases. *Eur Heart J*, 16, 12, 1975–1980.

Basset, C., Holton, J., Bazeos, A., Vaira, D. & Bloom, S. (2004). Are *Helicobacter* species and enterotoxigenic *Bacteroides fragilis* involved in inflammatory bowel disease? *Dig Dis Sci*, 49, 9, 1425–1432.

Beeching, N. J., Christmas, T. I., Ellis-Pegler, R. B. & Nicholson, G. I. (1985). *Streptococcus bovis* bacteraemia requires rigorous exclusion of colonic neoplasia and endocarditis. *Q J Med*, 56, 220, 439–450.

Biarc, J., Nguyen, I. S., Pini, A., Gosse, F., Richert, S., Thierse, D., Van Dorsselaer, A., Leize-Wagner, E., Raul, F., Klein, J. P. & Schöller-Guinard, M. (2004). Carcinogenic properties of proteins with pro-inflammatory activity from *Streptococcus infantarius* (formerly *S.bovis*). *Carcinogenesis*, 25, 8, 1477-1484.

Bodaghi, S., Yamanegi, K., Xiao, S. Y., Da Costa, M., Palefsky, J. M. & Zheng, Z. M. (2005). Colorectal papillomavirus infection in patients with colorectal cancer. *Clin Cancer Res*, 11, 8, 2862–2867.

Boguszakova, L., Hirsch, I., Brichacek, B., Faltýn, J., Fric, P., Dvoráková, H. & Vonka, V. (1988). Absence of cytomegalovirus, Epstein-Barr virus, and papillomavirus DNA from adenoma and adenocarcinoma of the colon. *Acta Virol*, 32, 4, 303–308.

Bonnet, M., Guinebretiere, J. M., Kremmer, E., Grunewald, V., Benhamou, E., Contesso, G. & Joab, I. (1999). Detection of Epstein-Barr virus in invasive breast cancers. *J Natl Cancer Inst*, 91, 16, 1376–1381.

Breuer-Katschinski, B., Nemes, K., Marr, A., Rump, B., Leiendecker, B., Breuer, N. & Goebell, H. (1999). *Helicobacter pylori* and the risk of colonic adenomas. Colorectal Adenoma Study Group. *Digestion*, 60, 3, 210–215.

Bulajic, M., Stimec, B., Jesenofsky, R., Kecmanovic, D., Ceranic, M., Kostic, N., Schneider-Brachert, W., Lowenfels, A., Maisonneuve, P. & Löhr, J. M. (2007). *Helicobacter pylori* in colorectal carcinoma tissue. *Cancer Epidemiol Biomarkers Prev*, 16, 3, 631 – 633.

Burns, C.A., McCaughey, R. & Lauter, C. B. (1985). The association of *Streptococcus bovis* fecal carriage and colon neoplasia: possible relationship with polyps and their premalignant potential. *Am J Gastroenterol*, 80, 1, 42–46.

Butel, J. S. (2000). Viral carcinogenesis: revelation of molecular mechanisms and etiology of human disease. *Carcinogenesis*, 21, 3, 405–426.

Buyru, N., Budak, M., Yazici, H. & Dalay, N. (2003). *p53* gene mutations are rare in human papillomavirus-associated colon cancer. *Oncol Rep*, 10, 6, 2089–2092.

Buyru, N., Tezol, A. & Dalay, N. (2006). Coexistence of K-ras mutations and HPV infection in colon cancer. *BMC Cancer*, 6, 115.

Caldarelli-Stefano, R., Boldorini, R., Monga, G., Meraviglia, E., Zorini, E. O. & Ferrante, P. (2000). JC virus in human glial-derived tumors. *Hum Pathol*, 31, 3, 394–395.

Campello, C., Comar, M., Zanotta, N., Minicozzi, A., Rodella, L. & Poli A. (2010). Detection of SV40 in colon cancer: a molecular case-control study from northeast Italy. *J Med Virol*, 82, 7, 1197-1200.

Casini, B., Borgese, L., Del Nonno, F., Galati, G., Izzo, L., Caputo, M., Perrone Donnorso, R., Castelli, M., Risuleo, G. & Visca, P. (2005). Presence and incidence of DNA sequences of human polyomaviruses BKV and JCV in colorectal tumor tissues. *Anticancer Res*, 25, 2A, 1079-1085.

Castro, C. Y., Ostrowski, M. L., Barrios, R., Green, L. K., Popper, H. H., Powell, S., Cagle, P. T. & Ro, J. Y. (2001). Relationship between Epstein-Barr virus and lymphoepithelioma-like carcinoma of the lung: a clinicopathologic study of 6 cases and review of the literature. *Hum Pathol*, 32, 8, 863–872.

Chaturvedi, A. K., Engels, E. A., Gilbert, E. S., Chen, B. E., Storm, H., Lynch, C. F., Hall, P., Langmark, F., Pukkala, E., Kaijser, M., Andersson, M., Fosså, S. D., Joensuu, H., Boice, J. D., Kleinerman, R. A. & Travis, L. B. (2007). Second cancers among 104,760 survivors of cervical cancer: evaluation of long-term risk. *J Natl Cancer Inst*, 99, 21, 1634–1643.

Cheever, A. W., Kamel, I. A., Elwi, A. M., Mosimann, J. E., Danner, R. & Sippel, J. E. (1987). *Schistosoma mansoni* and *S. haematobium* infections in Egypt. III. Extrahepatic pathology. *Am J Trop Med Hyg*, 27, 1, 55-75

Chen, J., Campbell, T. C., Li, J. & Peto, R. (1990). *Diet, Life-style, and Mortality in China. A Study of the Characteristics of 65 Chinese Counties*, Oxford University Press, Oxford.

Cheng, J. Y., Sheu, L. F., Lin, J. C. & Meng, C. L. (1995). Detection of human papillomavirus DNA in colorectal adenomas. *Arch Surg*, 130, 1, 73–76.

Chieffi, P. P. (1992). Interrelationship between schistosomiasis and concomitant diseases. *Mem Inst Oswaldo Cruz*, 87, Suppl 4, 291-296.

Ciccotosto, G. D., McLeish, A., Hardy, K. J. & Shulkes. A. (1995). Expression, processing, and secretion of gastrin in patients with colorectal carcinoma. *Gastroenterology*, 109, 4, 1142–1153

Corredoira, J., Alonson, M. P., Coira, A. & Varela, J. (2008). Association between *Streptococcus infantarius* (formerly *S. bovis* II/1) bacteremia and noncolonic cancer. *J Clin Microbiol*, 46, 4, 1570.

Coykendall, A. L. & Gustafson, K. B. (1985). Deoxyribonucleic acid hybridization among strains of *Streptococcus salivarius* and *Streptococcus bovis*. *Int J Syst Bacteriol*, 35, 3, 274-280.

Curren, R. D., Putman, D. L., Yang, L, L., Haworth, S. R., Lawlor, T. E., Plummer, S. M. & Harris, C. C. (1987). Genotoxicity of fecapentaene-12 in bacterial and mammalian cell assay systems. *Carcinogenesis*, 8, 2, 349-352.

D'Onghia, V., Leoncini, R., Carli, R., Santoro, A., Giglioni, S., Sorbellini, F., Marzocca ,G., Bernini, A., Campagna, S., Marinello, E. & Vannoni, D. (2007). Circulating gastrin and ghrelin levels in patients with colorectal cancer: correlation with tumour stage, Helicobacter pylori infection and BMI. *Biomed Pharmacother*, 61, (2-3), 137–141.

D'Souza, G., Kreimer, A. R., Viscidi, R., Pawlita, M., Fakhry, C., Koch, W. M., Westra, W. H. & Gillison, M. L. (2007). Case-control study of human papillomavirus and oropharyngeal cancer. *N Engl J Med*, 356, 19, 1944–1956.

Darjee, R. & Gibb, A. P. (1993). Serological investigation into the association between *Streptococcus bovis* and colonic cancer. *J Clin Pathol*, 46, 12, 1116–1119.

de Kok, T. M., Pachen, D., van Iersel, M. L., Baeten, C. G., Engels, L. G., ten Hoor, F. & Kleinjans, J.C. (1993). Case-control study on fecapentaene excretion and adenomatous polyps in the colon and rectum. *J Natl Cancer Inst*, 85, 15, 1241-1244.

Del Valle, L., Gordon, J., Assimakopoulou, M., Enam, S., Geddes, J. F., Varakis, J. N., Katsetos, C. D., Croul, S. & Khalili, K. (2001). Detection of JC virus DNA sequences and expression of the viral regulatory protein T-antigen in tumors of the central nervous system. *Cancer Res*, 61, 10, 4287–4293.

Del Valle, L., White, M. K., Enam, S., Piña Oviedo, S., Bromer, M. Q., Thomas, R. M., Parkman, H. P. & Khalili, K. (2005). Detection of JC virus DNA sequences and expression of viral T antigen and agnoprotein in esophageal carcinoma. *Cancer*, 103, 3, 516–527.

Dickinson, C. J. (1995). Relationship of gastrin processing to colon cancer. *Gastroenterology*, 109, 4, 1384–1388

Dimmette, R. M., Elwi, A. M. & Sproate, H. F. (1956). Relationship of schistosomiasis to polyposis and adenocareinoma of large intestine. *Am J Clin Patho*, 26, 3, 266-276

Dubrow, R., Edberg, S., Wikfors, E., Callan, D., Troncale, F., Vender, R., Brand, M. & Yapp, R. (1991). Fecal carriage of *Streptococcus bovis* and colorectal adenomas. *Gastroenterology*, 101, 3, 721–725.

Ellmerich, S., Djouder, N., Scholler, M. & Klein, J. P. (2000b). Production of cytokines by monocytes, epithelial and endothelial cells activated by *Streptococcus bovis*. *Cytokine*, 12, 1, 26-31.

Ellmerich, S., Scholler, M., Duranton, B., Gosse, F., Galluser, M., Klein, J. P. & Raul, F. (2000a). Promotion of intestinal carcinogenesis by *Streptococcus bovis*. *Carcinogenesis*, 21, 4, 753-756.

Enam, S., Del Valle, L., Lara, C., Gan, D. D., Ortiz-Hidalgo, C., Palazzo, J. P. & Khalili K. (2002). Association of human polyomavirus JCV with colon cancer: evidence for interaction of viral T-antigen and beta-catenin. *Cancer Res*, 62, 23, 7093–7101.

EUROGAST Study Group. (1993). An international association between *Helicobacter pylori* infection and gastric cancer. *Lancet*, 341, 8857, 1359 – 1362.

Fina, F., Romain, S., Ouafik, L., Palmari, J., Ben Ayed, F., Benharkat, S., Bonnier, P., Spyratos, F., Foekens, J. A., Rose, C., Buisson, M., Gérard, H., Reymond, M. O., Seigneurin, J. M. & Martin, P. M. (2001). Frequency and genome load of Epstein-Barr virus in 509 breast cancers from different geographical areas. *Br J Cancer*, 84, 6, 783–790.

Fireman, Z., Trost, L., Kopelman, Y., Segal, A. & Sternberg, A. (2000). *Helicobacter pylori*: seroprevalence and colorectal cancer. *Isr Med Assoc J*, 2, 1, 6–9.

Friedrich, I. A., Wormser, G. P. & Gottfried, E. B. (1982a). The association of recent *Streptococcus bovis* bacteremia with colonic neoplasia. Mil Med, 147,7, 584 – 5.

Friedrich, I.A., Wormser, G. P. & Gottfried, E. B. (1982b). The association of remote *Streptococcus bovis* bacteremia with colonic neoplasia. *Am J Gastroenterol*, 77, 2, 82-84.

Fujimori, S., Kishida, T., Kobayashi, T., Sekita, Y., Seo, T., Nagata, K., Tatsuguchi, A., Gudis, K., Yokoi, K., Tanaka, N., Yamashita, K., Tajiri, T., Ohaki, Y. & Sakamoto, C. (2005). Helicobacter pylori infection increases the risk of colorectal adenoma and adenocarcinoma, especially in women. J Gastroenterol, 40, 9, 887–893

Georgopoulos, S. D., Polymeros, D., Triantafyllou, K., Spiliadi, C., Mentis, A., Karamanolis, D. G. & Ladas, S. D. (2006). Hypergastrinemia is associated with increased risk of distal colon adenomas. *Digestion*, 74, 1, 42–46.

Goel, A., Li, M. S., Nagasaka, T., Shin, S. K., Fuerst, F., Ricciardiello, L., Wasserman, L. & Boland CR. (2006). Association of JC virus T-antigen expression with the methylator phenotype in sporadic colorectal cancers. *Gastroenterology*, 130, 7, 1950–1961.

Gold, J. S., Bayar, S. & Salem, R. R. (2004). Association of *Streptococcus bovis* bacteremia with colonic neoplasia and extracolonic malignancy. *Arch Surg*, 139, 7, 760 – 765.

Goodman, J. E., Hofseth, L. J., Hussain, S. P. & Harris, C. C. (2004). Nitric oxide and p53 in cancer-prone chronic inflammation and oxyradical overload disease. *Environ Mol Mutagen*, 44, 1, 3-9.

Grahn, N., Hmani-Aifa, M., Fransen, K., Soderkvist, P. & Monstein, H. J. (2005). Molecular identification of *Helicobacter* DNA present in human colorectal adenocarcinomas by 16S rDNA PCR amplification and pyrosequencing analysis. *J Med Microbiol*, 54, 11, 1031 – 1035.

Grinstein, S., Preciado, M. V., Gattuso, P., Chabay, P. A., Warren, W. H., De Matteo, E. & Gould, V. E. (2002). Demonstration of Epstein-Barr virus in carcinomas of various sites. *Cancer Res*, 62, 17, 4876–4878.

Guo, W., Zheng, W., Li, J. Y., Chen, J. S. & Blot, W. J. (1993). Correlations of colon cancer mortality with dietary factors, serum markers, and schistosomiasis in China. *Nutr Cancer*, 20, 1, 13-20

Hakanson, R., Axelson, J., Ekman, R. & Sundler, F. (1988). Hypergastrinaemia evoked by omeprazole stimulates growth of gastric mucosa but not of pancreas or intestines in hamster, guinea pig and chicken. *Regul Pept*, 23, 1, 105-115.

Hakanson, R., Blom, H., Carlsson, E., Larsson, H., Ryberg, B. & Sundler, F. (1986). Hypergastrinaemia produces trophic effects in stomach but not in pancreas and intestine. *Regul Pept*, 13, (3-4), 225-233.

Han, A. J., Xiong, M., Gu, Y. Y., Lin, S. X. & Xiong, M. (2001). Lymphoepithelioma-like carcinoma of the lung with a better prognosis. A clinicopathologic study of 32 cases. *Am J Clin Pathol*, 115, 6, 841-850.

Hart, H., Neill, W. A. & Norval, M. (1982). Lack of association of cytomegalovirus with adenocarcinoma of the colon. *Gut*, 23, 1, 21-30.

Hartwich J, Konturek SJ, Pierzchalski P, Zuchowicz M, Konturek PC, Bielański W, Marlicz K, Starzyńska T, Ławniczak M. (2001b). Molecular basis of colorectal cancer - role of gastrin and cyclooxygenase-2. *Med Sci Monit*, 7, 6, 1171-1181.

Hartwich, A., Konturek, S. J., Pierzchalski, P., Zuchowicz, M., Labza, H., Konturek, P. C., Karczewska, E., Bielanski, W., Marlicz, K., Starzynska, T., Lawniczak, M. & Hahn, E. G. (2001a). *Helicobacter pylori* infection, gastrin, cyclooxygenase-2, and apoptosis in colorectal cancer. *Int J Colorectal Dis* 16, 4, 202-210.

Hashiro, G. M., Horikami, S. & Loh, P. C. (1979). Cytomegalovirus isolations from cell cultures of human adenocarcinomas of the colon. *Intervirology*, 12, 2, 84-88.

Herrera, L. A., Benitez-Bribiesca, L., Mohar, A. & Ostrosky-Wegman, P. (2005). Role of infectious diseases in human carcinogenesis. *Environ Mol Mutagen*, 45, (2-3), 284-303.

Herrero, I. A., Rouse, M. S., Piper, K. E, Alyaseen, S. A., Steckelberg, J. M. & Patel, R. (2002). Reevaluation of *Streptococcus bovis* endocarditis cases from 1975 to 1985 by 16S ribosomal DNA sequence analysis. *J Clin Microbiol*, 40, 10, 3848-3850.

Hoen, B., Briancon, S., Delahaye, F., Terhé, V., Etienne, J., Bigard, M. A., Canton, P. (1994). Tumors of the colon increase the risk of developing *Streptococcus bovis* endocarditis: case-control study. *Clin Infect* Dis, 19, 2, 361 - 362.

Hope, M.E., Hold, G.L., Kain, R. & El-Omar, E.M. (2005). Sporadic colorectal cancer — role of the commensal microbiota. *FEMS Microbiol Lett*, 244, 1, 1-7.

Hori, R., Murai, Y., Tsuneyama, K., Abdel-Aziz, H. O., Nomoto, K., Takahashi, H., Cheng, C. M., Kuchina, T., Harman, B. V. & Takano, Y. (2005). Detection of JC virus DNA sequences in colorectal cancers in Japan. *Virchows Arch*, 447, 4, 723-730.

Hori, T., Matsumoto, K., Sakaitani, Y., Sato, M. & Morotomi, M. (1998). Effect of dietary deoxycholic acid and cholesterol on fecal steroid concentration and its impact on the colonic crypt cell proliferation in azoxymethane-treated rats. *Cancer Lett*, 124, 1, 79-84.

Huang, E. S. & Roche, J. K. (1978). Cytomegalovirus D.N.A. and adenocarcinoma of the colon: evidence for latent viral infection. *Lancet*, 1, 8071, 957-960.

Huycke, M. M., Abrams, V. & Moore, D. R. (2002). *Enterococcus faecalis* produces extracellular superoxide and hydrogen peroxide that damages colonic epithelial cell DNA. *Carcinogenesis*, 23, 3, 529–536.

IARC (1994). Monograph on the evaluation of carcinogenic risks to humans: Schistosomes, liver flukes and *Helicobacter pylori*. WHO: *International Agency for Research on Cancer* 61, 9–240.

IARC (1997). Monograph on the evaluation of carcinogenic risks to humans: Epstein-Barr Virus and Kaposi's Sarcoma Herpesvirus/Human Herpesvirus 8. WHO: *International Agency for Research on Cancer* 70, 47–374.

Inaba, Y. (1984). A cohort study on the causes of death in an endemic area of schistosomiasis japonica in Japan. *Ann Acad Med Singapore*, 13, 2, 142–148.

Ishii, A., Matsuoka, H., Aji, T., Hayatsu, H., Wataya, Y., Arimoto, S. & Tokuda, H. (1989). Evaluation of the mutagenicity and the tumor-promoting activity of parasite extracts: *Schistosoma japonicum* and *Clonorchis sinensis*. *Mutat Res*, 224, 2, 229-233.

Ishii, A., Matsuoka, H., Aji, T., Ohta, N., Arimoto, S., Wataya, Y. & Hayatsu, H. (1994). Parasite infection and cancer: with special emphasis on *Schistosoma japonicum* infections (Trematoda). A review. *Mutat Res*, 305, 2, 273-281.

Itzkowitz, S. H. & Yio, X. Inflammation and cancer IV. Colorectal cancer in inflammatory bowel disease: the role of inflammation. (2004). *Am J Physiol Gastrointest Liver Physiol*, 287, 1, G7–17

Jones, M., Helliwell, P., Pritchard, C., Tharakan, J. & Mathew, J. (2007). *Helicobacter pylori* in colorectal neoplasms: is there an aetiological relationship? *World J Surg Oncol*, 5, 51.

Jung, W. T., Li, M. S., Goel, A. & Boland, C. R. (2008). JC virus T-antigen expression in sporadic adenomatous polyps of the colon. *Cancer*, 112, 5, 1028–1036.

Kanno, T., Matsuki, T., Oka, M., Utsunomiya, H., Inada, K., Magari, H., Inoue, I., Maekita, T., Ueda, K., Enomoto, S., Iguchi, M., Yanaoka, K., Tamai, H., Akimoto, S., Nomoto, K., Tanaka, R. & Ichinose, M. (2009). Gastric acid reduction leads to an alteration in lower intestinal microflora. *Biochem Biophys Res Commun*, 381, 4, 666–670.

Karpinski, P., Myszka, A., Ramsey, D., Kielan, W. & Sasiadek, M. M. (2011). Detection of viral DNA sequences in sporadic colorectal cancers in relation to CpG island methylation and methylator phenotype. *Tumour Biol*, 32, 4, 653-659.

Kawano, A., Ishikawa, H., Kamano, T., Kanoh, M., Sakamoto, K., Nakamura, T., Otani, T., Sakai, T. & Kono, K. (2010). Significance of fecal deoxycholic Acid concentration for colorectal tumor enlargement. *Asian Pacific J Cancer Prev*, 11, 6, 1541-1546

Kean, J. M., Rao, S., Wang, M. & Garcea, R. L. (2009). Seroepidemiology of Human Polyomaviruses. *PLoS Pathog*, 5, 3, e1000363.

Keenan, J. I., Beaugie, C. R., Jasmann, B., Potter, H. C., Collett, J. A., Frizelle, F. A. (2010). *Helicobacter* species in the human colon. *Colorectal Dis*, 12, 1, 48-53

Kermorgant, S. & Lehy, T. (2001). Glycine-extended gastrin promotes the invasiveness of human colon cancer cells. *Biochem Biophys Res Commun*, 285, 1, 136–141.

Keusch, G. T. (1974). Opportunistic infections in colon carcinoma *Am J Clin Nutr*, 27, 12, 1481-1485.

Khalili, K., Del Valle, L., Otte, J., Weaver, M. & Gordon, J. (2003a). Human neurotropic polyomavirus, JCV, and its role in carcinogenesis. *Oncogene*, 22, 33, 5181–5191.

Kim, J. H., Park, H. J., Cho, J. S., Lee, K. S., Lee, S. I., Park, I. S., & Kim, C. K. (1999). Relationship of CagA to serum gastrin concentrations and antral G, D cell densities in *Helicobacter pylori* infection. *Yonsei Med J*, 40, 4, 301–306.

Kim, J. M., Cho, S. J., Oh, Y. K., Jung, H. Y., Kim, Y. J. & Kim, N. (2002). Nuclear factor-kappa B activation pathway in intestinal epithelial cells is a major regulator of chemokine gene expression and neutrophil migration induced by *Bacteroides fragilis* enterotoxin. *Clin Exp Immunol*, 130, 1, 59-66

Kim, J. M., Oh, Y.K., Oh, H. B. & Cho, Y. J. (2001). Polarized secretion of CXC chemokines by human intestinal epithelial cells in response to *Bacteroides fragilis* enterotoxin: NF-jB plays a major role in the regulation of IL-8 expression. *Clin Exp Immunol*, 123, 3, 421–427.

Kim, S. C., Tonkonogy, S. L., Karrasch, T., Jobin, C. & Sartor, R. B. (2007). Dual-association of gnotobiotic IL-10-/- mice with 2 nonpathogenic commensal bacteria induces aggressive pancolitis. *Inflamm Bowel Dis*, 13, 12, 1457-1466.

Kim, S. C., Tonkonogy, S.L., Albright, C.A., Tsang, J., Balish, E. J., Braun, J., Huycke, M. M. & Sartor, R. B. (2005). Variable phenotypes of enterocolitis in interleukin 10-deficient mice monoassociated with two different commensal bacteria. *Gastroenterology*, 128, 4, 891–906.

Kirgan, D., Manalo, P., Hall, M. & McGregor, B. (1990). Association of human papillomavirus and colon neoplasms. *Arch Surg*, 125, 7, 862–865.

Klein, R. S., Catalano, M. T., Edberg, S. C., Casey, J. I., Steigbigel, N. H. (1979). *Streptococcus bovis* septicemia and carcinoma of the colon. *Ann Intern Med*, 91, 4, 560 – 562.

Klein, R. S., Recco, R. A., Catalano, M. T., Edberg, S. C., Casey, J. I., Steigbigel, N. H. (1977). Association of *Streptococcus bovis* with carcinoma of the colon. *N Engl J Med*, 297, 15, 800–802.

Koh, T. J., Dockray, G. J., Varro, A., Cahill, R. J., Dangler, C. A., Fox, J. G. & Wang, T. C. (1999). Overexpression of glycine-extended gastrin in transgenic mice results in increased colonic proliferation. *J Clin Invest*, 103, 8, 1119–1126.

Konda, A. & Duffy, M. C. (2008). Surveillance of patients at increased risk of colon cancer: inflammatory bowel disease and other conditions. *Gastroenterol Clin North Am*, 37, 1, 191-213

Koriyama, C., Akiba, S., Iriya, K., Yamaguti, T., Hamada, G. S., Itoh, T., Eizuru, Y., Aikou, T., Watanabe, S., Tsugane, S. & Tokunaga, M. (2001). Epstein-Barr virus-associated gastric carcinoma in Japanese Brazilians and non-Japanese Brazilians in Sao Paulo. *Jpn J Cancer Res*, 92, 9, 911–917.

Koulos, J., Symmans, F., Chumas, J. & Nuovo, G. (1991). Human papillomavirus detection in adenocarcinoma of the anus. *Mod Pathol*, 4, 1, 58–61.

Koutsky, L. (1997). Epidemiology of genital human papillomavirus infection. *Am J Me*, 102, 5A, 3–8.

Kupferwasser, I., Darius, H., Muller, A. M., Mohr-Kahaly, S., Westermeier, T., Oelert, H., Erbel, R. & Meyer, J. (1998). Clinical and morphological characteristics in *Streptococcus bovis* endocarditis: a comparison with other causative microorganisms in 177 cases. *Heart*, 80, 3, 276–280.

Labrecque, L. G., Barnes, D. M., Fentiman, I. S. & Griffin, B. E. (1995). Epstein-Barr virus in epithelial cell tumors: a breast cancer study. *Cancer Res*, 55, 1, 39–45.

Laghi, L., Randolph, A. E., Chauhan, D. P., Marra, G., Major, E. O., Neel, J. V., Boland, C. R. (1999). JC virus DNA is present in the mucosa of the human colon and in colorectal cancers. *Proc Natl Acad Sci U S A*, 96, 13, 7484–7489.

Lee, Y. M., Leu, S. Y., Chiang, H., Fung, C. P. & Liu, W. T. (2001). Human papillomavirus type 18 in colorectal cancer. *J Microbiol Immunol Infect*, 34, 2, 87–91.

Legakis, N., Ioannides, H., Tzannetis, S., Golematis, B. & Papavassiliou, J. (1981). Faecal bacterial flora in patients with colon cancer and control subjects. *Zentralbl Bakteriol Mikrobiol Hyg A*, 251, 1, 54-61

Li, A., Varney, M. L. & Singh, R. K. (2001). Expression of interleukin 8 and its receptors in human colon carcinoma cells with different metastatic potentials. *Clin Cancer Res*, 7, 10, 3298–3304

Limburg, P. J., Stolzenberg-Solomon, R. Z., Colbert, L.H., Perez-Perez, G. I., Blaser, M. J., Taylor, P. R., Virtamo, J. & Albanes, D. (2002). *Helicobacter pylori* seropositivity and colorectal cancer risk: a prospective study of male smokers. *Cancer Epidemiol Biomarkers Prev*, 11, 10, 1095–1099.

Lin, M., Hanai, J. & Gui, L. (1998). Peanut lectin-binding sites and mucins in benign and malignant colorectal tissues associated with schistomatosis. *Histol Histopathol*, 1998, 13, 4, 961-966.

Lin, P. Y., Fung, C. Y., Chang, F. P., Huang, W. S., Chen, W. C., Wang, J. Y. & Chang, D. (2008). Prevalence and genotype identification of human JC virus in colon cancer in Taiwan. *J Med Virol*, 80, 10, 1828–1834.

Lin, Y. L., Chiang, J. K., Lin, S. M. & Tseng, C. E. (2010). *Helicobacter pylori* infection concomitant with metabolic syndrome further increase risk of colorectal adenomas. *World J Gastroenterol*, 16, 30, 3841-3846.

Link, A., Shin, S. K., Nagasaka, T., Balaguer, F., Koi, M., Jung, B., Boland, C. R. & Goel, A. (2009). JC virus mediates invasion and migration in colorectal metastasis. *PLoS One*, 4, 12, e8146.

Liou, J. M., Lin, J. W., Huang, S. P., Lin, J. T. & Wu, M. S. (2006). *Helicobacter pylori* infection is not associated with increased risk of colorectal polyps in Taiwanese. *Int J Cancer*, 119, 8, 1999 – 2000

Little, J., Owen, R. W., Femandez, F., Hawtin, P. G., Hill, M. J., Logan, R. F., Thompson, M. H. & Hardcastle, J. D. (2002). Asymptomatic colorectal neoplasia and fecal characteristics: a case-control study of subjects participating in the Nottingham fecal occult blood screening trial. *Dis Colon Rectum*, 45, 9, 1233-1241.

Liu, H. X., Ding, Y. Q., Li, X. & Yao, K. T. (2003). Investigation of Epstein-Barr virus in Chinese colorectal tumors. *World J Gastroenterol*, 9, 11, 2464–2468.

Liu, H. X., Ding, Y. Q., Sun, Y. O., Liang, L., Yang, Y. F., Qi, Z. L., Liu, J. H. & Xiong, P. X. (2002). Detection of Epstein-Barr virus in human colorectal cancer by in situ hybridization. *Di Yi Jun Yi Da Xue Xue Bao*, 22, 10, 915–917.

Long, X. C., Bahgat, M., Chlichlia, K., Ruppel, A. & Li, Y. L. (2004). Detection of inducible nitric oxide synthase in *Schistosoma japonicum* and *S. mansoni*. *J Helminthol*, 78, 1, 47-50.

Ludlow, J. W. (1993). Interactions between SV40 large-tumor antigen and the growth suppressor proteins *pRB* and *p53*. *FASEB J*, 7, 866–871.

Lundstig, A., Stattin, P., Persson, K., Sasnauskas, K., Viscidi, R. P., Gislefoss, R. E. & Dillner, J. (2007). No excess risk for colorectal cancer among subjects seropositive for the JC polyomavirus. *Int J Cancer*, 121, 5, 1098–1102.

Machida-Montani, A., Sasazuki, S., Inoue, M., Natsukawa, S., Shaura, K., Koizumi, Y., Kasuga, Y., Hanaoka, T. & Tsugane, S. (2007). Atrophic gastritis, Helicobacter pylori, and colorectal cancer risk: a case-control study. *Helicobacter*, 12, 4, 328–332.

Madbouly, K. M., Senagore, A. J., Mukerjee, A., Hussien, A. M., Shehata, M. A., Navine. P., Delaney, C. P. & Fazio, V. W. (2007). Colorectal cancer in a population with endemic *Schistosoma mansoni*: is this an at-risk population?. *Int J Colorectal Dis*, 22, 2, 175-181

Maddocks, O. D., Short, A. J., Donnenberg, M. S., Bader, S. & Harrison, D. J. (2009). Attaching and effacing *Escherichia coli* downregulate DNA mismatch repair protein in vitro and are associated with colorectal adenocarcinomas in humans. *PLoS One*, 4, 5, e5517.

Martin, H. M., Campbell, B. J., Hart, C. A., Mpofu, C., Nayar, M., Singh, R., Englyst, H., Williams, H. F. & Rhodes, J. M. (2004). Enhanced *Escherichia coli* adherence and invasion in Crohn's disease and colon cancer. *Gastroenterology*, 127, 1, 80–93.

Matsuda, K., Masaki, T., Ishii, S., Yamashita, H., Watanabe, T., Nagawa, H., Muto, T., Hirata, Y., Kimura, K. & Kojima, S. (1999). Possible associations of rectal carcinoma with *schistosoma japonicum* infection and membranous nephropathy: a case report with a review. *Jpn J Clin Oncol*, 29, 11, 576-578.

Mayer, D. A. & Fried, B. (2007). The Role of Helminth Infections in Carcinogenesis, In: *Advances in Parasitology*, Vol 65, Muller, R., Rollinson, D., & Hay, S. I., 239-296, Academic Press, London.

McGregor, B., Byrne, P., Kirgan, D., Albright, J., Manalo, P. & Hall, M. (1993). Confirmation of the association of humanpapillomavirus with human colon cancer. *Am J Surg*, 166, 6, 738–740.

McLaughlin-Drubin, M. E. & Munger, K. (2008). Viruses associated with human cancer. *Biochim Biophys Acta*, 1782, 3, 127-150.

Meucci, G., Tatarella, M., Vecchi, M., Ranzi, M. L., Biguzzi, E., Beccari, G., Clerici, E. & de Franchis, R. (1997). High prevalence of *Helicobacter pylori* infection in patients with colonic adenomas and carcinomas. *J Clin Gastroenterol*, 25, 4, 605–607.

Militello, V., Trevisan, M., Squarzon, L., Biasolo, M. A., Rugge, M., Militello, C., Palù, G. & Barzon, L. (2009). Investigation on the presence of polyomavirus, herpesvirus, and papillomavirus sequences in colorectal neoplasms and their association with cancer. *Int J Cancer*, 124, 10, 2501-2503.

Ming-Chai, C., Chang, P. Y., Chuang, C. Y., Chen, Y. J., Wang, F. P., Tang, Y. C. & Chou, S. C. (1981). Colorectal cancer and schistomiasis. *Lancet*, 1, 8227, 971-973.

Ming-Chai, C., Chi-Yuan, C., Pei-Yu, C. & Jen-Chun, H. (1980). Evolution of colorectal cancer in schistosomiasis: transitional mucosal changes adjacent to large intestinal carcinoma in colectomy specimens. *Cancer*, 46, 7, 1661-1675

Ming-Chai, C., Hu, J. C., Chang, P. Y., Chuang, C. Y., Tsao, P. F., Chang, S. H., Wang, F. P., Ch'en, T. L. & Chou, S. C. (1965), Pathogenesis of carcinoma of the colon and rectum in schistosomiasis japonica: a study on 90 cases. *Chin Med J*, 84, 8, 513-525.

Mizuno, S., Morita, Y., Inui, T., Asakawa, A., Ueno, N., Ando, T., Kato, H., Uchida, M., Yoshikawa, T. & Inui, A. (2005) *Helicobacter pylori* infection is associated with colon adenomatous polyps detected by high-resolution colonoscopy. *Int J Cancer*, 117, 6, 1058-1059.

Mohamed, A. R., Al Karawi, M. A. & Yasawy, M. I. (1990). Schistosomal colonic disease. *Gut*, 31,4, ,439-442

Moore, W. E. & Moore, L. H. (1995). Intestinal flora of populations that have a high risk for colon cancer. *Appl Env Microbiol*, 61, 9, 3202-3207.

Moss, S. F., Neugut, A. I., Garbowski, G. C., Wang, S., Treat, M. R. & Forde, K. A. (1995). *Helicobacter pylori* seroprevalence and colorectal neoplasia: evidence against an association. *J Natl Cancer Inst*, 87, 10, 762-763.

Muhlemann, K., Graf, S. & Tauber, M. G. (1999). *Streptococcus bovis* clone causing two episodes of endocarditis 8 years apart. *J Clin Microbiol*, 37, 3, 862-863.

Munoz, N., Bosch, F. X., de Sanjose, S., Herrero, R., Castellsagué, X., Shah, K.mV., Snijders, P. J. & Meijer, C. J. (2003). Epidemiologic classification of human papillomavirus types associated with cervical cancer. *N Engl J Med*, 348, 6, 518-527.

Murray, H. W. & Roberts, R. B. (1978). *Streptococcus bovis* bacteremia and underlying gastrointestinal disease. *Arch Intern Med*, 138, 7, 1097 - 1099.

Newcomb, P. A., Bush, A. C., Stoner, G. L., Lampe, J. W., Potter, J. D. & Bigler, J. (2004). No evidence of an association of JC virus and colon neoplasia. Cancer Epidemiol Biomarkers Prev, 13, 4, 662-666.

Nguyen, I., Biarc, J., Pini, A., Gosse, F., Richert, S., Thierse, D., Van Dorsselaer, A., Leize-Wagner, E., Raul, F., Klein, J. P., Scholler-Guinard, M. (2006). *Streptococcus infantarius* and colonic cancer: Identification and purification of cell wall proteins putatively involved in colorectal inflammation and carcinogenesis in rats. *International Congress Series*, 1289, 257-261.

Niv, Y., Vilkin, A. & Levi, Z. (2010b). Patients with sporadic colorectal cancer or advanced adenomatous polyp have elevated anti-JC virus antibody titer in comparison with healthy controls: a cross-sectional study. *J Clin Gastroenterol*, 44, 7, 489-494.

Niv, Y., Vilkin, A., Brenner, B., Kendel, Y., Morgenstern, S. & Levi, Z. (2010a). hMLH1 promoter methylation and JC virus T antigen presence in the tumor tissue of colorectal cancer Israeli patients of different ethnic groups. *Eur J Gastroenterol Hepatol*, 22, 8, 938-941.

Norfleet, R. G. & Mitchell, R. G. (1993). *Streptococcus bovis* does not selectively colonize colorectal cancer and polyps. *J Clin Gastroenterol*, 17, 1, 25-28.

Nosho, K., Shima, K., Kure, S., Irahara, N., Baba, Y., Chen, L., Kirkner, G. J., Fuchs, C. S. & Ogino, S. (2009). JC virus T-antigen in colorectal cancer is associated with p53 expression and chromosomal instability, independent of CpG island methylator phenotype. *Neoplasia*, 11, 1, 87-95.

Nosho, K., Yamamoto, H., Takahashi, T., Mikami, M., Hizaki, K., Maehata, T., Taniguchi, H., Yamaoka, S., Adachi, Y., Itoh, F., Imai, K. & Shinomura, Y. (2008). Correlation of laterally spreading type and JC virus with methylator phenotype status in colorectal adenoma. *Hum Pathol*, 39, 5, 767–775.

Ogino, S., Nosho, K., Irahara, N., Shima, K., Baba, Y., Kirkner, G. J., Meyerhardt, J. A. & Fuchs, C. S. (2009). Prognostic significance and molecular associations of 18q loss of heterozygosity: a cohort study of microsatellite stable colorectal cancers. *J Clin Oncol*, 27, 27, 4591–4598.

Ohshima, H. & Bartsch, H. (1994). Chronic infections and inflammatory processes as cancer risk factors: possible role of nitric oxide in carcinogenesis. *Mutat Res*, 305, 2, 253–264.

Ojo, O. S., Odesanmi, W. O. & Akinola, O. O. (1991). The surgical pathology of colorectal carcinoma in Nigerians. *Trop Gastroenterol*, 13, 2, 180-184.

Osada, Y., Kumagai, T., Masuda, K., Suzuki, T. & Kanazawa, T. (2005). Mutagenicity evaluation of *Schistosoma* spp. extracts by the umu-test and V79/HGPRT gene mutation assay. *Parasitol Int*, 54, 1, 29-34.

Pagano, J. S., Blaser, M., Buendia, M. A., Damania, B., Khalili, K., Raab-Traub, N. & Roizman, B. (2004). Infectious agents and cancer: criteria for a causal relation. *Semin Cancer Biol*, 14, 6, 453-471

Parkin, D. M. (2006). The global health burden of infection-associated cancers in the year 2002. *Int J Cancer*, 118, 12, 3030–3044.

Parkin, D. M., Arslan, A., Bieber, A., Bouvy, O., Muir, C.S., Owor, R. & Whelan, S. (1986). Cancer Occurrence in Developing Countries, In: *International Agency for Research on Cancer (IARC) Scientific Publication No. 75*, IARC Press, Lyon, France.

Parsonnet, J. (1995). Bacterial infection as a cause of cancer. *Environ Health Perspect*, 103, Suppl 8, 263-268.

Peek, R. M., Jr., Miller, G. G., Tham, K. T., Perez-Perez, G. I., Zhao, X., Atherton, J. C., and Blaser, M. J. (1995). Heightened inflammatory response and cytokine expression in vivo to cagA+ *Helicobacter pylori* strains. *Lab Investig*, 73, 6, 760–770.

Peiffer, L. P., Peters, D. J. & McGarrity, T. J. (1997). Differential effects of deoxycholic acid on proliferation of neoplastic and differentiated colonocytes in vitro. *Dig Dis Sci*, 42, 11, 2234-2240.

Penman, I. D., el-Omar, E., Ardill, J. E., McGregor, J. R., Galloway, D. J., O'Dwyer, P. J., McColl, K. E. (1994). Plasma gastrin concentrations are normal in patients with colorectal neoplasia and unaltered following tumour resection. *Gastroenterology*, 106, 5, 1263–1270.

Perez, L. O., Abba, M. C., Laguens, R. M. & Golijow, C. D. (2005). Analysis of adenocarcinoma of the colon and rectum: detection of human papillomavirus (HPV) DNA by polymerase chain reaction. *Colorectal Dis*, 7, 5, 492–495.

Pergola, V., Di Salvo, G., Habib, G., Avierinos, J. F., Philip, E., Vailloud, J. M., Thuny, F., Casalta, J. P., Ambrosi, P., Lambert, M., Riberi, A., Ferracci, A., Mesana, T., Metras, D., Harle, J. R., Weiller, P. J., Raoult, D. & Luccioni, R. (2001). Comparison of clinical and echocardiographic characteristics of *Streptococcus bovis* endocarditis with that caused by other pathogens. *Am J Cardiol*, 88, 8, 871–875.

Pigrau, C., Lorente, A., Pahissa, A. & Martinez-Vazquez, J. M. (1988) *Streptococcus bovis* bacteremia and digestive system neoplasms. *Scand J Infect Dis*, 20, 4, 459–460.

Plummer, S.M., Grafstrom, R.C., Yang, L. L., Curren, R. D., Linnainmaa, K. & Harris, C. C. (1986). Fecapentaene-12 causes DNA damage and mutations in human cells. *Carcinogenesis*, 7, 9, 1607-1609.

Potter, M. A., Cunliffe, N. A., Smith, M., Miles, R. S., Flapan, A. D. & Dunlop, M. G. (1998). A prospective controlled study of the association of *Streptococcus bovis* with colorectal carcinoma. *J Clin Pathol*, 51, 6, 473 -474.

Prindiville, T. P., Sheikh, R. A., Cohen, S. H., Tang, Y. J., Cantrell, M. C. & Silva, J. Jr. (2000). *Bacteroides fragilis* enterotoxin gene sequences in patients with inflammatory bowel disease. *Emerg Infect Dis*, 6, 2, 171–174.

Qiu, D. C., Hubbard, A. E., Zhong, B., Zhang, Y. & Spear, R. C. (2005). A matched, case control study of the association between *Schistosoma japonicum* and liver and colon cancers, in rural China. *Ann Trop Med Parasitol*, 99, 1, 47-52

Reddy, B. S. & Wynder, E.L.. (1977). Metabolic epidemiology of colon cancer: fecal bile acids and neutral sterols in colon cancer patients and patients with adenomas polyps. *Cancer*, 39, 6, 1533-1539.

Renga, M., Brandi, G., Paganelli, G. M., Calabrese, C., Papa, S., Tosti, A., Tomassetti, P, Miglioli, M. & Biasco, G. (1997). Rectal cell proliferation and colon cancer risk in patients with hypergastrinaemia. *Gut*, 41, 3, 330–332.

Rex, D. (2000). Should we colonoscope women with gynecologic cancer? *Am J Gastroenterol*, 95, 3, 812–813.

Reynolds, J. G., Silva, E. & McCormack, W. M. (1983). Association of *Streptococcus bovis* bacteremia with bowel disease. *J Clin Microbiol*, 17, 4, 696–697.

Rhee, K. J., Wu, S., Wu, X., Huso, D. L., Karim, B., Franco, A. A., Rabizadeh, S., Golub, J. E., Mathews, L. E., Shin, J., Sartor, R. B., Golenbock, D., Hamad, A. R., Gan, C. M., Housseau, F. & Sears, C. L. (2009). Induction of persistent colitis by a human commensal, enterotoxigenic *Bacteroides fragilis*, in wild-type C57BL/6 mice. *Infect Immun*, 77, 4, 1708–1718.

Ricciardiello, L., Baglioni, M., Giovannini, C., Pariali, M., Cenacchi, G., Ripalti, A., Landini, M. P., Sawa, H., Nagashima, K., Frisque, R. J., Goel, A., Boland, C. R., Tognon, M., Roda, E. & Bazzoli, F. (2003). Induction of chromosomal instability in colonic cells by the human polyomavirus JC virus. *Cancer Res*, 63, 21, 7256–7262.

Ricciardiello, L., Chang, D. K., Laghi, L., Goel, A., Chang, C. L. & Boland, C. R. (2001). Mad-1 is the exclusive JC virus strain present in the human colon, and its transcriptional control region has a deleted 98-base-pair sequence in colon cancer tissues. *J Virol*, 75, 4, 1996–2001.

Ricciardiello, L., Laghi, L., Ramamirtham, P., Chang, C. L., Chang, D. K., Randolph, A. E. & Boland, C. R. (2000). JC virus DNA sequences are frequently present in the human upper and lower gastrointestinal tract. *Gastroenterology*, 119, 5, 1228–1235.

Robbins, N. & Klein, R. S. (1983). Carcinoma of the colon 2 years after endocarditis due to *Streptococcus bovis*. *Am J Gastroenterol*, 78, 3, 162–163.

Robertson, D. J., Sandler, R. S., Ahnen, D. J., Greenberg, E. R., Mott, L. A., Cole, B. F. & Baron, J. A. (2009). Gastrin, *Helicobacter pylori*, and colorectal adenomas, 7, 2, 163-167.

Rollison, D. E., Helzlsouer, K. J., Lee, J. H., Fulp, W., Clipp, S., Hoffman-Bolton, J. A., Giuliano, A. R., Platz, E. A. & Viscidi, R. P. (2009). Prospective study of JC virus seroreactivity and the development of colorectal cancers and adenomas. *Cancer Epidemiol Biomarkers Prev*, 18, 5, 1515-1523.

Rosin, M. P., Anwar, W. A. & Ward, A. J. (1994). Inflammation, chromosomal instability, and cancer: the schistosomiasis model. *Cancer Res*, 54, Suppl 7, 1929-1933.

Ross, A. G., Bartley, P. B., Sleigh, A. C., Olds, G. R., Li, Y., Williams, G. M. & McManus, D. P. (2002). Schistosomiasis. *N Engl J Med*, 346, 16, 1212-1220.

Ruger, R. & Fleckenstein, B. (1985). Cytomegalovirus DNA in colorectal carcinoma tissues. *Klin Wochenschr*, 63, 9, 405–408.

Ruoff, K. L., Miller, S. I., Garner, C. V., Ferraro, M. J. & Calderwood S. B. (1989). Bacteremia with *Streptococcus bovis* and *Streptococcus salivarius*: clinical correlates of more accurate identification of isolates. *J Clin Microbiol*, 27, 2, 305–308.

Ruoff, K.L., Whiley, R. A. & Beighton, D. (1999). Streptococcus, In: *Manual of Clinical Microbiology*, 7th edn. P. R. Murray, E. J. Baron, M. A. Pfaller, F. C. Tenover, and R. H. Yolken (ed.), 283–296, ASM press, Washington, D.C.

Sanfiloppo, L., Li, C. K., Seth, R., Balwin, T. J., Menozzi, M. G. & Mahida, Y. R. (2000). *Bacteroides fragilis* enterotoxin induces the expression of IL-8 and transforming growth factor beta by human colonic epithelial cells. *Clin Exp Immunol*, 119, 3, 456–463.

Schiffman, M. H., Van Tassell, R. L., Robinson, A., Smith, L., Daniel, J., Hoover, R. N., Weil, R., Rosenthal, J., Nair, P. P., Schwartz, S. (1989). Case-control study colorectal cancer and fecapentaene excretion. *Cancer Res*, 49, 5, 1322–1326.

Schlegel, L., Grimont, F., Ageron, E., Grimont, P. A. & Bouvet, A. (2003). Reappraisal of the taxonomy of the *Streptococcus bovis/Streptococcus equines* complex and related species: description of *Streptococcus gallolyticus* subsp. *gallolyticus* subsp. nov., *S. gallolyticus* subsp. *macedonicus* subsp. nov. and *S. gallolyticus* subsp. *pasteurianus* subsp. nov. *Int J Syst Evol Micribiol*, 53, 3, 631–645.

Sears, C. L., Islam, S., Saha, A., Arjumand, M., Alam, N. H., Faruque, A. S., Salam, M. A., Shin, J., Hecht, D., Weintraub, A., Sack, R. B. & Qadri, F. (2008). Association enterotoxigenic *Bacteroides fragilis* infection with inflammatory diarrhea. *Clin Infect Dis*, 47, 6, 797–803.

Selgrad, M., Koornstra, J. J., Fini, L., Blom, M., Huang, R., Devol, E. B., Boersma-van Ek, W., Dijkstra, G., Verdonk, R. C, de Jong, S., Goel, A., Williams, S. L., Meyer, R. L., Haagsma, E. B., Ricciardiello, L. & Boland, C. R. (2008). JC virus infection in colorectal neoplasia that develops after liver transplantation. *Clin Cancer Res*, 14, 20, 6717–6721.

Shah, K. V. (1996). Polyomaviruses, In: *Fields Virology*, B. N. Fields, D. M. Knipe, P. M. Howley, (Eds), 2027–2043, Lippincott-Raven, Philadelphia, USA.

Shah, K. V., Daniel, R. W., Simons, J. W. & Vogelstein, B. (1992). Investigation of colon cancers for human papillomavirus genomic sequences by polymerase chain reaction. *J Surg Oncol*, 51, 1, 5–7.

Shin, S. K., Li, M. S., Fuerst, F., Hotchkiss, E., Meyer, R., Kim, I. T., Goel, A. & Boland, C. R. (2006). Oncogenic T-antigen of JC virus is present frequently in human gastric cancers. *Cancer*, 107, 3, 481-488.

Shindo, K. (1976). Significance of schistosomiasis japonica in the development of cancer of the large intestine: Report of a case and review of the literature. *Dis Colon Rectum*, 19, 5, 460-469.

Shmuely, H., Passaro, D., Figer, A., Niv, Y., Pitlik, S., Samra, Z., Koren, R. & Yahav, J. (2001). Relationship between *Helicobacter pylori* CagA status and colorectal cancer. *Am J Gastroenterol*, 96, 12, 3406-3410.

Shroyer, K. R., Kim, J. G., Manos, M. M., Greer, C. E., Pearlman, N. W. & Franklin, W. A. (1992). Papillomavirus found in anorectal squamous carcinoma, not in colon adenocarcinoma. *Arch Surg*, 127, 6, 741-744.

Siddheshwar, R. K., Muhammad, K. B., Gray, J. C. & Kelly, S. B. (2001). Seroprevalence of *Helicobacter pylori* in patients with colorectal polyps and colorectal carcinoma. *Am J Gastroenterol*, 96, 1, 84-88.

Singh, P., Velasco, M., Given, R., Varro, A. & Wang T. C. (2000a). Progastrin expression predisposes mice to development of colon carcinomas and adenomas in response to AOM. *Gastroenterology*, 119, 1, 162-171.

Singh, P., Velasco, M., Given, R., Wargovich, M., Varro, A. & Wang, T. C. (2000b). Mice overexpressing progastrin are predisposed for developing aberrant colonic crypt foci in response to AOM. *Am J Physiol Gastrointest Liver Physiol*, 278, 3, G390-399.

Slattery, M. L., Curtin, K., Schaffer, D., Anderson, K. & Samowitz, W. (2002). Associations between family history of colorectal cancer and genetic alterations in tumors. *Int J Cancer*, 97, 6, 823-827.

Soliman, A. S., Bondy, M. L., El-Badawy, S. A., Mokhtar, N., Eissa, S., Bayoumy, S., Seifeldin, I. A., Houlihan, P. S., Lukish, J. R., Watanabe, T., Chan, A. O., Zhu, D., Amos, C. I., Levin, B. & Hamilton, S. R. (2001). Contrasting molecular pathology of colorectal carcinoma in Egyptian and Western patients. *Br J Cancer*, 85, 7, 1037-1046.

Song, L. B., Zhang, X., Zhang, C. Q., Zhang, Y., Pan, Z. Z., Liao, W. T., Li, M. Z. & Zeng, M. S. (2006). Infection of Epstein-Barr virus in colorectal cancer in Chinese. *Ai Zheng*, 25, 11, 1356-1360.

Soylu, A., Ozkara, S., Alis, H., Dolay, K., Kalayci, M., Yasar, N. & Kumbasar, A. B. (2008). Immunohistochemical testing for *Helicobacter Pylori* existence in neoplasms of the colon. *BMC Gastroenterol*, 14, 8, 35.

Steenbergen, R. D., de Wilde, J., Wilting, S. M., Brink, A. A., Snijders, P. J., Meijer, C. J. (2005). HPV-mediated transformation of the anogenital tract. *J Clin Virol*, 2005; 32, 1, S25-33.

Swidsinski, A., Khilkin, M., Kerjaschki, D., Schreiber, S., Ortner, M., Weber, J. & Lochs H. (1998). Association between intraepithelial *Escherichia coli* and colorectal cancer. *Gastroenterology*, 115, 2, 281-286.

Takada, K. (2000). Epstein-Barr virus and gastric carcinoma. *Mol Pathol*, 53, 5, 255-261.

Takeda, H. & Asaka, M. (2005) *Helicobacter pylori* and colorectal neoplasm: a mysterious link? *J Gastroenterol*, 40, 9, 919-920.

Theodoropoulos, G., Panoussopoulos, D., Papaconstantinou, I., Gazouli, M., Perdiki, M., Bramis, J. & Lazaris, A. Ch. (2005). Assessment of JC polyoma virus in colon neoplasms. *Dis Colon Rectum*, 48, 1, 86–91.

Thorburn, C. M., Friedman, G. D., Dickinson, C. J., Vogelman, J. H., Orentreich, N. & Parsonnet, J. (1998). Gastrin and colorectal cancer: a prospective study. *Gastroenterology*, 115, 2, 275–280.

Tjalsma, H., Scholler-Guinard, M., Lasonder, E., Ruers, T. J., Willems, H. L. & Swinkels, D. W. (2006). Profiling the humoral immune response in colon cancer patients: diagnostic antigens from *Streptococcus bovis*. *Int J Cancer*, 119, 9, 2127–2135.

Toprak, N. U., Yagci, A., Gulluoglu, B. M., Akin, M. L., Demirkalem, P., Celenk, T. and Soyletir. G. (2006). A possible role of *Bacteroides fragilis* enterotoxin in the aetiology of colorectal cancer. *Clin Microbiol Infect*, 12, 8, 782–786.

Trakatelli, C., Frydas, S., Hatzistilianou, M., Papadopoulos, E., Simeonidou, I., Founta, A., Paludi, D., Petrarca, C., Castellani, M. L., Papaioannou, N., Salini, V., Conti, P., Kempuraj, D. & Vecchiet, J. (2005). Chemokines as markers for parasiteinduced inflammation and tumors. *Int J Biol Markers*, 20, 4, 197-203

Tripodi, M. F., Adinolfi, L. E., Ragone, E., Durante-Mangoni, E., Fortunato, R., Iarussi, D., Ruggiero, G. & Utili, R. (2004). *Streptococcus bovis* endocarditis and its association with chronic liver disease: an underestimated risk factor. *Clin Infect Dis*, 38, 10, 1394–1400.

Tuazon, C. U., Nash, T., Cheever, A. & Neva, F. (1985). Interaction of *Schistosoma japonicum* with *Salmonellae* and other gram-negative bacteria. *J Infect Dis*, 152, 4, 722-726.

van Riet, E., Hartgers, F. C. & Yazdanbakhsh, M. (2007). Chronic helminth infections induce immunomodulation: consequences and mechanisms. *Immunobiology*, 212, 6, 475-490

Vaska, V. L. & Faoagali, J. L. (2009) *Streptococcus bovis* bacteraemia: identification within organism complex and association with endocarditis and colonic malignancy. *Pathology*, 41, 2, 183-186.

Vennervald, B. J. & Polman, K. (2009). Helminths and malignancy. *Parasite Immunol*, 31, 11, 686-696.

Waku, M., Napolitano, L., Clementini, E., Staniscia, T., Spagnolli, C., Andama, A., Kasiriye, P. & Innocenti, P. (2005). Risk of cancer onset in sub-Saharan Africans affected with chronic gastrointestinal parasitic diseases. *Int J Immunopathol Pharmacol*, 18, 3, 503-511.

Wang, L., Yi, T., Kortylewski, M., Pardoll, D. M., Zeng, D. & Yu, H. (2009). IL-17 can promote tumor growth through an IL-6-Stat3 signaling pathway. *J Exp Med*, 206, 7, 1457-1464

Wang, S., Liu, Z., Wang, L. & Zhang, X. (2009). NF-kappaB signaling pathway, inflammation and colorectal cancer. *Cell Mol Immunol*, 6, 5, 327-334.

Wang, T. C., Koh, T. J., Varro, A., Cahill, R. J., Dangler, C. A., Fox, J. G., Dockray, G. J. (1996). Processing and proliferative effects of human progastrin in transgenic mice. *J Clin Invest*, 98, 8, 1918–1929.

Wang, X. & Huycke, M. M. (2007). Extracellular superoxide production by *Enterococcus faecalis* promotes chromosomal instability in mammalian cells. *Gastroenterology*, 132, 2, 551–561.

Wang, X., Allen, T. D., May, R. J., Lightfoot, S., Houchen, C. W. & Huycke, M. M. (2008). *Enterococcus faecalis* induces aneuploidy and tetraploidy in colonic epithelial cells through a bystander effect. *Cancer Res*, 68, 23, 9909–9917.

Weinberg, D. S., Newschaffer, C. J. & Topham, A. (1999). Risk for colorectal cancer after gynecologic cancer. *Ann Intern Med*, 131, 3, 189–193.

Wexler, H. M. (2007). Bacteroides: the good, the bad, and the nitty-gritty. *Clin Microbiol Rev*, 20, 4, 593–621.

Wiley, D. & Masongsong, E. (2006). Human papillomavirus: the burden of infection. *Obstet Gynecol Surv*, 61, 6, S3–14.

Winters, M. D., Schlinke, T. L., Joyce, W. A., Glore, S. R. & Huycke, M. M. (1998). Prospective case-cohort study of intestinal colonization with enterococci that produce extracellular superoxide and the risk for colorectal adenomas or cancer. *Am J Gastroenterol*, 93, 12, 2491–2500.

Wong, M. P., Chung, L, P., Yuen, S. T., Leung, S. Y., Chan, S. Y., Wang, E. & Fu, K. II. (1995). In situ detection of Epstein-Barr virus in nonsmall cell lung carcinomas. *J Pathol*, 177, 3, 233–240.

Wong, N. A., Herbst, H., Herrmann, K., Kirchner, T., Krajewski, A. S., Moorghen, M., Niedobitek, F., Rooney, N., Shepherd, N. A. & Niedobitek, G. (2003). Epstein-Barr virus infection in colorectal neoplasms associated with inflammatory bowel disease: detection of the virus in lymphomas but not in adenocarcinomas. *J Pathol*, 201, 2, 312–318.

World Health Organization. (2003). The global burden of cancer, In: *World Cancer Report*, B. W. Stewart, P. Kleihues, (ed.), pp. 13, IARC Press, Lyon, France.

Wu, S., Lim, K. C., Huang, J., Saidi, R. F. & Sears, C. L. (1998). *Bacteroides fragilis* enterotoxin cleaves the zonula adherens protein, E-cadherin. *Proc Natl Acad Sci*, 95, 25, 14979–14984.

Wu, S., Morin, P. J., Mauyo, D. & Sears, C. (2003). *Bacteroides fragilis* enterotoxin induces c-*myc* expression and cellular proliferation. *Gastroenterology*, 124, 2, 392–400.

Wu, S., Rhee, K. J., Albesiano, E., Rabizadeh, S., Wu, X., Yen, H. R., Huso, D. L., Brancati, F. L., Wick, E., McAllister, F., Housseau, F., Pardoll, D. M. & Sears, C. L. (2009). A human colonic commensal promotes colon tumorigenesis via activation of T helper type 17 T cell responses. *Nat Med*, 15, 9, 1016–1022.

Xu, Z. & Su, D. (1984). *Schistosoma japonicum* and colorectal cancer: an epidemiological study in the People's Republic of China. *Int J Cancer*, 34, 3, 315-318.

Yu, X. R., Chen, P. H., Xu, J. Y., Xiao, S., Shan, Z. J. & Zhu, S. J. (1991). Histological classification of schistosomal egg induced polyps of colon and their clinical significance. An analysis of 272 cases. *Chin Med J(Engl)* 104, 1, 64-70

Yuen, S. T., Chung, L. P., Leung, S. Y., Luk, I. S., Chan, S. Y. & Ho, J. (1994). In situ detection of Epstein-Barr virus in gastric and colorectal adenocarcinomas. *Am J Surg Pathol*, 18, 11, 1158–1163.

Zalata, K. R., Nasif, W. A., Ming, S. C., Lotfy, M., Nada, N. A., El-Hak, N. G & Leech, S. H. (2005). *p53, Bcl-2* and *C-myc* expressions in colorectal carcinoma associated with schistosomiasis in Egypt. *Cell Oncol*, 27, 4, 245-253

Zarkin, B. A., Lillemoe, K. D., Cameron, J. L., Effron, P. N., Magnuson, T. H. & Pitt, H. A. (1990). The triad of *Streptococcus bovis* bacteremia, colonic pathology, and liver disease. *Ann Surg*, 211, 6, 786 – 791

Zhang, R., Takahashi, S., Orita, S., Yoshida, A., Maruyama, H., Shirai, T. & Ohta, N. (1998). *p53* gene mutations in rectal cancer associated with schistosomiasis japonica in Chinese patients. *Cancer Lett*, 131, 2, 215-221.

Zhao, E. S. (1981). Cancer of the colon and schistosomiasis. *J R Soc Med*, 74, 9, 645.

Zhao, Y. S., Wang, F., Chang, D., Han, B. & You, D. Y. (2008). Meta-analysis of different test indicators: *Helicobacter pylori* infection and the risk of colorectal cancer. *Int J Colorectal Dis*, 23, 9, 875-882.

Zumkeller, N., Brenner, H., Chang-Claude, J., Hoffmeister, M., Nieters, A., Rothenbacher, D. (2007). *Helicobacter pylori* infection, interleukin-1 gene polymorphisms and the risk of colorectal cancer: evidence from a case-control study in Germany. *Eur J Cancer*, 43, 8, 1283–1289.

Zumkeller, N., Brenner, H., Zwahlen, M. & Rothenbacher, D. (2006). *Helicobacter pylori* infection and colorectal cancer risk: a meta-analysis. *Helicobacter*, 11, 2, 75 – 80.

7

Adaptive and Innate Immunity, Non Clonal Players in Colorectal Cancer Progression

Lucia Fini, Fabio Grizzi and Luigi Laghi

Laboratory of Molecular Gastroenterology and Department of Gastroenterology,
IRCCS Istituto Clinico Humanitas, Rozzano, Milan,
Italy

1. Introduction

The progression of colorectal cancer (CRC), like that of other solid tumors, has been first conceptualized by pathological staging (initially according to Dukes and later by the AJCC/UICC TNM staging system) as a step-wise invasion of bowel layers, followed by lymph-node involvement, to culminate into distant organ metastasis [1]. Additionally, the recognition of pre-cancerous lesions (*i.e.*, adenoma) set up the notion that cancer develops from a benign lesion, according to an adenoma-to-adenocarcinoma sequence. In the last two decades, the anatomic frame of progression has been embraced by the molecular genetic model of CRC, according to which accumulation of gene damage drives progression from adenoma to cancer, subsequently leading to the emergence of invasive and spreading clones [2]. Gene damage is known to be driven from two types of genetic instabilities: microsatellite (MSI) and chromosomal (CIN) instability. More recently, the epigenetic silencing of tumor suppressor genes, namely CpG island methylator phenotype (CIMP), has been claimed as a distinct pathway of colorectal carcinogenesis **(Table 1)** [3].

Moving from this cornerstone, current research is exploring non-clonal determinants of tumor progression **(Table 1)**[4,5]. Collectively referred to as "tumor microenvironment" these factors can restrain or fuel tumor development and fate, and comprise infiltrating immune cells, neo-vessels, activated fibroblasts, and mesenchymal stem cells [6]. Not acting like a tumor scaffold, rather actively signaling with neoplastic cells, microenvironment influences the selection and emergence of aggressive clones, as well as their dissemination. In a bi-directional way, tumor molecular features influence the nearby environment by expressing tumor antigens, while tumor microenvironment influences the molecular changes, controlling the tumor growth. Additionally, chemokines and their receptors can be expressed as well by cancer cells and by non-neoplastic cells, influencing clonal expansion and cancer spread [4]. The role of microenvironment in cancer promoting dynamics is well established, providing cancer cells with oxygen, growth factors and nutrients, which can impact on tumor growth, progression and dissemination. However, the contribution of persistent inflammation in the carcinogenesis process encourages anti-inflammatory drug administration as the most effective chemopreventive strategy. More recently, a growing body of evidence suggests a dual role of immunity in cancer pathogenesis **(Figure 1)**, including tumor protective functions, tightly linked to patient's prognosis. Endogenous responses may inhibit tumor growth and modulate the clinical course of disease [7,8].

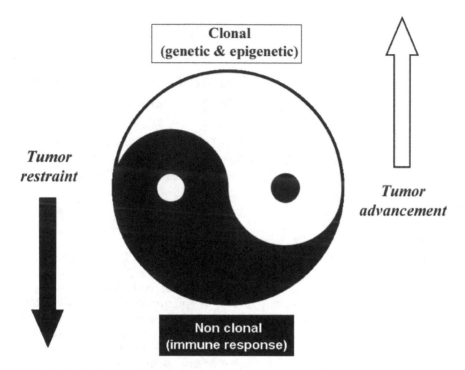

Fig. 1. Elements fueling and braking colorectal cancer progression

---

Genetic or Clonal Determinants

Genetic Instability

        Microsatellite Instability (MSI)

        Chromosomal Instability (CIN)

        CpG Island Methylator Phenotype (CIMP)

Non-Clonal Determinants

Adaptive Immunity

        CD4$^+$ lymphocytes

        CD8$^+$ lymphocytes

        T regulatory lymphocytes

        B lymphocytes

Innate Immunity

        Macrophages

        Mast Cells

        Neutrophils

        Natural Killer cells

        Dendritic Cells

Table 1. Sub-anatomical determinants of colorectal carcinogenesis

We review the builders of the CRC microenvironment, focusing on innate immunity and adaptive immunity. Although there is enormous heterogeneity of results and many open issues in methodological standardization strongly limit definitive conclusions, promising evidences support the clinical utility of tumor infiltrating subpopulations, in particular as prognostic biomarkers and potential therapeutic targets.

2. The players

2.1 Innate immunity

It is well known that innate immunity, not involving specific recognition of immunogenic peptides, represents the first defense to pathological stresses, including cancer. Innate immune cells orchestrate an inflammatory response that may stimulate or inhibit cancer growth. A number of innate immune cells have been implicated in CRC development and progression, including macrophages, mast cells (MC), neutrophils, natural killer (NK) cells and dendritic cells (DC) [9-12].

Macrophages. They are a heterogeneous cell population of the myeloid linage derived from monocytes. These cells show two different polarization states, M1 and M2, in response to different micro environmental signals [13]. M1-macrophages, involved in cancer protecting mechanism, interface susceptible target cells through several different mechanisms, including secretion of tumor necrosis factor-α (TNF-α), nitric oxide, interleukin-1β (IL-1β) and reactive oxygen intermediates. Additionally, M1s can support T-helper 1 (Th1) adaptive immunity. Conversely, M2 macrophages can secrete factors stimulating the growth and migration of tumor cells, such as platelet-derived growth factor (PDGF), epidermal growth factor (EGF), and transforming growth factor-β (TGF- β), and angiogenesis-promoting factors like vascular endothelial growth factor (VEGF) and TNF-α, as well as produce proteases (such as metalloproteinases, MMPs) that potentially could facilitate tumor invasion and metastasis [13-16].

In patients with CRC, tumor associated macrophages (TAM) are usually found located around necrotic areas and the advancing tumor margin. It was originally thought that the main function of TAMs was a direct cytotoxic effect on tumor cells, phagocytosis apoptotic/necrotic *cell debris*, and present *tumor-associated antigens* to T lymphocytes. Current associative evidence is in line with this view, as a high density of TAM at the CRC invasion front, particularly the highest TAM density scored as a "hot-spot", is associated with a better patient outcome [17]. More data are likely still needed as to TAM role in CRC, as well as on the state of their activation (M1 *versus* M2) [10].

Among the M2 population, TAMs have been shown as capable of secreting proteases that enhance invasion and metastases, together with a range of cytokines inhibiting an adaptive tumor-specific immune response, and angiogenic factors that increase neovascularity. The pro-angiogenetic ability of M2-macrophages has been well characterized and it is mediated by secretion of specific factors, including VEGF, IL-1β, TNF-α, angiogenin or, indirectly, by the release of MMPs. MMPs are responsible for extracellular matrix degradation and invasiveness through the connective tissue. They are released by TAMs after cancer cell stimulation and they can act locally or be recruited to cancer cell membrane for their trip toward progression and invasion [6]. Increased frequencies of intra-tumoural TAMs have mainly been associated with high levels of MMP type 2 and 9 expression in CRC cells. These findings are in accord with a previous cell-line study showing that co-culturing of tumor cells with macrophages enhances cancer cell migration, invasiveness, and MMP-2 and MMP-9 secretion [18].

Several authors have also shown that macrophages can release various cytokines. Kaler *et al.* have recently established that macrophages promote Wnt signaling pathway in CRC cells and enhance their proliferation, and demonstrated that macrophages exert their protumorigenic activity mainly through the release of IL-1β. The same authors demonstrated that Tumor Necrosis Factor Related Apoptosis Inducing Ligand (TRAIL) induced apoptosis of CRC cells is inhibited by macrophage derived IL-1β, and showed that macrophages and recombinant IL-1β counteract TRAIL-induced apoptosis through activation of Wnt signaling and stabilization of the nuclear transcription factor Snail in tumor cells [19]. Li *et al.* first reported that IL-6 released by macrophage directly promotes CRC cell progression, also suggesting that the interaction between IL-6 and IL-10 released from macrophages is involved in CRC progression and prognosis [20]. The above findings suggest that TAMs might play a regulatory role in the tumor microenvironment, supporting cancer cells to manipulate their microenvironment and facilitate cancer growth.

Among M1 population, TAM secreting IL-12 and IL-23, infiltrating the tumor invasive front are positively correlated with a favorable outcome. As mentioned above, Forssell *et al.* showed that the higher CD68+ macrophage infiltration along the tumor invasive front correlated with improved survival in colon cancer compared to rectal cancer. They concluded that a dense macrophage infiltration at the tumor invasive front positively influences prognosis in colon cancer and that the degree of cell-to-cell contact may influence the balance between pro-tumorigenic and anti-tumorigenic properties of macrophages [17]. High levels of tissue macrophages have been also associated with earlier disease stage, absence of nodal and lympho-vascular metastases and an overall better prognosis. Zhou *et al.* by analyzing the relationship between the density of TAMs and the potential of hepatic metastasis and survival have shown that a higher density of macrophages along the tumor invasive front of CRC was associated with a higher 5-year survival rate [21]. In addition, according to Forssell's scoring system that defines CD68 *hot-spots* as small areas among which the infiltration of macrophages is above the average level of CD68-positive cells, the highest CD68 hot-spot is associated with the lowest incidence of hepatic metastasis and a long interval between colon resection and the occurrence of hepatic metastasis [17, 21].

The mechanisms behind the anti-tumor effects of TAMs have still not been fully elucidated, and seem to potentially be ascribed to the M1 phenotype, which is in part controlled by the CD4+T-lymphocytes and the death of cancer cells [22]. It has been ascertained that recruitment of TAMs contributes to the development of an adaptive immune response against cancer, and the balance between antigen availability and clearance through phagocytosis and subsequent degradation of senescent or apoptotic cells.

Mast Cells (MC) originate from the bone-marrow hematopoietic progenitors and migrate to peripheral tissue close to the blood vessels, nerves and mucosal surfaces, in order to provide a quick defense against any external attack. They participate in tissue remodeling, wound healing and angiogenesis, but also they are responsible for pathological conditions such as acute and chronic allergic disorders or autoimmune disorders. Recently, increasing evidences in animal models and humans support their involvement in cancer. In APC deficient and KitW-KitW-v mice, polyps contain significantly higher amount of MC [23], while depletion of MC, either pharmacologically or in MC deficient mice, correspond to tumor suppression[24]. In accordance, MC infiltration has been reported in human CRC. MC are involved in angiogenesis as well as in tumor microenvironment remodeling. Based on the close association between MC and vasculature, their role in angiogenesis is intuitive, and it is supported by the evidence of increasing densities of MC during tumor growth, which goes with neo-vessels. Although MC tryptase has been claimed as the major player in this association, human MC also constitutively expresses VEGF isoforms. Beyond the angiogenesis, MC can play other functions in tumor microenvironment, mainly through stimulatory signals, such as Fc receptors and Toll-like receptors (TLR). When activated MC release mediators involved in inflammation, matrix destruction and tissue remodeling, promoting cancer invasion and metastasis [10, 25, 26]. Accordingly, it has been reported that the increase in MC count correlated with a worse prognosis in patients. Gulubova and Vlaykova proposed the MCs density along the tumor invasive front as a helpful tool for prognosis of patients after surgical therapy, showing a correlation between high MCs density and poor prognosis [27]. Moreover, interactions between MC and regulatory T cells (Treg) have been reported [28]. MCs have been reported to mobilize T cells and antigen-presenting dendritic cells. They modulate Treg-induced tolerance, shifting the local balance of immune surveillance toward pro-inflammatory Treg activation and cancer progression[29]. In light of these evidences, modulating mast cell recruitment, viability, activity, or mediator release patterns could also have important implication in cancer therapy strategies.

However, some conflicting data still need to be solved. Analyzing a old large cohort of patients, MC infiltration resulted an independent prognostic marker of favorable outcome [30], and in a recent report by *Xia et al.* there was no association between MC and prognosis in stage IIIB CRCs [24]. More studies are required to solve contradictions and validate the role of MC as potential prognostic markers and therapeutic target.

Neutrophils may form up to 15% of the inflammatory infiltrate associated with CRCs (tumor associated neutrophils, TAN) and this proportion increases within areas of tumor necrosis. Neutrophils secrete substances such as reactive oxygen species and proteinases that are capable of altering cell behavior and tumor microenvironment, with both pro-host and pro-tumor effects.

In patients with rectal cancer a high density of neutrophils has been shown as an independent predictor of improved prognosis, especially when microscopic abscesses form [10, 31]. On the other hand, an elevated neutrophil/lymphocyte ratio was found by Halazun *et al.* to contribute to a poorer survival time and higher rate of recurrence in CRC patients undergoing surgery for liver metastasis [10, 32]. It has been proposed that TANs impact on tumor growth depends on their activation state. When moderately activated, they promote tumor growth and remodel extra cellular matrix *via* Reactive Oxygen Species (ROS) and proteinases. In contrast, when TANs are highly activated they release higher concentrations of the same mediators with toxic consequences on tumor cells[31].

Natural killer (NK) cells are granular lymphocytes that form part of the innate cellular immune response. In CRC, high numbers of NK cells in the inflammatory infiltrate are associated with better prognosis. The number of NK cells decreases with increasing cancer stage [10]. Similarly, low preoperative levels of NK cell activity in patients undergoing curative resections are associated with disease recurrence. Because of these effects, it has been suggested that NK cells can rapidly eliminate tumor cells without prior exposure, whereas cytotoxic T cells require prior sensitization and therefore more time to become effective [10]. The ratio of NK cells in the peripheral blood has also been proposed as a prognostic indicator in patients with colon cancer and it is of interest to note that 5 fluorouracil (FU)-based chemotherapy increases the numbers of NK cells [33].

Dendritic cells (DCs), antigen-presenting cells (APCs) that are critical to the stimulation of effective anti-tumor adaptive immune responses, can become defective in the tumor microenvironment and aid in tumor immune evasion by failing to stimulate T lymphocytes.

It has been suggested that the presence of DCs may be of significant benefit in patients with CRC [34]. Xie *et al.* also demonstrated that the presence of DCs was found predominantly in early compared to later disease stages and mostly located in tumor surrounding tissue [35].

2.2 Adaptive immunity

It is well known that the adaptive, or specific, immunity, occurs several days after the exposure to a particular antigen, and it is distinct from the innate immunity with respect to: *a)* the specificity towards the different macromolecules, *b)* the immunological memory, *c)* the ability to respond in a more powerful and effective way in case of repeated exposure to a single pathogen, and *d)* immunological tolerance *i.e.* the ability to discriminate between *self* and *non-self*.

The adaptive immunity consists of a cellular component represented by T- and B-lymphocytes, and soluble components represented by the immunoglobulin (Ig) or *antibodies*. From a functional point of view, it can be distinguished between an adaptive humoral immunity and a cell-mediated immunity. The antibodies represent the humoral effectors and are produced following the activation of specific bone marrow derived B-lymphocytes, while cell-mediated effectors are represented by T-lymphocytes.

T-lymphocytes participate in inflammation, cancer development and progression, as well as in anticancer immunity [4, 9]. In colitis-associated tumors (CAC) the adaptive immune system seems to have mainly a pro-tumorigenic role, while in CRC it may play a double-faced role, being the balance between *immune-surveillance* (carried out by CD8+ and CD4+ T-lymphocytes) and tumor-promoting inflammation (by various sub-types of T-lymphocytes) to change over time, and eventually dictating disease progression.

Cytotoxic T lymphocytes (CD8+ T-lymphocytes, or CTL) constitute one of the leading effectors of antitumor immunity. In order for CD8+ T cells to recognize antigens, these need to be exposed on the tumor cells in association with the human leukocyte antigen (HLA) class I proteins [36]. Upon encounter of a tumor cell antigen/HLA I complex for which their T cell receptor (TCR) is specific, CD8+ T-lymphocytes clonally expand and differentiate [36]. Once activated, cytotoxic T-lymphocytes can mediate specific destruction of tumor cells through the release of lytic components via cell-cell interaction [36, 37]. Perforin, a cytolytic protein found in the granules of CD8+ T-lymphocytes and NK cells, and enzymatic proteases, including granzyme B, are secreted determining cell death by disruption of the cell membrane and activation of the apoptotic pathway respectively.

CD4+ T-lymphocytes, which only respond to antigens presented by the HLA class II proteins expressed by DCs, are important for antitumor immunity. CD4+ T-lymphocytes are mainly subdivided into T helper-1 (Th1) or -2 (Th2) lymphocytes [38]. Th1 cells secrete cytokines such as interferon-gamma (IFN-γ) and TNF-α, and support cytotoxic T-lymphocytes by producing IL-2, required for CD8+ T cells proliferation. Conversely, Th2 cells principally secrete IL-10, IL-4, and IL-5, and limit cytotoxic T-lymphocytes proliferation.

Regulatory T cells (Treg cells) have been defined as a T-cell population that functionally suppresses an immune response by influencing the activity of another cell type. Treg cells have been mainly categorized into two classes based on their ontogeny: naturally occurring Treg (nTreg), which develop in the thymus and are present in mice and healthy humans from an early postnatal period, and Treg which can arise in the periphery (or *in vitro*). nTreg are characterized by their high expression of CD25 (CD4+CD25+) and co-expression of the FoxP3 [39].

Although the role of **B-lymphocytes** in cancer has been overshadowed by the interest in developing T-cell-mediated cellular responses, it is now apparent that B-lymphocytes can play a complementary role in the host response against tumor. B-lymphocytes represent a cell population that express clonally diverse cell surface Ig receptors recognizing specific antigenic epitopes [40]. In addition to the role of B-lymphocytes in antibody production, these cells mediate/regulate several other functions fundamental for immune homeostasis. Of significant importance is the antigen-presenting role of B-lymphocytes in the initiation of T-cell immune responses. Moreover, B-lymphocytes can play a significant role in infection and autoimmunity as regulatory cells (indicated as Breg) via the elaboration of suppressive cytokines, such as IL-10, TGF-β, or IL-4. The role played by B cells in cancer immunology remains still complex and somewhat controversial. Depending upon their state of activation, B-lymphocytes have had divergent roles on T-cell differentiation and effector function. Oversimplifying, *resting B-lymphocytes* have been reported to suppress T-cell-mediated antitumor immunity, by acting on both CD4+ and CD8+ T-lymphocytes. In contrast, a number of reports suggest the efficacy of *activated B-lymphocytes* in cellular immunotherapy of malignancies. In particular, activated B-lymphocytes have been reported to enhance the ability to generate tumor-infiltrating lymphocytes *in vitro* involving anti-CD3 and IL-2.

The therapeutic targeting of tumors or components of the immune system with molecule-specific monoclonal antibodies (mAb) is now considered a viable treatment option for cancer patients [41]. One of the currently applied antibodies in clinics is represented by rituximab (Rituxan) that targets B cells for elimination by binding the B cell-associated marker CD20. Interestingly, Haynes *et al.* have recently developed a C57BL/6 TRAIL-sensitive tumor model with the aim of being able to use gene-targeted mice to better evaluate the innate and adaptive immune cells contributing to the tumoricidal activity of the MD5-1 mAb (*i.e.* an anti-mDR5 mAb) in more clinically relevant established tumors. C57BL/6 gene-targeted or immune cell-depleted mice were used to examine the antitumor activity of MD5-1 against the TRAIL-sensitive mouse MC38 colon adenocarcinoma. They found that an intact B cell compartment was critical for the therapeutic activity of MD5-1 against established tumors. B cells were confirmed to trigger tumor cell apoptosis by FcR-mediated cross-linking of the MD5-1 mAb *in vitro* and *in vivo* B lymphocytes were critical for directly triggering MD5-1–mediated tumor cell apoptosis.

Although the role of B-cells in human CRCs is still not completely characterized, B-cell-deficient mice exhibit spontaneous regression of MC38 colon carcinoma cells. Studies involving BCR transgenic mice indicated that B-cells might inhibit antitumor T-lymphocytes responses by antigen-nonspecific mechanisms. Shah *et al.* investigated the role of B cells in tumor immunity by studying immune responses of mice genetically lacking B cells to primary tumors. They highlight that although the effects of B-lymphocytes on anti-tumor response warrant further study, adoptive transfer of CD40(-/-) B cells into B cell-deficient mice resulted in restored growth of MC38 colon carcinoma cells suggesting additional factors other than CD40 are involved in dampening anti-tumor responses [42].

3. Immune cells in the colorectal cancer playground

Nowadays, it is well accepted that the host mounts both an innate and adaptive immune response against the cancer with variable effects. The strength of this response can be measured and has prognostic significance [43]. Dendritic cells, M1 macrophages, Th1 CD4+ T lymphocytes, cytotoxic CD8+ T-lymphocytes and NK cells are associated with a tumor protective behavior, while M2 macrophages, neutrophils, Th2 and Th17 CD4+ T cells, and Treg stimulate cancer progression [34] **(Table 2)**.

	PRO-TUMORIGENIC IMMUNITY	ANTI-TUMORIGENIC IMMUNITY
Cell sub-population	M2-polarized macrophages Myeloid-derived suppressor cells Moderately activated neutrophils FOXP3⁺ T-regulatory lymphocytes	M1-polarized macrophages Dendritic cells Highly activated neutrophils Cytotoxic T-lymphocytes Natural Killer cells
Cytokine profiles	T-lymphocytes helper-2 T-lymphocytes helper-17	T-lymphocytes helper-1 CX3CL1 CX3CL9 CX3CL10
Tissue distrution	Peritumoral	Intratumoral Close to cancer cells Invasive tumor front
Associated features	STAT 3 phosphorylation	High endothelial venules
Clinical impact	Negative *prognostic* impact	Positive *prognostic* and *predictive* impact

Table 2. Dula role of immunity in colorectal cancer

Chronic inflammation, mediated by infections, autoimmune disorders or inflammatory disease (*i.e.* Inflammatory Bowel Disease, IBD), is a well recognized cancer-trigger and represents the conceptual basis for using anti inflammatory drugs in CRC prevention. Macrophages (M2 subtype), secreting growth-, angiogenic- and chemotactic-factors, are the main determinant of this process and they are associated with poor patients' survival. Growing evidence suggests that other factors take part in this process, with negative consequences on prognosis, such as the pro-inflammatory Th17 cells or Treg [44]. However, expression of the transcription factor STAT3 was correlated with higher disease specific mortality in CRC [45]. In stage IIIB CRC, abnormal expression of the High Motility Group Box 1 protein (HMGB1) predicted poor survival [46]. It has been postulated that STAT3 and HMGB1 may have negative effects on the recruitment of anti-cancer effectors.

In contrast to chronic inflammation, immunosurveillance protects against cancer formation and progression. In this scenario, the presence of high numbers of T-lymphocytes has been reported to be a positive prognostic factor. The first reports on the beneficial effect of lymphocytic infiltration in CRC appeared already in the 1980's. They were subsequently confirmed until recent studies highlighting a prominent function for memory T-lymphocytes and CD8+ T-lymphocytes in predicting disease-free survival (DFS) and overall survival (OS) [47].

In general terms, it has been suggested that prognosis in patients with cancer is mainly positively affected by *a*) the presence of a tumor gene signature consistent with a type I adaptive immune response (*i.e.*, increased antigen presentation, IFN-γ signaling, and TCR signaling), and *b*) the presence of T cells that penetrate through tumor stroma and deeply infiltrate the parenchyma to become intra-tumoural T cells [9]. Thus, besides a Th-1 response signature, the other key feature of an effective immune response is the ability of T cells to reach the site of the tumor and to infiltrate it (Table 2).

A number of studies have reported that MSI, CIMP, BRAF mutation, PIK3CA mutation, and tumor LINE-1 hypomethylation are associated with CRC prognosis and that lymphocytic infiltration is associated with many of these molecular variables. The association of a prognostic biomarker with a given disease, strongly suggests its stage-dependency as outcome predictor. This is best exemplified by MSI CRC, whose overall prognostic advantage is associated with a low frequency of stage III and IV cases at diagnosis as compared to MSS counterpart [48]. Most MSI CRCs show a pronounced intra-tumoral inflammatory infiltrate (which remains a criterion for MSI testing), the mechanistic explanation of which, however, is still incompletely understood. Within these tumors, infiltrating lymphocytes have been identified as predominantly activated CD8+ T-lymphocytes. The presence of CTLs has been attributed to the inherently greater production of abnormal peptides as a result of unreliable DNA repair in MSI-positive tumors. It is known that truncated peptides produced by frameshift mutations due to MSI may be immunogenic and contribute to the host immune response. However, the interrelationship between tumor-infiltrating T-lymphocytes, MSI status, and other tumor molecular features is still unknown. In any event, the data concerning the prognostic implications of T cells have reached now a large volume and support a clear positive correlation between the density of T cells and a better prognosis. In this respect, most seminal work has been produced by Galon et al. [49], who first showed that a given immunological signature was associated with the absence of pathological evidence of early metastasis and with better survival. Such signature featured a high number of CD8+ T cells (including early and effector memory T cells). The presence of a high density of infiltrating memory CD45RO+ cells, at immunohistochemical analysis of tumor samples, was associated with the absence of signs of early metastatic invasion, a less advanced pathological stage, and increased survival [47]. Subsequently, the same group showed that a high density of CD3+ T cells at the tumor invasion front or located in the center of the tumor, once combined, can predict patient outcome better than the AJCC stage in patients with stage I to III CRC [49]. The question as to whether infiltrating T cells are such a powerful prognostic marker to overrun the prognostic predictive value of AJCC staging system was faced even by other groups. Laghi et al. [50] found that, in the absence of node metastasis, CD3+ T infiltrating cells at the tumor invasive front were associated with a low risk of metachronous metastasis and consequent survival advantage, independently of the MS-status. This finding challenged the view that the density of the T cell infiltrate is a stage independent predictor of survival in CRC, and that the positive prognostic value of T cells is dependent upon the CRC MS-status. More relevant, is the issue of the real relevance of the adaptive immune cell infiltrate in the clinical field. Overall, one would like to know whether the density of T-cells can predict patient's outcome, and at what stage of the disease it can be safely applied, rather than whether this is a stage-dependent or independent prognostic factor. It now appears that the density of T cells, whether CD3+, CD8+, or CD45RO+, can predict outcome in early stage CRC [49-51]. Inherently new issues arise from these data. One concerns the CD marker with the strongest prognostic value, and the other the standardization of the methods to assess T-cell density and their location with respect to CRC (i.e., within the tumor or at its invasive margin). It remains controversial whether the T cells infiltration has a prognostic impact beyond the stage of lymph-node invasion, a point at which immunoevasion may overcome immunosurveillance, although recent data still support the view that even at this disease stage T-cells retain a positive prognostic impact [52].

Recently, Nosho *et al.* examined the prognostic role of tumor-infiltrating T-cell subsets in a database of 768 CRCs from two prospective cohort studies. They concurrently assessed the densities of CD3+, CD8+, CD45RO+, and FoxP3+ lymphocytes as well as other relevant molecular (including KRAS, BRAF, and PIK3CA mutations, MSI, CIMP, and LINE-1 hypomethylation) and pathological features, therefore making possible to estimate the independent effect of each T-cell subset density on patient survival. They found that the density of CD45RO+ cells, but not that of CD3+, CD8+, or FoxP3+ cells, was an independent prognostic biomarker of longer survival in CRC patients, while MSI-high and tumor LINE-1 methylation level are independent predictors of CD45RO+-cell density [53]. In contrast, Salama *et al.* [54] by analyzing T-cell infiltrates in 967 CRCs including 593 stage II and 374 stage III cases, reported that FoxP3+ lymphocytes density had stronger prognostic significance than CD8+ and CD45RO+ cells, and predicted a better outcome. FoxP3+ lymphocytes were found not associated with any histopathological features. At multivariate analysis, stage, vascular invasion, and FoxP3+ cell density in tumoural tissue were found to be independent prognostic indicators. These results led Salama *et al.* to conclude that the inclusion of FoxP3+ cell density may help to improve the prognostication of early-stage CRC. Again, some contradiction exists, as data by other authors suggest that a high density of intraepithelial FoxP3+ is associated with a worse survival [55]. It should be mentioned that in the study by Salama, tissue sampling was obtained randomly, while in the study by Sinicrope *et al.* the density of FoxP3+ cells was measured within the tumor. Thus a low ratio of CD3+/FoxP3+ and a low CD3+ numbers were associated with a poor outcome, underscoring that even the interplay between effector and Treg cells might be relevant for cancer progression [55]. However, it is surprising how density of FoxP3+ resulted to be a positive prognostic factor when assessed in unspecified tumor regions and a negative one when assessed within the tumor. This contradiction calls for further studies aimed to re-appraise FoxP3+ cells role in CRC, but also underlines the methodological issue of T cells topographic assessment [56]. More recently, Chew *et al.* investigated whether Secreted Protein Acidic and Rich in Cysteine (SPARC), a matricellular protein involved in tissue remodeling, cell migration and angiogenesis, FoxP3, CD8 and CD45RO expression levels were associated with CRC stage, disease outcome and long-term cancer specific survival (CSS) in stage II and III [57]. They found that high levels of SPARC and FoxP3 protein (which seems to have an anti-tumorigenic role in cancer progression) were associated with better disease outcome in stage II CRC and may be prognostic indicators of CSS.

As a concluding remark, it should be pointed out that the prognostic value of a given CD set likely overlaps with that of a neighbor or subset, and that the overall prognostic value is likely the sum of different action exerted by each subset, including the balance between effector and regulatory arms.

It might not exist a T-cell marker that has the highest performance, as the overlapping nature of CD includes more than one cell subset.

Targeting the immune system represents an attractive strategy for the new frontiers in colon cancer treatment. *Strategy interfering cancer-promoting inflammation:* it has been widely recognized that the use of anti-inflammatory agents reduces the risk of developing CRC. In randomized clinical trials, the administration of celecoxib diminished the cumulative adenoma incidence and the frequency of advanced adenomas, suggesting their efficacy in both polyp formation and progression. In patients with familial adenomatous polyposis, celecoxib and sulindac decrease the incidence of colorectal and duodenal polyps. It is unlikely that anti-inflammatory drugs alone can represent effective monotherapies for CRC patients, but they might find place in combination withchemo- or radio-therapy or in chemoprevention. The non- selective cyclooxygenase (COX) inhibitor sulindac resulted effective in CRC prevention and treatment, while aspirin, which reduces CRC risk in a dose- and time-dependent manner, is mostly considered as chemopreventive agent. However, a more complete understanding of the mechanisms underlying tumor-promoting/protecting inflammation has identified more selective targets for intervention. Among non-steroidal anti-inflammatory drugs, specific COX2 inhibitors, such as celecoxib and rofecoxib, reduced CRC risk and slowed progression of colorectal adenomatous polyps to carcinomas, interfering with the COX isoform whose increased activity is specifically associated with CRC pathogens. In the late Nineties and early 2000s, a great deal of expectations arose from COX-2 inhibitors as tools for primary prevention that were lately banned from clinical practice, due to the burden of cardiovascular side effects. Highly selective inhibitors of prostaglandin E2 (PGE2) signaling, such as ONO-8711 receptor antagonists, are expected to reduce the cardiovascular risks associated with COX inhibition but still prevent CRC [58, 59]. Recently biologic agents have been introduced in clinical practice in combination with classical chemotherapy for some subtype of disease, as a form of passive immunotherapy [60]. In contrast to traditional chemotherapeutic drugs, they target specific signaling pathways.   For example, VEGF inhibition (i.e. bevacizumab) blocks tumor angiogenesis while the interfering with the EGF receptor signaling (i.e. cetuximab) reduces survival and growth of cancer cells. Bevacizumab and cetuximab are currently approved in the metastatic disease treatment [61]. Additionally, it has recently demonstrated that Bevacizumab-based therapy is able to increase B- and T-lymphocytes compartments [62]. It is known that the expansion of T lymphocytes could imply an amelioration of dendritic cell-presenting capacity. These effects correlate with a more favorable clinical outcome and could be taken into account in clinical protocols aimed at combining anti-angiogenetic-therapy with immunotherapy in metastatic CRC.

Inhibitors of pro-inflammatory cytokines might also be developed to block inflammation. A number of studies have been conducted using anti-IL6, anti-TNF, anti-IL-1, anti- IL-17, or anti-IL-23, but, although some of them have already been approved in IBD or autoimmune disorders (i.e. infliximab, etanercept), there is a lack of clinical trials in oncologic settings. Similarly, anti-adhesion molecules drugs, currently applied for IBD and rheumatologic disorders (i.e. the α (4)-integrin subunit inhibitor Natalizumab) could be potential cancer protective agents, preventing an excessive inflammatory response. A monoclonal antibody against CD3 (visilizumab), which prevents T-cell activation, had promising preliminary results in patients with active Crohn disease [10, 61, 63]. In this scenario, colitis associated cancer represents an ideal model where such drugs can be helpfully tested. Of notice, the mentioned strategies interfere with the tumor promoting inflammation. In the light of the dual role of inflammation in CRC, it is important to determine which agents block tumor-promoting inflammation without reducing antitumor immunity.

Strategy enhancing cancer-protective inflammation: the immune system in cancer patients can be stimulated by active specific immunotherapy (vaccine) in order to eradicate tumor cells. Vaccines are expected to be specific for the tumor cells, self sustaining and systemic. However a successful vaccine strategy should address and overcome the suppressor response that tumor cells are able to mount [10].

So far, vaccines to treat cancer have been largely investigated with disappointing results in terms of clinical response. In advanced CRC patients, although some measurable immune response can be registered, the current trails failed to obtain meaningful improvement in survivals. Similarly, in adjuvant setting randomized control trials did not show promising result; in this setting, only the autologous tumor cell vaccines combined with Bacilles Calmette-Guerin (BCG) seems to significantly improve patients' survival [64].

Finally, among passive immunotherapies, a novel charming strategy consists in removing anti-tumor T cells from the body for *ex vivo* culture, followed by reinfusion (adoptive T cell transfer)[65]. Although the first trial failed mostly due to technical issues, the researcher remains optimistic that increasing competences will make this strategy a feasible form of immunotherapy in the future.

4. Open issues

Although the well established role of immune system provides concrete opportunities for clinical applications, the heterogeneity of results among studies suggest that many issues need to be solved before moving into clinical practice.

The existing discrepancies in literature may be due to a number of factors such as intra-tumor distribution of the immune cells and type of subpopulations, type of organ, tumor genetic background, and the assessment methods employed. Recent studies have reported that different macrophage phenotypes localized to different regions of the carcinoma have variable effects on tumor cells [49, 66]. Furthermore, evidence has shown that the relationship between TAMs and tumor progression is tumor type-dependent. Nevertheless, since the tumor microenvironment includes different T-cell sub-populations **(Figure 2)**, which do not display a homogeneous infiltration of tumor tissues, potential different impact on prognosis may depend on type of sub-population and peri/intra tumor distribution. Because T cell infiltration is not spatially homogeneous in CRC, attention has been focused on the predictive values of T-lymphocytes located in the center of the tumor, along the invasive margin and in lymphoid aggregate (*i.e.* tertiary lymphoid structures) mainly detectable in proximity of the tumor [43, 67]. However, the interrelationship between tumor-infiltrating T-lymphocytes, MSI status, and other tumor molecular features remains to be elucidated. It is indubitable that to define the prognostic effect of tumor-infiltrating T cells, large studies of CRC with extensive molecular characterization are needed. Additionally, caution is needed before incorporating tumor-infiltrating T cells into tumor staging. To minimize the risk of inappropriate tumor down-staging at diagnosis, survival data need to be confirmed in independent series of patients studied in the past decade. Moreover, the association has to be conclusively proven between low densities of tumor-infiltrating T cells and the clinical detection of metachronous metastases, which remains the most appropriate outcome measure for recognizing a role of the local immune response in micrometastasis suppression. Laghi *et al.* [50] investigated the relationship between the density of CD3+ T infiltrating lymphocytes along the tumor invasive margin, and the occurrence of metachronous distant-organ metastases after potentially curative resection, in a large, consecutive series of patients with deeply invading (pT3 or pT4) MSI-typed CRC, and no evidence of distant organ metastasis at diagnosis. They found that large areas covered by CD3+ cells at the tumor invasive front are associated with a low risk of metachronous metastasis and consequently a survival advantage, only in patients with node-negative cancers, but not in patients whose cancers involved lymph nodes. The prognostic advantage conferred by a high density of CD3+ cells was independent of tumor MS-status in patients with stage II CRC. CD3-immunostaining of CRC tissue might therefore be useful for selecting stage II patients who, because they are at very low risk for cancer progression, could be spared adjuvant treatments. The usefulness in the clinical scenario of T-cell density in patients with more advanced disease, who are subject to chemotherapy remains to be assessed. With respect to this, the relationship between T-cells and current chemotherapy regimens for CRC should be also explored, a field in which very few data are currently available.

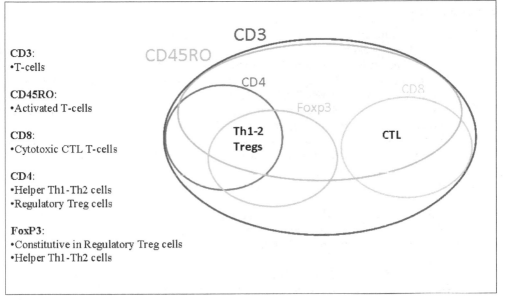

Fig. 2. Adaptive immunity: different Clusters of Differentiation (CD) are expressed by subsets of T-lymphocytes

It is clear that as tumors are heterogeneous cell populations that show distinctive genetic and epigenetic profiles, there may not be a single biomarker that will prove sufficient information for predicting treatment response and patient outcome. However, it remains to be solved, several critical issues related to the heterogeneity and complexity between the actual studies, in terms of sample size; study setting; disease stage; the presence *versus* absence of treatment data; and treatment modality (no therapy to chemotherapy, radiation therapy, or both) [8]. Laboratory methods to assess immune response (tissue microarray *versus* whole tissue; objective image analysis *versus* subjective pathologist qualitative or semi-quantitative interpretation); immunophenotyping markers; covariates and potential confounders assessed (in particular the presence versus absence of tumor molecular characteristics); and statistical method and multivariate analysis models all represent issues to take in account when comparing results from different laboratories. It is clear that to standardize research methods and appropriately evaluate evidence, we need to develop general and specific consensus on immune-cell evaluation in oncology research.

In conclusion, it can be stressed that the standardized analysis of the *type, quantity, location* and the *functions* of the immune infiltrate becomes a primary step in understanding CRC natural history, and, in a clinical perspective, its prognostic determinants. A comprehensive analysis of all components of the lymphocytic infiltrates in the context of their localization, organization and impact at various steps of tumor progression remains largely, if not entirely, to be reported to prospective studies. In parallel, understanding the mechanisms of efficient immune reactions, the place where they are initiated, the cells and key cytokines and chemokines involved, and their impact at different stages of the disease should provide new tools and goals for more effective and less toxic targeted therapies.

5. References

[1] Burke HB. Outcome prediction and the future of the TNM staging system. J Natl Cancer Inst 2004;96:1408-1409.

[2] Vogelstein B, Fearon ER, Hamilton SR, Kern SE, Preisinger AC, Leppert M, Nakamura Y, White R, Smits AM, Bos JL. Genetic alterations during colorectal-tumor development. N Engl J Med 1988;319:525-532.

[3] Grady WM, Carethers JM. Genomic and epigenetic instability in colorectal cancer pathogenesis. Gastroenterology 2008;135:1079-1099.

[4] Mantovani A, Romero P, Palucka AK, Marincola FM. Tumour immunity: effector response to tumour and role of the microenvironment. Lancet 2008;371:771-783.

[5] Ogino S, Chan AT, Fuchs CS, Giovannucci E. Molecular pathological epidemiology of colorectal neoplasia: an emerging transdisciplinary and interdisciplinary field. Gut 2011;60:397-411.

[6] Ungefroren H, Sebens S, Seidl D, Lehnert H, Hass R. Interaction of tumor cells with the microenvironment. Cell Commun Signal 2011;9:18.

[7] Ferrone C, Dranoff G. Dual roles for immunity in gastrointestinal cancers. J Clin Oncol 2010;28:4045-4051.

[8] Ogino S, Galon J, Fuchs CS, Dranoff G. Cancer immunology-analysis of host and tumor factors for personalized medicine. Nat Rev Clin Oncol 2011;8:711-719.

[9] Disis ML. Immune regulation of cancer. J Clin Oncol 2010;28:4531-4538.

[10] Salama P, Platell C. Host response to colorectal cancer. ANZ J Surg 2008;78:745-753.

[11] Saleh M, Trinchieri G. Innate immune mechanisms of colitis and colitis-associated colorectal cancer. Nat Rev Immunol 2011;11:9-20.

[12] Secher T, Gaillot O, Ryffel B, Chamaillard M. Remote control of intestinal tumorigenesis by innate immunity. Cancer Res 2010;70:1749-1752.

[13] Biswas SK, Mantovani A. Macrophage plasticity and interaction with lymphocyte subsets: cancer as a paradigm. Nat Immunol 2010;11:889-896.

[14] Mantovani A, Schioppa T, Porta C, Allavena P, Sica A. Role of tumor-associated macrophages in tumor progression and invasion. Cancer Metastasis Rev 2006;25:315-322.

[15] Mantovani A, Sica A, Locati M. New vistas on macrophage differentiation and activation. Eur J Immunol 2007;37:14-16.

[16] Sica A, Larghi P, Mancino A, Rubino L, Porta C, Totaro MG, Rimoldi M, Biswas SK, Allavena P, Mantovani A. Macrophage polarization in tumour progression. Semin Cancer Biol 2008;18:349-355.

[17] Forssell J, Oberg A, Henriksson ML, Stenling R, Jung A, Palmqvist R. High macrophage infiltration along the tumor front correlates with improved survival in colon cancer. Clin Cancer Res 2007;13:1472-1479.

[18] Kang JC, Chen JS, Lee CH, Chang JJ, Shieh YS. Intratumoral macrophage counts correlate with tumor progression in colorectal cancer. J Surg Oncol 2010;102:242-248.

[19] Kaler P, Galea V, Augenlicht L, Klampfer L. Tumor associated macrophages protect colon cancer cells from TRAIL-induced apoptosis through IL-1beta-dependent stabilization of Snail in tumor cells. PLoS One 2010;5:e11700.

[20] Li YY, Hsieh LL, Tang RP, Liao SK, Yeh KY. Interleukin-6 (IL-6) released by macrophages induces IL-6 secretion in the human colon cancer HT-29 cell line. Hum Immunol 2009;70:151-158.

[21] Zhou Q, Peng RQ, Wu XJ, Xia Q, Hou JH, Ding Y, Zhou QM, Zhang X, Pang ZZ, Wan DS, Zeng YX, Zhang XS. The density of macrophages in the invasive front is inversely correlated to liver metastasis in colon cancer. J Transl Med 2010;8:13.

[22] Umemura N, Saio M, Suwa T, Kitoh Y, Bai J, Nonaka K, Ouyang GF, Okada M, Balazs M, Adany R, Shibata T, Takami T. Tumor-infiltrating myeloid-derived suppressor cells are pleiotropic-inflamed monocytes/macrophages that bear M1- and M2-type characteristics. J Leukoc Biol 2008;83:1136-1144.

[23] Heijmans J, Büller NV, Muncan V, van den Brink GR. Role of mast cells in colorectal cancer development, the jury is still out. Biochim Biophys Acta. 2012;1822:9-13.

[24] Xia Q, Wu XJ, Zhou Q, Jing Z, Hou JH, Pan ZZ, Zhang XS. No relationship between the distribution of mast cells and the survival of stage IIIB colon cancer patients. J Transl Med 2011;9:88.

[25] Liu J, Zhang Y, Zhao J, Yang Z, Li D, Katirai F, Huang B. Mast cell: insight into remodeling a tumor microenvironment. Cancer Metastasis Rev 2011;30:177-184.

[26] Ribatti D, Crivellato E, Roccaro AM, Ria R, Vacca A. Mast cell contribution to angiogenesis related to tumour progression. Clin Exp Allergy 2004;34:1660-1664.

[27] Gulubova M, Vlaykova T. Prognostic significance of mast cell number and microvascular density for the survival of patients with primary colorectal cancer. J Gastroenterol Hepatol 2009;24:1265-1275.

[28] Blatner NR, Bonertz A, Beckhove P, Cheon EC, Krantz SB, Strouch M, Weitz J, Koch M, Halverson AL, Bentrem DJ, Khazaie K. In colorectal cancer mast cells contribute to systemic regulatory T-cell dysfunction. Proc Natl Acad Sci U S A 2010;107:6430-6435.

[29] Khazaie K, Blatner NR, Khan MW, Gounari F, Gounaris E, Dennis K, Bonertz A, Tsai FN, Strouch MJ, Cheon E, Phillips JD, Beckhove P, Bentrem DJ. The significant role of mast cells in cancer. Cancer Metastasis Rev 2011;30:45-60.

[30] Nielsen HJ, Hansen U, Christensen IJ, Reimert CM, Brunner N, Moesgaard F. Independent prognostic value of eosinophil and mast cell infiltration in colorectal cancer tissue. J Pathol 1999;189:487-495.

[31] Houghton AM. The paradox of tumor-associated neutrophils: fueling tumor growth with cytotoxic substances. Cell Cycle 2010;9:1732-1737.

[32] Halazun KJ, Aldoori A, Malik HZ, Al-Mukhtar A, Prasad KR, Toogood GJ, Lodge JP. Elevated preoperative neutrophil to lymphocyte ratio predicts survival following hepatic resection for colorectal liver metastases. Eur J Surg Oncol 2008;34:55-60.

[33] Vesely P, Touskova M, Melichar B. Phenotype of peripheral blood leukocytes and survival of patients with metastatic colorectal cancer. Int J Biol Markers 2005;20:126-133.

[34] Fridman WH, Galon J, Pages F, Tartour E, Sautes-Fridman C, Kroemer G. Prognostic and predictive impact of intra- and peritumoral immune infiltrates. Cancer Res 2011;71:5601-5605.

[35] Xie ZJ, Jia LM, He YC, Gao JT. Morphological observation of tumor infiltrating immunocytes in human rectal cancer. World J Gastroenterol 2006;12:1757-1760.

[36] Paschen A, Eichmuller S, Schadendorf D. Identification of tumor antigens and T-cell epitopes, and its clinical application. Cancer Immunol Immunother 2004;53:196-203.

[37] Loose D, Van de WC. The immune system and cancer. Cancer Biother Radiopharm 2009;24:369-376.

[38] Barnas JL, Simpson-Abelson MR, Yokota SJ, Kelleher RJ, Bankert RB. T cells and stromal fibroblasts in human tumor microenvironments represent potential therapeutic targets. Cancer Microenviron 2010;3:29-47.

[39] Saurer L, Mueller C. T cell-mediated immunoregulation in the gastrointestinal tract. Allergy 2009;64:505-519.

[40] Namm JP, Li Q, Lao X, Lubman DM, He J, Liu Y, Zhu J, Wei S, Chang AE. B lymphocytes as effector cells in the immunotherapy of cancer. J Surg Oncol 2011.

[41] Haynes NM, Hawkins ED, Li M, McLaughlin NM, Hammerling GJ, Schwendener R, Winoto A, Wensky A, Yagita H, Takeda K, Kershaw MH, Darcy PK, Smyth MJ. CD11c+ dendritic cells and B cells contribute to the tumoricidal activity of anti-DR5 antibody therapy in established tumors. J Immunol 2010;185:532-541.

[42] Shah S, Divekar AA, Hilchey SP, Cho HM, Newman CL, Shin SU, Nechustan H, Challita-Eid PM, Segal BM, Yi KH, Rosenblatt JD. Increased rejection of primary tumors in mice lacking B cells: inhibition of anti-tumor CTL and TH1 cytokine responses by B cells. Int J Cancer 2005;117:574-586.

[43] Pages F, Galon J, eu-Nosjean MC, Tartour E, Sautes-Fridman C, Fridman WH. Immune infiltration in human tumors: a prognostic factor that should not be ignored. Oncogene 2010;29:1093-1102.

[44] Tosolini M, Kirilovsky A, Mlecnik B, Fredriksen T, Mauger S, Bindea G, Berger A, Bruneval P, Fridman WH, Pages F, Galon J. Clinical impact of different classes of infiltrating T cytotoxic and helper cells (Th1, th2, treg, th17) in patients with colorectal cancer. Cancer Res 2011;71:1263-1271.

[45] Morikawa T, Baba Y, Yamauchi M, Kuchiba A, Nosho K, Shima K, Tanaka N, Huttenhower C, Frank DA, Fuchs CS, Ogino S. STAT3 expression, molecular features, inflammation patterns, and prognosis in a database of 724 colorectal cancers. Clin Cancer Res 2011;17:1452-1462.

[46] Peng RQ, Wu XJ, Ding Y, Li CY, Yu XJ, Zhang X, Pan ZZ, Wan DS, Zheng LM, Zeng YX, Zhang XS. Co-expression of nuclear and cytoplasmic HMGB1 is inversely associated with infiltration of CD45RO+ T cells and prognosis in patients with stage IIIB colon cancer. BMC Cancer 2010;10:496.

[47] Pages F, Berger A, Camus M, Sanchez-Cabo F, Costes A, Molidor R, Mlecnik B, Kirilovsky A, Nilsson M, Damotte D, Meatchi T, Bruneval P, Cugnenc PH, Trajanoski Z, Fridman WH, Galon J. Effector memory T cells, early metastasis, and survival in colorectal cancer. N Engl J Med 2005;353:2654-2666.

[48] Malesci A, Laghi L, Bianchi P, Delconte G, Randolph A, Torri V, Carnaghi C, Doci R, Rosati R, Montorsi M, Roncalli M, Gennari L, Santoro A. Reduced likelihood of metastases in patients with microsatellite-unstable colorectal cancer. Clin Cancer Res 2007;13:3831-3839.

[49] Galon J, Costes A, Sanchez-Cabo F, Kirilovsky A, Mlecnik B, Lagorce-Pages C, Tosolini M, Camus M, Berger A, Wind P, Zinzindohoue F, Bruneval P, Cugnenc PH, Trajanoski Z, Fridman WH, Pages F. Type, density, and location of immune cells within human colorectal tumors predict clinical outcome. Science 2006;313:1960-1964.

[50] Laghi L, Bianchi P, Miranda E, Balladore E, Pacetti V, Grizzi F, Allavena P, Torri V, Repici A, Santoro A, Mantovani A, Roncalli M, Malesci A. CD3+ cells at the invasive margin of deeply invading (pT3-T4) colorectal cancer and risk of post-surgical metastasis: a longitudinal study. Lancet Oncol 2009;10:877-884.

[51] Pages F, Kirilovsky A, Mlecnik B, Asslaber M, Tosolini M, Bindea G, Lagorce C, Wind P, Marliot F, Bruneval P, Zatloukal K, Trajanoski Z, Berger A, Fridman WH, Galon J. In situ cytotoxic and memory T cells predict outcome in patients with early-stage colorectal cancer. J Clin Oncol 2009;27:5944-5951.

[52] Mlecnik B, Tosolini M, Kirilovsky A, Berger A, Bindea G, Meatchi T, Bruneval P, Trajanoski Z, Fridman WH, Pages F, Galon J. Histopathologic-based prognostic factors of colorectal cancers are associated with the state of the local immune reaction. J Clin Oncol 2011;29:610-618.

[53] Nosho K, Baba Y, Tanaka N, Shima K, Hayashi M, Meyerhardt JA, Giovannucci E, Dranoff G, Fuchs CS, Ogino S. Tumour-infiltrating T-cell subsets, molecular changes in colorectal cancer, and prognosis: cohort study and literature review. J Pathol 2010;222:350-366.

[54] Salama P, Phillips M, Grieu F, Morris M, Zeps N, Joseph D, Platell C, Iacopetta B. Tumor-infiltrating FOXP3+ T regulatory cells show strong prognostic significance in colorectal cancer. J Clin Oncol 2009;27:186-192.

[55] Sinicrope FA, Rego RL, Ansell SM, Knutson KL, Foster NR, Sargent DJ. Intraepithelial effector (CD3+)/regulatory (FoxP3+) T-cell ratio predicts a clinical outcome of human colon carcinoma. Gastroenterology 2009;137:1270-1279.

[56] Laghi L, Bianchi P, Grizzi F, Malesci A. How dense, how intense? Role of tumour-infiltrating lymphocytes across colorectal cancer stages. Re: Nosho et al. Tumour-infiltrating T-cell subsets, molecular changes in colorectal cancer, and prognosis: cohort study and literature review. J Pathol 2010; 222: 350-366. J Pathol 2011;225:628.

[57] Chew A, Salama P, Robbshaw A, Klopcic B, Zeps N, Platell C, Lawrance IC. SPARC, FOXP3, CD8 and CD45 correlation with disease recurrence and long-term disease-free survival in colorectal cancer. PLoS One 2011;6:e22047.

[58] Chan AT, Ogino S, Fuchs CS. Aspirin use and survival after diagnosis of colorectal cancer. JAMA 2009;302:649-658.

[59] Keller JJ, Giardiello FM. Chemoprevention strategies using NSAIDs and COX-2 inhibitors. Cancer Biol Ther 2003;2:S140-S149.

[60] Cohen DJ, Hochster HS. Rationale for combining biotherapy in the treatment of advanced colon cancer. Gastrointest Cancer Res 2008;2:145-151.

[61] Terzic J, Grivennikov S, Karin E, Karin M. Inflammation and colon cancer. Gastroenterology 2010;138:2101-2114.

[62] Manzoni M, Rovati B, Ronzoni M, Loupakis F, Mariucci S, Ricci V, Gattoni E, Salvatore L, Tinelli C, Villa E, Danova M. Immunological effects of bevacizumab-based treatment in metastatic colorectal cancer. Oncology 2010;79:187-196.

[63] Stenson WF. Prostaglandins and epithelial response to injury. Curr Opin Gastroenterol 2007;23:107-110.

[64] Hanna MG, Jr., Hoover HC, Jr., Vermorken JB, Harris JE, Pinedo HM. Adjuvant active specific immunotherapy of stage II and stage III colon cancer with an autologous tumor cell vaccine: first randomized phase III trials show promise. Vaccine 2001;19:2576-2582.

[65] June CH. Adoptive T cell therapy for cancer in the clinic. J Clin Invest 2007;117:1466-1476.

[66] Galon J, Fridman WH, Pages F. The adaptive immunologic microenvironment in colorectal cancer: a novel perspective. Cancer Res 2007;67:1883-1886.

[67] Zlobec I, Lugli A. Invasive front of colorectal cancer: dynamic interface of pro-/anti-tumor factors. World J Gastroenterol 2009;15:5898-5906.

8

Streptococcus bovis/gallolyticus Induce the Development of Colorectal Cancer

A.S. Abdulamir[1,2], R.R. Hafidh[1,3] and F. Abu Bakar[1]
[1]*Institute of Bioscience, University Putra Malaysia, Serdang, Selangor,*
[2]*Microbiology Department, College of Medicine, Alnahrain University PO, Baghdad,*
[3]*Microbiology Department, College of Medicine, Baghdad University,*
[1]*Malaysia*
[2,3]*Iraq*

1. Introduction

The role, of microbial agents and the infection of the intestinal mucosa in the carcinogenesis, or the development of colorectal cancer (CRC) is one of the hot topics in the field of CRC where much research has been done. However, this topic has long been underestimated by most of the related books. This chapter is intended to cover the relationship of CRC development with bacteria implicated in the development of CRC such as *S. bovis*, *S. gallolyticus*, *S. equines*, *S. infantarius*, *E .coli*, *C. difficile*...etc. However, *S. gallolyticus* and *S. bovis* will be discussed thoroughly in this chapter as they are considered the prototype for intestinal microorganisms related to CRC and colorectal premalignant lesions.

Studying CRC association with infection of intestinal mucosa is not complete without studying the underlying mechanisms. There is compelling evidence that CRC is largely affected by the status of intestinal bioflora. CRC has been found to be affected by certain microbial agents that have particular characteristics capable of inducing dysplastic changes in intestinal mucosa. However, the underlying mechanisms of the association of implicated infective agents with CRC development are yet not clear. In addition, the role of oncogenic factors, cell growth factors, and pro-inflammatory cytokines in the association of bacterial infection in intestinal mucosa with CRC has not yet been clarified well. Therefore, the current chapter attempts to scrutinize the nature and the underlying mechanisms of the association of infective agents represented by *S. bovis/gallolyticus* with CRC. Nevertheless, the association of *S. bovis/gallolyticus* with CRC is still under controversy regarding whether the bacterial infection of intestine, along with associated bacteremia/endocarditis, is a consequence or the etiological factor of CRC. Hence, this chapter also attempts to explore the facts available in the field to assess which scenario is more favorable for the association of *S. bovis/gallolyticus* with CRC namely, the consequence or the etiology scenario.

One of the bacterial agents that have been most associated with cancer is *Streptococcus bovis* (*S. bovis*). *S. bovis* has been shown to be important in human health because 25 to 80% of patients with *S. bovis* bacteremia had also colorectal tumor, and the incidence of association of colonic neoplasia with *S. bovis* endocarditis was shown to be 18 to 62% (Gupta et al., 2009; Kok et al., 2007; Leport et al., 1987; Malkin et al., 2008; Reynolds et al., 1983; Wilson et al.,

1981; Zarkin et al., 1990). Later, it was shown that a new species resembling *S. bovis* is actually most implicated in CRC development; *S. bovis* infecting human intestine has been named as *S. gallolyticus* (Osawa et al., 1995). More precisely, *S. bovis* biotype I and II/2 isolates were shown to be *S. gallolyticus* (Devriese et al., 1998). Accordingly, *S. bovis* biotype I was replaced by *S. gallolyticus* subspecies *gallolyticus* and biotype II/2 was replaced by *S. gallolyticus* subspecies *pasterianus* and *S. gallolyticus* subspecies *macedonicus* (Schlegel et al., 2003). *S. gallolyticus* subspecies *gallolyticus*, rather than other related taxa, have been found to be constantly associated with underlying colorectal cancer.

2. The association of colorectal cancer with *S. bovis/gallolyticus* bacteremia/endocarditis

S. bovis, has long been linked to the development of CRC. However, the extent, nature, and basis of this association are still not completely understood. *S. bovis/gallolyticus* became important in human health since it was shown that 25 to 80% of patients who presented *S. bovis/gallolyticus* bacteremia had also a colorectal tumor and the incidence of association of colonic neoplasia with *S. bovis/gallolyticus* endocaditis was shown to be 18 to 62% (Gupta et al., 2009; Kok et al., 2007; Leport et al., 1987; Malkin et al., 2008; Murray & Roberts, 1978; Reynolds et al., 1983; Wilson et al., 1981; Zarkin et al., 1990). The knowledge that there is an association between endocarditis from *S. bovis/gallolyticus* and carcinoma of the colon has important clinical implications (Boleij et al., 2009a; Kok et al., 2007). The majority of the studies that found clues on the association of *S. bovis/gallolyticus* with CRC was in Europe and North America. Actually, it is true that the association of *S. bovis/gallolyticus* bacteremia with colorectal cancer has been found variable among different geographical and ethnic groups (Boleij et al., 2009a), but this association is not restricted to certain geographical region. A recent study done in Malaysia found that 48.6% of *S. bovis* isolates was found in patients with colonic polyps, adenocarcinomas, inflammatory bowel diseases. It was also found that colorectal cancer incidence was 24.7%, adenocarinomas accounting for 51% with the highest incidence in the sigmoid part of the colon(Al-Jashamy et al., 2010). This study indicates a strong relationship between *S. bovis/gallolyticus* and colonic premalignant as well as malignant lesions in a geographical region that was considered of low incidence for CRC cases associated with bacterial infections. Moreover, an epidemiological study conducted in Hong Kong on *S. bovis* bacteremia and its relation to colorectal cancer, confirmed the association of *S. bovis/gallolyticus* with CRC and found that *S. bovis* biotype II/2 is the dominant in Hong Kong rather than biotype I (*S. gallolyticus*) which is dominant in Western countries (Lee et al., 2003).

Thorough studies on *S. bovis* have shown that associations between *S. bovis* bacteraemia and carcinoma of the colon and infective endocarditis were biotype-specific. It was shown that there is 94% association between *S. bovis* biotype I bacteraemia and infective endocarditis and 71% association between *S. bovis* biotype I bacteraemia and colonic carcinoma. On the other hand, it is only 18% association between *S. bovis* biotype II bacteraemia and infective endocarditis and 17% association between *S. bovis* biotype II bacteraemia and colonic carcinoma (Murray & Baron, 2007). Following the description of *S. gallolyticus*, Devriese team used whole-cell protein analysis to show that all six bacterial isolates studied, which were derived from patients with endocarditis and identified by conventional techniques as *S. bovis*, were in fact *S. gallolyticus*. Therefore, they suggested that *S. gallolyticus* is more likely to be involved in human infections than is *S. bovis* (Devriese et al., 1998).

The underlying mechanisms for the association of CRC with *S. bovis/gallolyticus* bacteremia/endocarditis have been obscure for a long time. The possible reason behind that, maybe, *S. bovis/gallolyticus* is a member of intestinal flora in 2.5 to 15% of individuals which usually make scientists counteract any malicious role of this bacteria (Burns et al., 1985; Murray & Roberts, 1978). It was conceived in the beginning that the ulceration of neoplastic lesions might form a pathway for the microorganism to enter the bloodstream (Gupta et al., 2009). However, the latter scenario of bacterial access into the circulation does not explain the cases of patients with infectious endocarditis and non-ulcerated colonic polyps (Cutait et al., 1988). Furthermore, colonic neoplasia may arise years after the presentation of the condition of bacterial bacteremia or infectious endocarditis (Fagundes et al., 2000; Zarkin et al., 1990). For this reason, patients with infectious endocarditis and normal colonoscopy may be included in the group who present risk for developing colonic cancer because of the late appearance of such lesions after the infectious episode *of S. bovis/gallolyticus* (Fagundes et al., 2000). Moreover, in supporting the second scenario, it has been shown that the relative risk of developing infectious endocarditis from *S. bovis/gallolyticus* in the presence of carcinoma of the colon is merely 3 to 6% (Bisno & 12.ed. New York: , 1991) while 60 to 75% of patients with endocarditis by *S. bovis/gallolyticus* simultaneously present malignant gastrointestinal disease that was not previously diagnosed (Grinberg et al., 1990).

3. The association of premalignant colorectal lesions with *S. bovis/gallolyticus*

There is a high incidence of colorectal cancer in individuals with polyps; about 90% of preinvasive neoplastic lesions of the colorectum are polyps or polyp precursors, namely aberrant crypt foci (Nielsen et al., 2007). Neoplastic polyps are often referred to more specifically as adenomas or adenomatous polyps (Srivastava et al., 2001). Adenomatous polyps are considered as good and few surrogate end point markers for colorectal cancer (Kelly et al., 1989; Nielsen et al., 2007).

It would be of interest to substantiate any relationship between bacterial colonic carriage, colonic polyps and the type of polyp and its malignant potential (Boleij et al., 2009a; Schlegel et al., 2003). Contrary to the more commonly reported association between *S. bovis/gallolyticus* bacteremia and colorectal cancer, a link to pre-neoplastic adenomatous polyps was less frequently reported (Burns et al., 1985; Ellmerich et al., 2000a). Nevertheless, the relationship between colorectal bacterial infection and the progressive development of malignant disease in pre-neoplastic adenomatous polyps was supported by recent reports (Abdulamir et al., 2009; Kahveci et al., 2010; Murinello et al., 2006). Interestingly, benign lesions (diverticulosis, inflammatory bowel disease, cecal volvulus, perirectal abscess hemorrhoids, benign polyps) were found to be mildly associated with intestinal bacterial infections such as *S. bovis/gallolyticus* while a strong relationship between more malignant diseases of the colon (cancer and neoplastic polyps) and *S. bovis/gallolyticus* was found (Abdulamir et al., 2009; Burns et al., 1985; Klein et al., 1979; Nielsen et al., 2007; Reynolds et al., 1983; Smaali et al., 2008). It was also revealed that *S. bovis/gallolyticus* septicemia and/or endocarditis is selectively related to the presence of villous or tubulovillous adenomas in the large intestine (Fagundes et al., 2000; Smaali et al., 2008). In fact, Villous and tubulovillous adenomas, which have risk of malignant transformation about 15-25%, were found to be associated with *S. bovis/gallolyticus* bacteria more often than other types of adenomas (Bond, 2005). For example, Hoen team performed a case-control study on subjects underwent colonoscopy comparing between patients with *S. bovis/gallolyticus* endocarditis and sex- and age- matched unaffected patients. This study showed that colonic adenomatous polyps were present in twice as many cases as controls (15 of 32 *vs* 15 of 64), and colorectal cancer was present approximately 3 times as often (3 of 32 *vs* 2 of 64) (Hoen et al., 1994). However, surprisingly, another study (Devis et al., 1989) found that the association between *S. bovis/gallolyticus* and adenoma was more evident than that with colorectal cancer; they reported that 36% of positive blood cultures of *S. bovis/gallolyticus* were found in proliferative lesions (15% of cancers and 21% of adenomas). A recent study (Abdulamir et al., 2009) supported this concept showing that the level of *S. bovis/gallolyticus* IgG antibodies in adenoma patients is much higher than in both colorectal cancer patients and control subjects. However, other reports did not reveal the same thing. (Burns et al., 1985) stated that the incidence of *S. bovis/gallolyticus* carriage in all colons with polyps was intermediary between normal colons and colons with carcinoma although the difference did not achieve statistical significance.

Regarding the fecal carriage of *S. bovis/gallolyticus*, (Burns et al., 1985) demonstrated that highly premalignant polyps were found to be more often associated with *S. bovis/gallolyticus* carriage than were benign polyps. A clue for the active role of intestinal bacteria in the development of CRC, *S. bovis/gallolyticus* endocarditis, rather than other members of group D Streptococcus, showed special predilection to colonic lesions. It was found that of 77 infections with group D Streptococcus endocarditis, colonic polyps and colonic carcinoma were significantly more frequent in the *S. bovis/gallolyticus* group (67 and 18%) respectively than in the Enterococcus group (21 and 2%) respectively (Leport et al., 1987). This indicates that certain bacteria have role in the etiology of CRC development from premalignant poly lesions.

The remarkable association between adenomatous polyps and *S. bovis/gallolyticus* seems to be of importance due to the compelling evidence that colon cancer progresses from normal tissue to adenoma and then to carcinoma through an accumulation of genetic alterations (Baron & Sandler, 2000). Although ulceration of the neoplastic lesion might form a pathway for the *S. bovis/gallolyticus* to enter the bloodstream (Gupta et al., 2009), the association of *S. bovis/gallolyticus* bacteremia with non-ulcerated colonic polyps indicates an etiological/promoter role of these bacteria in polyps progression (Cutait et al., 1988; Konda & Duffy, 2008). The possibility of *S. bovis/gallolyticus* to act as a promoter for the preneoplastic lesions is worthy to be considered. A remarkable study supported this hypothesis using rats treated with *S. bovis* wall extracted antigens (WEA), rats treated with a chemical carcinogen, rats treated with both WEA and chemical carcinogen, and untreated rats. All groups of rats did not develop hyperplastic colonic crypts except for the group treated with both WEA and the chemical carcinogen; about 50 % rats of this group developed neoplastic lesions (Ellmerich et al., 2000a). This indicated that *S. bovis* bacteria might exert their pathological activity in the colonic mucosa only when preneoplastic lesions are established. Another model supporting the promoter effect of *S. bovis/gallolyticus*, H. pylori infection and subsequent inflammation seem most likely to be promoters in the multistep development of carcinoma (from chronic gastritis to atrophy, intestinal metaplasia, dysplasia, and, ultimately, cancer) rather than the causative agents (Leung, 2006). Therefore, the association of *S. bovis/gallolyticus* in etiology and/or acceleration of the transformation of aberrant crypts to adenoma and to cancer is now being reconsidered.

Accordingly, the knowledge of association of colorectal adenoma with *S. bovis/gallolyticus* has important clinical implications. If the lesion can be discovered at an early stage, curative resection may become possible (Waisberg et al., 2002). Thus, bacteremia due to *S. bovis/gallolyticus* should prompt rigorous investigation to exclude both endocarditis and tumors of the large bowel (Beeching et al., 1985; Konda & Duffy, 2008). Therefore, it was concluded that the discovery of a malignant or premalignant proliferative lesion in one third of the cases justifies the exploration of the colon by barium enema and/or colonoscopy in the case of *S. bovis/gallolyticus* septicemia (Beeching et al., 1985; Konda & Duffy, 2008). This would empirically aid for the early detection of adenoma in the gastrointestinal tract before its progression to cancer.

4. The proposed mechanisms for the development of colorectal cancer by *S. bovis/gallolyticus*

Chronic inflammation is associated with malignant changes. Host genetic polymorphisms of the adaptive and innate immune response play an important role in bacteria-induced cancer formation (El-Omar, 2006; Hou et al., 2007; Karin & Greten, 2005). Therefore, studying the immunological responses to chronic bacterial infections is likely to yield important clues on both the mechanisms of persistent infection and the relationship between inflammation and cancer formation (Ernst et al., 2006; Monack et al., 2004). Clinical studies have shown that the use of non-steroidal anti-inflammatory drugs is associated with a reduced risk of gastric cancer (Dai & Wang, 2006). However, bacteria implicated in carcinogenesis, like *S. bovis/gallolyticus*, might use several mechanisms for carcinogenesis such as the colonization of epithelial surfaces and the use of virulence factors to chronically affect host cell cycle control, apoptosis, cell junction integrity or cell polarity ((Vogelmann & Amieva, 2007).

4.1 Clues for etiological role

The big question is whether bacteria play an etiological role in the carcinoma of colon or it is merely marker of the disease. There are many clues collectively provide evidence for the etiological role of bacteria in colon cancer development. The striking association between bacteremia caused by *S. bovis* biotype I and both colonic neoplasia (71%) and bacterial endocarditis (94%), rather than bacteremia caused by closely related organisms such as *S. bovis* variant and *S. salivarius*, suggests the possibility of specific bacterium-host interactions (Ruoff et al., 1989). Moreover, the appearance of new colonic lesions 2-4 after the incidence of *S. bovis/gallolyticus* bacteremia/endocarditis, provides more evidence that *S. bovis/gallolyticus* is not merely a consequence of the tumor lesion (Wentling et al., 2006). In terms of pathogenesis, as *S. bovis/gallolyticus* is a transient normal flora in the gut, researchers have postulated that the increased bacterial load of *S. bovis/gallolyticus* in colon might be responsible for its association with colon cancer. Several studies have shown that increased stool carriage of *S. bovis/gallolyticus* is particularly found in patients with inflammatory bowel diseases or malignant/premalignant lesions of the colon while *S. bovis/gallolyticus* bacteria were rarely isolated from normal subjects (Teitelbaum & Triantafyllopoulou, 2006). Another clue supporting the etiological role of *S. bovis/gallolyticus*, patients diagnosed with colon cancer have only 3–6% chance to develop *S. bovis/gallolyticus* endocarditis (zur Hausen, 2006), which is far lower than the percentage of the detection of colorectal cancer in patients with *S. bovis/gallolyticus* bacteremia/endocarditis, which his more than 70%.

4.2 Mechanisms of the proposed etiological role of *S. bovis/gallolyticus* in the development of colorectal cancer

4.2.1 Selective adherence to intestinal tumor cells

Some bacteria such as *S. bovis/gallolyticus* are frequent colonizers of the intestinal tract, which can also cause endocarditis. However, their ability to adhere to and colonize host tissues is largely unknown. It was found that *S. bovis/gallolyticus* bacteria possess collagen-binding proteins and pili that are responsible for adhesion to colorectal mucosa as well as to endocardium (Sillanpaa et al., 2009). On the other hand, another study (Boleij et al., 2009b) found a histone-like protein A on the surface of *S. bovis/gallolyticus* able to bind heparan sulfate proteoglycans at the colon tumor cell surface during the first stages of infection; this cell surface protein in *S. gallolyticus* acts as one of the main heparin-binding proteins that is largely responsible for bacteria selective adhesive potential as well as entry to the blood circulation. Another study assessing 17 endocarditis-derived human isolates, identified 15 *S. gallolyticus* subspecies *gallolyticus*, one *S. gallolyticus* subspecies *pasteurianus* (biotype II/2) and one *S. infantarius* subspecies *coli* (biotype II/1) for their in vitro adherence to components of the extracellular matrix; this study provided evidence that *S. gallolyticus* subspecies *gallolyticus* bacteria possess very efficient adherence characteristics to the host extracellular matrix; this bacteria showed powerful adherence to collagen type I and type IV, fibrinogen, collagen type V, and fibronectin (Sillanpaa et al., 2008). These adherence merits render these bacteria successful colonizers in both intestinal and cardiac tissues which might explain the association between *S. bovis/gallolyticus* endocarditis and intestinal lesions.

4.2.2 Changing the intestinal bacterial flora and alterations in the local vascular attributes

Increased incidence of hepatic dysfunction has been reported in patients with bacterial infectious endocarditis (Fagundes et al., 2000). It has been speculated that *S. bovis/gallolyticus* affects portal circulation through bacterial translocation, thereby determining hepatic alterations. Modifications in the hepatic secretion of bile salts and the production of immunoglobulins contribute towards increasing the participation of S. bovis/gallolyticus in abnormal changes in the bacterial flora of the colonic lumen which might then promote carcinogenesis of the intestinal mucosa (Beeching et al., 1985; Gupta et al., 2009).

It has been suggested that alterations in local conditions and disruption of capillary channels at the site of neoplasm allowed S. bovis/gallolyticus to proliferate and gain entry into blood stream (Biarc et al., 2004; Ellmerich et al., 2000a; Nguyen et al., 2006). The local action of cytokines or of chemical mediators able to promote vasodilatation and the enhancement of capillary permeability, may support the bacterial entry at tumor sites, and increase bacterial adherence to various cells (Biarc et al., 2004; Ellmerich et al., 2000b).

4.2.3 Promoting/propagating effect on preneoplastic lesions and inflammation-driven carcinogenesis

A series of interesting experiments was conducted for investigating the role of *S. bovis/gallolyticus* in the initiation and development of colorectal cancer. Chemical carcinomas were induced by giving adult rats intraperitonial injections of azoxymethane (15 mg/kg body weight) once per week for 2 weeks. Fifteen days (week 4) after the last injection of the carcinogen, the rats received, by gavage twice per week during 5 weeks, either *S. bovis* (10^{10} bacteria) or wall-extracted antigens (WEAs) (100 µg). One week after the last gavage (week 10), it was found that administration of either *S. bovis* or its antigens promoted the progression of preneoplastic lesions into neoplastic lesions through the increased formation of hyperproliferative aberrant colonic crypts, which enhanced the expression of proliferation markers and increased the production of IL-8 in the colonic mucosa (Biarc et al., 2004; Ellmerich et al., 2000b). Therefore, this study suggests that *S. bovis/gallolyticus* bacteria act as potential promoters of early preneoplastic lesions in the colon of rats, and their cell wall proteins are more potent inducers of neoplastic transformation than the intact bacteria. This study also revealed that the development of colonic adenomas increased remarkably in 50% of the tested rats and the expression level of proliferation markers, the polyamine content and proliferating cell nuclear antigen was also increased (Biarc et al., 2004; Ellmerich et al., 2000a; Nguyen et al., 2006). This provided extra evidence that *S. bovis/gallolyticus* acts more likely as promoter/propagator of colorectal carcinoma rather than just a consequence of the tumor lesion. These studies might suggest that bacteria, in general, are often not capable to induce cancer without the presence of other predisposing factors for carcinogenesis. In this regard, it was conceived that the transformation process of colorectal tumors associated with *S. bovis/gallolyticus* is more likely accompanied with long-lasting bacterial promoting/propagating effect along with chronic inflammation status in intestinal mucosa. This conclusion was supported by Balkwill et al. stating that tumor formation might require independent mutations in oncogenic signaling pathways in addition to chronic inflammatory conditions which are needed to promote transformation process (Balkwill et al., 2005).

In vitro experiments showed that the binding of *S. bovis* wall extracted antigens to various cell lines including human colonic cancer cells (Caco-2) stimulated the production of inflammatory cytokines by those cells (Biarc et al., 2004; Nguyen et al., 2006). Earlier it was found that the production of inflammatory cytokines in response to *S. bovis/gallolyticus*, such as TNF-α, IL-1ß and IL-6, and the chemokine IL-8, were found to contribute to the normal defense mechanisms of the host (Ellmerich et al., 2000b; Travers & Rosen, 1997) leading to the formation of nitric oxide and free radicals such as superoxide, peroxynitrites, hydroxyl radicals as well as alkylperoxy radicals (Nguyen et al., 2006; Ohshima & Bartsch, 1994). Owing to their potent mutagenicity, all these molecular species can contribute to the neoplastic processes by modifying cellular DNA. On the other hand, in the colonic mucosa, the production of angiogenic factors, such as IL-8, triggered by *S. bovis/gallolyticus* antigens may also favor the progression of colon carcinogenesis (Eisma et al., 1999; Ellmerich et al., 2000b; Norrby, 1996). This resembles *H. pylori* infection for the development of chronic inflammation in the gastric mucosa (Dixon et al., 1996); therefore, it seems that chronic infection and subsequent chronic inflammation are responsible for the maintenance and development of pre-existing neoplastic lesions (Shacter & Weitzman, 2002).

Moreover, it was found that WEAs of *S. bovis* induced *in vitro* overexpression of cyclooxygenase-2 (COX-2) (Biarc et al., 2004; Nguyen et al., 2006) COX-2, via prostaglandins, promotes cellular proliferation and angiogenesis and inhibits apoptosis, thus acting as a promoter in the cancer pathway (Tafte & Ruoff, 2007). It is noteworthy to mention that non-steroidal anti-inflammatory drugs (NSAIDS) were found to decrease the relative risk of gastrointestinal carcinomas and their main target was found to be cyclooxygenase 2 (COX-2) that is over-expressed in up to 85% of colorectal adenocarcinomas (Kargman et al., 1995). Moreover, (Haqqani et al., 2000) revealed that the activation of leukocytes by *S. bovis/gallolyticus* was found to release various other inflammatory mediators (NO, free radicals, peroxynitriles, etc.) which could interfere directly or indirectly with the cell proliferation process. A recent study conducted by our team, *S. gallolyticus* has shown a specific association with colorectal cancer and colorectal adenoma when compared with the more dominant intestinal bacteria, *B. fragilis*. This provided evidence for a possible important role of *S. gallolyticus* in the carcinogenesis of colorectal cancer from pre-malignant polyps. In addition, it was also found that NF-κB and IL-8 rather than other transformation factors p21, p27 and p53 act as important mediators for the *S. gallolyticus*-associated transformation of adenoma to carcinoma (Abdulamir et al., 2009). Moreover, it was concluded that NF-κB exerts most probably a promoting carcinogenic effect and IL-8 exerts mainly an angiogenic-based propagating effect on colorectal mucosal cells (Abdulamir et al., 2009). In addition, a more recent study done by our team showed a direct and active role of *S. bovis/gallolyticus* in colorectal cancer development through inflammation-based sequel of tumor development or propagation via IL-1, COX-2, and IL-8 (Abdulamir et al., 2010). By these studies, a strong relationship was shown to be evident between the proinflammatory potential of *S. bovis/gallolyticus* bacteria and their carcinogenic properties confirming the linkage between inflammation and colon carcinogenesis.

In the presence of WEAs proteins of *S. bovis/gallolyticus*, Caco-2 cells exhibited enhanced phosphorylation of 3 classes of mitogen activated protein kinases (MAPKs) (Biarc et al., 2004). Several reports showed that MAPKs activation stimulates cells to undergo DNA synthesis and cellular uncontrolled proliferation (Hirata et al., 2001; Ihler, 1996; Smith & Lawson, 2001). Therefore *S. bovis/gallolyticus* proteins could promote cell proliferation by triggering MAPKs which might increase the incidence of cell transformation and the rate of genetic mutations. Furthermore MAPKs, particularly p38 MAPK, can induce COX-2 which is an important factor in tumorogenesis (Lasa et al., 2002; Wang & Dubois, 2010) and up-regulate the expression of NFkB which is considered the central link between inflammation and carcinogenesis (Karin & Greten, 2005). Accordingly, the pro-inflammatory potential of *S. bovis/gallolyticus* proteins and their pro-carcinogenic properties as well as the chronic inflammation and the leucocytic recruitment driven by *S. bovis/gallolyticus* provide strong evidence on the possible causal link between *S. bovis/gallolyticus* inflammation and colonic carcinogenesis. Therefore, the above data support the hypothesis that colonic bacteria can contribute to cancer development particularly via chronic infection/inflammation where bacterial components may interfere with cell function for long time (Biarc et al., 2004; Wang & Dubois, 2010).

5. Selective colonization of *S. bovis/gallolyticus* in colorectal mucosa

The association of bacteria with colorectal cancer has always been described through the incidence of *S. bovis/gallolyticus* bacteremia and/or endocarditis (Leport et al., 1987; Murray & Roberts, 1978; Reynolds et al., 1983; Wilson et al., 1981; Zarkin et al., 1990). On the other hand, little bacteriological research has been done on elucidating the colonization of *S. bovis/gallolyticus* in tumor lesions of colorectal cancer in order to confirm or refute, on solid bases, the direct link between colorectal cancer and *S. bovis/gallolyticus* (Norfleet & Mitchell, 1993; Potter et al., 1998). A recent study of by our team was conducted to assess the colonization of *S. bovis/gallolyticus* bacteria in colon by detecting *S. bovis/gallolyticus* DNA in colorectal cancer tumors using advanced molecular assays (Abdulamir et al., 2010). In Abdulamir et al. study, *S. bovis/gallolyticus*-specific primers and probes were used in PCR and in situ hybridization (ISH) assays, respectively, to detect *S. bovis/gallolyticus* DNA from feces, tumor mucosal surfaces, and from the inside of tumor lesions. In addition, bacteriological isolation of *S. bovis/gallolyticus* was conducted to isolate *S. bovis/gallolyticus* cells from feces, tumor mucosal surfaces, and from the inside of tumor lesions. In this study, *S. bovis/gallolyticus* was successfully isolated, via bacteriological assays, from tumorous and non-tumorous tissues, of colorectal cancer patients with bacteremia, 20.5% and 17.3%, and of colorectal cancer patients without bacteremia, 12.8% and 11.5%, respectively while only 2% of control tissues revealed colonization of *S. bovis/gallolyticus*.

On the other hand, the positive detection of *S. bovis/gallolyticus* DNA, via PCR, in tumorous and non-tumorous tissues of colorectal cancer patients with bacteremia, 48.7 and 35.9%, and without bacteremia, 32.7 and 23%, respectively, was remarkably higher than that in control tissues, 4%. And the positive detection of *S. bovis/gallolyticus* DNA, via ISH, in tumorous and non-tumorous tissues of colorectal cancer patients with bacteremia, 46.1 and 30.7%, and without bacteremia 28.8 and 17.3%, respectively was remarkably higher than that in control tissues, 2%. In addition, by using absolute quantitative PCR for *S. bovis/gallolyticus* DNA, the *S. bovis/gallolyticus* count, in terms of copy number (CN), in tumorous and non-tumorous tissues of colorectal cancer patients with bacteremia, 2.96-4.72 and 1.29-2.81 $\log_{10}$ CN/g, respectively, and colorectal cancer patients without bacteremia, 2.16-2.92 and 0.67-2.07 $\log_{10}$ CN/g, respectively, showed significantly higher level of colonization in tumorous than in non-tumorous tissues and in colorectal cancer patients with bacteremia than in colorectal cancer patients without bacteremia. Accordingly, this study provided several new observations. First, *S. bovis/gallolyticus* colonizes selectively tumorous tissues of colorectal cancer patients rather than normal mucosal tissues. Second, the colonization of *S. bovis/gallolyticus* is mainly found inside tumor lesions rather than on mucosal surfaces of tumors. Third, the titer of the colonizing *S. bovis/gallolyticus* bacteria in colorectal cancer patients with bacteremia/endocarditis was much higher than in patients without bacteremia/endocarditis; this explains why some colorectal cancer patients develop concomitant bacteremia of *S. bovis/endocarditis* while others do not. Actually, the newly discovered selective colonization of *S. bovis/gallolyticus* explains the conclusions of an earlier report (Tjalsma et al., 2006) stating that colonic lesions provide a suitable microenvironment for *S. bovis/gallolyticus* colonization resulting in silent tumor-associated infections that only become apparent when cancer patients become immunocompromised, as in bacteraemia, or have coincidental cardiac valve lesions and develop endocarditis.

6. Using *S. bovis/gallolyticus* in the early detection of colorectal tumors

For a long time, it has been conceived that there is a need to establish a good screening test for colonic cancer patients, particularly a test which could detect early lesions. It has been suggested that the presence of antibodies to certain bacterial antigens or the presence of certain bacterial antigens in the bloodstream may act as markers for carcinogenesis of the colon (Beeching et al., 1985; Potter et al., 1998). The serology-based detection of colorectal cancer has advantage on other tests such as fecal occult blood which is neither sensitive nor specific or carcinoembryonic antigen which is regularly detectable in only advanced diseases (Tafte & Ruoff, 2007). Darjee and Gibb stated that it might be possible to develop a test to screen patients for the presence of colonic cancer by measuring IgG antibody titer of *S. bovis/gallolyticus* (Darjee & Gibb, 1993). Hence, since the association between slow evolving bacterial inflammation and colorectal cancer takes long time, it is prudent to seek specifically for IgG antibodies. Furthermore, IgG antibodies reflect an image of the past and the chronic presence of *S. bovis/gallolyticus* antigens in the circulation.

Some studies showed the possibility of constructing a serology test for the successful detection of colonic cancer based on the detection of antibody to *S. bovis/gallolyticus* or *Enterococcus faecalis* (Abdulamir et al., 2009; Groves, 1997). Therefore, a simple ELISA test with no more than 2 ml of patient's blood might be a good candidate for screening high risk individuals for the presence of premalignant neoplastic polyps, adenomas, and cancers. However, some other studies of antibody response to *S. bovis/gallolyticus* and other streptococci have found that antibody is detectable in endocarditis but not in either clinically insignificant bacteremias (Burnie et al., 1987), or colonic cancers ((Kaplan et al., 1983) by using immunoblotting, immunoflourescence and other techniques. In a recent study of our team (Abdulamir et al., 2009), the serum level of IgG antibodies against *S. gallolyticus* subspecies *gallolyticus* antigens adsorbed on solid phase of ELISA was found to be significantly higher in colorectal cancer patients than in control subjects. This is in full agreement with the study of (Darjee & Gibb, 1993) who showed that patients with colonic cancer had higher median IgG antibody titers to *S. bovis* and *E. faecalis* preparations than did the control samples. Accordingly, the applicability of using ELISA as a cheap and effective assay for the early detection of colorectal cancer using IgG antibodies against *S. bovis/gallolyticus* has been tested and proven (Abdulamir et al., 2009). Therefore, the early detection of colorectal cancer using simple means of testing opens doors to monitor high risk groups of colorectal cancer more efficiently.

7. Conclusions

Colorectal tumors, adenoma or carcinoma, are associated remarkably with bacterial infections of intestine. The manifestation of this association is usually observed as concurrent bacteremia or endocarditis of *S. bovis/gallolyticus*. The association of *S. bovis/gallolyticus* bacteria with colorectal cancer is more likely etiological in nature rather than a consequence of the disease. The proposed etiological role of *S. bovis/gallolyticus* in the development of colorectal cancer might be attributed to many factors including selective adhesion potential of *S. bovis/gallolyticus* to tumor tissues, the selective colonization of *S. bovis/gallolyticus* inside tumor tissues, the suitable microenvironment of tumors for *S. bovis/gallolyticus* proliferation, the local disruption of tumor tissues and capillaries which allow the entry of *S. bovis/gallolyticus* into blood circulation leading to bacteremia and endocarditis, and the bacterially-induced cytokines and transcriptional factors, such as IL-1, IFN-γ, IL-8, and NFkB, which induce and propagate the chronic inflammatory environment which promote/propagate premaligant intestinal lesions to malignant ones. This is a very important role of *S. bovis/gallolyticus* in the carcinogenesis of colorectal tissues since the majority of cases of colorectal cancer are sporadic cancers arising through the transformation of normal colorectal tissues to premalignant lesions, adenomas, and finally to malignant tissues. Besides, the early detection of colorectal adenomas or carcinomas via detection of *S. bovis/gallolyticus* DNA or their specific IgG antibodies might be of high value in screening the high risk groups for colorectal cancer. More in-depth research is needed to exploit the association of bacteria with colorectal cancer in terms of early diagnosis of the disease as well as understanding the bacterial carcinogenic potential to determine the appropriate means to prevent and/or treat bacterially-associated cancers.

8. References

Abdulamir, A.S., Hafidh, R.R., Bakar, F.A., (2010). Molecular detection, quantification, and isolation of Streptococcus gallolyticus bacteria colonizing colorectal tumors: inflammation-driven potential of carcinogenesis via IL-1, COX-2, and IL-8. *Mol Cancer*, Vol. 9, No. pp. 249, 1476-4598 (Electronic)1476-4598 (Linking)

Abdulamir, A.S., Hafidh, R.R., Mahdi, L.K., Al-jeboori, T., Abubaker, F., (2009). Investigation into the controversial association of Streptococcus gallolyticus with colorectal cancer and adenoma. *BMC Cancer*, Vol. 9, No. pp. 403, 1471-2407 (Electronic) 1471-2407 (Linking)

Al-Jashamy, K., Murad, A., Zeehaida, M., Rohaini, M., Hasnan, J., (2010). Prevalence of colorectal cancer associated with Streptococcus bovis among inflammatory bowel and chronic gastrointestinal tract disease patients. *Asian Pac J Cancer Prev*, Vol. 11, No. 6, pp. 1765-1768, 1513-7368 (Print) 1513-7368 (Linking)

Balkwill, F., Charles, K.A., Mantovani, A., (2005). Smoldering and polarized inflammation in the initiation and promotion of malignant disease. *Cancer Cell*, Vol. 7, No. 3, pp. 211-217, 1535-6108 (Print) 1535-6108 (Linking)

Baron, J.A., Sandler, R.S., (2000). Nonsteroidal anti-inflammatory drugs and cancer prevention. *Annu Rev Med*, Vol. 51, No. pp. 511-523, 0066-4219 (Print) 0066-4219 (Linking)

Beeching, N.J., Christmas, T.I., Ellis-Pegler, R.B., Nicholson, G.I., (1985). Streptococcus bovis bacteraemia requires rigorous exclusion of colonic neoplasia and endocarditis. *Q J Med*, Vol. 56, No. 220, pp. 439-450, 0033-5622 (Print) 0033-5622 (Linking)

Biarc, J., Nguyen, I.S., Pini, A., Gosse, F., Richert, S., Thierse, D., Van Dorsselaer, A., Leize-Wagner, E., Raul, F., Klein, J.P., Scholler-Guinard, M., (2004). Carcinogenic properties of proteins with pro-inflammatory activity from Streptococcus infantarius (formerly S.bovis). *Carcinogenesis*, Vol. 25, No. 8, pp. 1477-1484, 0143-3334 (Print) 0143-3334 (Linking)

Bisno, A., 12.ed. New York:, (1991). Streptococcal infection. In: *Harrison's principles of internal medicine*. Harrison, T., Stone, R.s (Eds.), pp. 563-569, McGraw-Hill, New York.

Boleij, A., Schaeps, R.M., de Kleijn, S., Hermans, P.W., Glaser, P., Pancholi, V., Swinkels, D.W., Tjalsma, H., (2009b). Surface-exposed histone-like protein a modulates adherence of Streptococcus gallolyticus to colon adenocarcinoma cells. *Infect Immun*, Vol. 77, No. 12, pp. 5519-5527, 1098-5522 (Electronic) 0019-9567 (Linking)

Boleij, A., Schaeps, R.M., Tjalsma, H., (2009a). Association between Streptococcus bovis and colon cancer. *J Clin Microbiol*, Vol. 47, No. 2, pp. 516, 1098-660X (Electronic) 0095-1137 (Linking)

Bond, J.H., (2005). Colon polyps and cancer. *Endoscopy*, Vol. 37, No. 3, pp. 208-212, 0013-726X (Print) 0013-726X (Linking)

Burnie, J.P., Holland, M., Matthews, R.C., Lees, W., (1987). Role of immunoblotting in the diagnosis of culture negative and enterococcal endocarditis. *J Clin Pathol*, Vol. 40, No. 10, pp. 1149-1158, 0021-9746 (Print) 0021-9746 (Linking)

Burns, C.A., McCaughey, R., Lauter, C.B., (1985). The association of Streptococcus bovis fecal carriage and colon neoplasia: possible relationship with polyps and their premalignant potential. *Am J Gastroenterol*, Vol. 80, No. 1, pp. 42-46, 0002-9270 (Print) 0002-9270 (Linking)

Cutait, R., Mansur, A., Habr-Gama, A., (1988). Endocardite por Streptococcus bovis e pólipos de cólon. *Rev Bras Coloproctol*, Vol. 8, No. pp. 109-110,

Dai, Y., Wang, W.H., (2006). Non-steroidal anti-inflammatory drugs in prevention of gastric cancer. *World J Gastroenterol*, Vol. 12, No. 18, pp. 2884-2889, 1007-9327 (Print) 1007-9327 (Linking)

Darjee, R., Gibb, A.P., (1993). Serological investigation into the association between Streptococcus bovis and colonic cancer. *J Clin Pathol*, Vol. 46, No. 12, pp. 1116-1119, 0021-9746 (Print) 0021-9746 (Linking)

Devis, A., Dony, A., De Boelpaepe, F., Verhulst, C., Serste, J.P., (1989). [Streptococcus bovis septicemia and colonic cancer]. *Acta Chir Belg*, Vol. 89, No. 1, pp. 58-60, 0001-5458 (Print) 0001-5458 (Linking)

Devriese, L.A., Vandamme, P., Pot, B., Vanrobaeys, M., Kersters, K., Haesebrouck, F., (1998). Differentiation between Streptococcus gallolyticus strains of human clinical and veterinary origins and Streptococcus bovis strains from the intestinal tracts of ruminants. *J Clin Microbiol*, Vol. 36, No. 12, pp. 3520-3523, 0095-1137 (Print) 0095-1137 (Linking)

Dixon, M.F., Genta, R.M., Yardley, J.H., Correa, P., (1996). Classification and grading of gastritis. The updated Sydney System. International Workshop on the Histopathology of Gastritis, Houston 1994. *Am J Surg Pathol*, Vol. 20, No. 10, pp. 1161-1181, 0147-5185 (Print) 0147-5185 (Linking)

Eisma, R.J., Spiro, J.D., Kreutzer, D.L., (1999). Role of angiogenic factors: coexpression of interleukin-8 and vascular endothelial growth factor in patients with head and neck squamous carcinoma. *Laryngoscope*, Vol. 109, No. 5, pp. 687-693, 0023-852X (Print) 0023-852X (Linking)

El-Omar, E.M., (2006). Role of host genes in sporadic gastric cancer. *Best Pract Res Clin Gastroenterol*, Vol. 20, No. 4, pp. 675-686, 1521-6918 (Print) 1521-6918 (Linking)

Ellmerich, S., Djouder, N., Scholler, M., Klein, J.P., (2000b). Production of cytokines by monocytes, epithelial and endothelial cells activated by Streptococcus bovis. *Cytokine*, Vol. 12, No. 1, pp. 26-31, 1043-4666 (Print) 1043-4666 (Linking)

Ellmerich, S., Scholler, M., Duranton, B., Gosse, F., Galluser, M., Klein, J.P., Raul, F., (2000a). Promotion of intestinal carcinogenesis by Streptococcus bovis. *Carcinogenesis*, Vol. 21, No. 4, pp. 753-756, 0143-3334 (Print) 0143-3334 (Linking)

Ernst, P.B., Peura, D.A., Crowe, S.E., (2006). The translation of Helicobacter pylori basic research to patient care. *Gastroenterology*, Vol. 130, No. 1, pp. 188-206; quiz 212-183, 0016-5085 (Print) 0016-5085 (Linking)

Fagundes, J., Noujain, H., Coy, C., Ayrizono, M., Góes, J., Martinuzzo, W., (2000). Associação entre endocardite bacteriana e neoplasias - relato de 4 casos. *Rev Bras Coloproctol*, Vol. 20, No. pp. 95-99,

Grinberg, M., Mansur, A., Ferreira, D., Bellotti, G., Pileggi, F., (1990). Endocardite por Streptococcus bovis e neoplasias de cólon e reto. *Arq Bras Cardiol*, Vol. 67, No. pp. 265-269,

Groves, C., (1997). Case presentation. *The Jhon Hokins Microbiology Newsletter*, Vol. 16, No. pp. 42-44,

Gupta, A., Madani, R., Mukhtar, H., (2009). Streptococcus bovis endocarditis; a silent sign for colonic tumour. *Colorectal Dis*, Vol., No. pp., 1463-1318 (Electronic) 1462-8910 (Linking)

Haqqani, A.S., Sandhu, J.K., Birnboim, H.C., (2000). Expression of interleukin-8 promotes neutrophil infiltration and genetic instability in mutatect tumors. *Neoplasia*, Vol. 2, No. 6, pp. 561-568, 1522-8002 (Print) 1476-5586 (Linking)

Hirata, Y., Maeda, S., Mitsuno, Y., Akanuma, M., Yamaji, Y., Ogura, K., Yoshida, H., Shiratori, Y., Omata, M., (2001). Helicobacter pylori activates the cyclin D1 gene through mitogen-activated protein kinase pathway in gastric cancer cells. *Infect Immun*, Vol. 69, No. 6, pp. 3965-3971, 0019-9567 (Print) 0019-9567 (Linking)

Hoen, B., Briancon, S., Delahaye, F., Terhe, V., Etienne, J., Bigard, M.A., Canton, P., (1994). Tumors of the colon increase the risk of developing Streptococcus bovis endocarditis: case-control study. *Clin Infect Dis*, Vol. 19, No. 2, pp. 361-362, 1058-4838 (Print) 1058-4838 (Linking)

Hou, L., El-Omar, E.M., Chen, J., Grillo, P., Rabkin, C.S., Baccarelli, A., Yeager, M., Chanock, S.J., Zatonski, W., Sobin, L.H., Lissowska, J., Fraumeni, J.F., Jr., Chow, W.H., (2007). Polymorphisms in Th1-type cell-mediated response genes and risk of gastric cancer. *Carcinogenesis*, Vol. 28, No. 1, pp. 118-123, 0143-3334 (Print) 0143-3334 (Linking)

Ihler, G.M., (1996). Bartonella bacilliformis: dangerous pathogen slowly emerging from deep background. *FEMS Microbiol Lett*, Vol. 144, No. 1, pp. 1-11, 0378-1097 (Print) 0378-1097 (Linking)

Kahveci, A., Ari, E., Arikan, H., Koc, M., Tuglular, S., Ozener, C., (2010). Streptococcus bovis bacteremia related to colon adenoma in a chronic hemodialysis patient. *Hemodial Int*, Vol. 14, No. 1, pp. 91-93, 1542-4758 (Electronic) 1492-7535 (Linking)

Kaplan, M.H., Chmel, H., Stephens, A., Hsieh, H.C., Tenenbaum, M.J., Rothenberg, I.R., Joachim, G.R., (1983). Humoral reactions in human endocarditis due to Streptococcus bovis: evidence for a common S bovis antigen. *J Infect Dis*, Vol. 148, No. 2, pp. 266-274, 0022-1899 (Print) 0022-1899 (Linking)

Kargman, S.L., O'Neill, G.P., Vickers, P.J., Evans, J.F., Mancini, J.A., Jothy, S., (1995). Expression of prostaglandin G/H synthase-1 and -2 protein in human colon cancer. *Cancer Res*, Vol. 55, No. 12, pp. 2556-2559, 0008-5472 (Print) 0008-5472 (Linking)

Karin, M., Greten, F.R., (2005). NF-kappaB: linking inflammation and immunity to cancer development and progression. *Nat Rev Immunol*, Vol. 5, No. 10, pp. 749-759, 1474-1733 (Print) 1474-1733 (Linking)

Kelly, C., Evans, P., Bergmeier, L., Lee, S.F., Progulske-Fox, A., Harris, A.C., Aitken, A., Bleiweis, A.S., Lehner, T., (1989). Sequence analysis of the cloned streptococcal cell surface antigen I/II. *FEBS Lett*, Vol. 258, No. 1, pp. 127-132, 0014-5793 (Print) 0014-5793 (Linking)

Klein, R.S., Catalano, M.T., Edberg, S.C., Casey, J.I., Steigbigel, N.H., (1979). Streptococcus bovis septicemia and carcinoma of the colon. *Ann Intern Med*, Vol 91, No 4, pp 560-562, 0003-4819 (Print) 0003-4819 (Linking)

Kok, H., Jureen, R., Soon, C.Y., Tey, B.H., (2007). Colon cancer presenting as Streptococcus gallolyticus infective endocarditis. *Singapore Med J*, Vol. 48, No. 2, pp. e43-45, 0037-5675 (Print) 0037-5675 (Linking)

Konda, A., Duffy, M.C., (2008). Surveillance of patients at increased risk of colon cancer: inflammatory bowel disease and other conditions. *Gastroenterol Clin North Am*, Vol. 37, No. 1, pp. 191-213, viii, 0889-8553 (Print) 0889-8553 (Linking)

Lasa, M., Abraham, S.M., Boucheron, C., Saklatvala, J., Clark, A.R., (2002). Dexamethasone causes sustained expression of mitogen-activated protein kinase (MAPK) phosphatase 1 and phosphatase-mediated inhibition of MAPK p38. *Mol Cell Biol*, Vol. 22, No. 22, pp. 7802-7811, 0270-7306 (Print) 0270-7306 (Linking)

Lee, R.A., Woo, P.C., To, A.P., Lau, S.K., Wong, S.S., Yuen, K.Y., (2003). Geographical difference of disease association in Streptococcus bovis bacteraemia. *J Med Microbiol*, Vol. 52, No. Pt 10, pp. 903-908, 0022-2615 (Print) 0022-2615 (Linking)

Leport, C., Bure, A., Leport, J., Vilde, J.L., (1987). Incidence of colonic lesions in Streptococcus bovis and enterococcal endocarditis. *Lancet*, Vol. 1, No. 8535, pp. 748, 0140-6736 (Print) 0140-6736 (Linking)

Leung, W.K., (2006). Helicobacter pylori and gastric neoplasia. *Contrib Microbiol*, Vol. 13, No. pp. 66-80, 1420-9519 (Print) 1420-9519 (Linking)

Malkin, J., Kimmitt, P.T., Ou, H.Y., Bhasker, P.S., Khare, M., Deng, Z., Stephenson, I., Sosnowski, A.W., Perera, N., Rajakumar, K., (2008). Identification of Streptococcus gallolyticus subsp. macedonicus as the etiological agent in a case of culture-negative multivalve infective endocarditis by 16S rDNA PCR analysis of resected valvular tissue. *J Heart Valve Dis*, Vol. 17, No. 5, pp. 589-592, 0966-8519 (Print) 0966-8519 (Linking)

Monack, D.M., Mueller, A., Falkow, S., (2004). Persistent bacterial infections: the interface of the pathogen and the host immune system. *Nat Rev Microbiol*, Vol. 2, No. 9, pp. 747-765, 1740-1526 (Print) 1740-1526 (Linking)

Murinello, A., Mendonca, P., Ho, C., Traverse, P., Peres, H., RioTinto, R., Morbey, A., Campos, C., Lazoro, A., Milheiro, A., Arias, M., Oliveira, J., Braz, S., (2006). Streptococcus gallolyticus bacteremia assoaiced with colonic adenmatous polyps. *GE-J-Port Gastrentrol* Vol. 13, No. pp. 152-156,

Murray, H.W., Roberts, R.B., (1978). Streptococcus bovis bacteremia and underlying gastrointestinal disease. *Arch Intern Med*, Vol. 138, No. 7, pp. 1097-1099, 0003-9926 (Print) 0003-9926 (Linking)

Murray, P.R., Baron, E.J., (2007). *Manual of clinical microbiology* (9th). ASM Press, 1555813712 (set) 9781555813710 (set) Washington, D.C.

Nguyen, I., Biarc, J., Pini, A., Gosse, F., Richert, S., Thierse, D., Van Dorsselaer, A., Leize-Wagner, E., Raul, F., Klein, J., Scholler-Guinard, M., (2006). Streptococcus infantarius and colonic cancer: Identification and purification of cell wall proteins putatively involved in colorectal inflammation and carcinogenesis in rats. *International Congress Series* Vol., No. pp. 257– 261,

Nielsen, S.D., Christensen, J.J., Laerkeborg, A., Haunso, S., Knudsen, J.D., (2007). [Molecular-biological methods of diagnosing colon-related Streptococcus bovis endocarditis]. *Ugeskr Laeger*, Vol. 169, No. 7, pp. 610-611, 1603-6824 (Electronic) 0041-5782 (Linking)

Norfleet, R.G., Mitchell, P.D., (1993). Streptococcus bovis does not selectively colonize colorectal cancer and polyps. *J Clin Gastroenterol*, Vol. 17, No. 1, pp. 25-28, 0192-0790 (Print) 0192-0790 (Linking)

Norrby, K., (1996). Interleukin-8 and de novo mammalian angiogenesis. *Cell Prolif*, Vol. 29, No. 6, pp. 315-323, 0960-7722 (Print) 0960-7722 (Linking)

Ohshima, H., Bartsch, H., (1994). Chronic infections and inflammatory processes as cancer risk factors: possible role of nitric oxide in carcinogenesis. *Mutat Res*, Vol. 305, No. 2, pp. 253-264, 0027-5107 (Print) 0027-5107 (Linking)

Osawa, R., Fujisawa, T., LI., S., (1995). Streptococcus gallolyticus sp. nov.: gallate degrading organisms formerly assigned to Streptococcus bovis. *Syst. Appl. Microbiol.*, Vol. 18, No. pp. 74-78,

Potter, M.A., Cunliffe, N.A., Smith, M., Miles, R.S., Flapan, A.D., Dunlop, M.G., (1998). A prospective controlled study of the association of Streptococcus bovis with colorectal carcinoma. *J Clin Pathol*, Vol. 51, No. 6, pp. 473-474, 0021-9746 (Print) 0021-9746 (Linking)

Reynolds, J.G., Silva, E., McCormack, W.M., (1983). Association of Streptococcus bovis bacteremia with bowel disease. *J Clin Microbiol*, Vol. 17, No. 4, pp. 696-697, 0095-1137 (Print) 0095 1137 (Linking)

Ruoff, K.L., Miller, S.I., Garner, C.V., Ferraro, M.J., Calderwood, S.B., (1989). Bacteremia with Streptococcus bovis and Streptococcus salivarius: clinical correlates of more accurate identification of isolates. *J Clin Microbiol*, Vol. 27, No. 2, pp. 305-308, 0095-1137 (Print) 0095-1137 (Linking)

Schlegel, L., Grimont, F., Ageron, E., Grimont, P.A., Bouvet, A., (2003). Reappraisal of the taxonomy of the Streptococcus bovis/Streptococcus equinus complex and related species: description of Streptococcus gallolyticus subsp. gallolyticus subsp. nov., S. gallolyticus subsp. macedonicus subsp. nov. and S. gallolyticus subsp. pasteurianus subsp. nov. *Int J Syst Evol Microbiol*, Vol. 53, No. Pt 3, pp. 631-645, 1466-5026 (Print) 1466-5026 (Linking)

Shacter, E., Weitzman, S.A., (2002). Chronic inflammation and cancer. *Oncology (Williston Park)*, Vol. 16, No. 2, pp. 217-226, 229; discussion 230-212, 0890-9091 (Print) 0890-9091 (Linking)

Sillanpaa, J., Nallapareddy, S.R., Qin, X., Singh, K.V., Muzny, D.M., Kovar, C.L., Nazareth, L.V., Gibbs, R.A., Ferraro, M.J., Steckelberg, J.M., Weinstock, G.M., Murray, B.E., (2009). A collagen-binding adhesin, Acb, and ten other putative MSCRAMM and pilus family proteins of Streptococcus gallolyticus subsp. gallolyticus (Streptococcus bovis Group, biotype I). *J Bacteriol*, Vol. 191, No. 21, pp. 6643-6653, 1098-5530 (Electronic) 0021-9193 (Linking)

Sillanpaa, J., Nallapareddy, S.R., Singh, K.V., Ferraro, M.J., Murray, B.E., (2008). Adherence characteristics of endocarditis-derived Streptococcus gallolyticus ssp. gallolyticus (Streptococcus bovis biotype I) isolates to host extracellular matrix proteins. *FEMS Microbiol Lett*, Vol. 289, No. 1, pp. 104-109, 0378-1097 (Print) 0378-1097 (Linking)

Smaali, I., Bachraoui, K., Joulek, A., Selmi, K., Boujnah, M.R., (2008). [Infectious endocarditis secondary to streptococcus bovis revealing adenomatous polyposis coli]. *Tunis Med*, Vol. 86, No. 7, pp. 723-724, 0041-4131 (Print) 0041-4131 (Linking)

Smith, D.G., Lawson, G.H., (2001). Lawsonia intracellularis: getting inside the pathogenesis of proliferative enteropathy. *Vet Microbiol*, Vol. 82, No. 4, pp. 331-345, 0378-1135 (Print) 0378-1135 (Linking)

Srivastava, S., Verma, M., Henson, D.E., (2001). Biomarkers for early detection of colon cancer. *Clin Cancer Res*, Vol. 7, No. 5, pp. 1118-1126, 1078-0432 (Print) 1078-0432 (Linking)

Tafte, L., Ruoff, K., (2007). Streptococcus bovis: Answers and Questions. *Clin microbial newslett*, Vol. 29, No. pp. 49-55,

Teitelbaum, J.E., Triantafyllopoulou, M., (2006). Inflammatory bowel disease and Streptococcus bovis. *Dig Dis Sci*, Vol. 51, No. 8, pp. 1439-1442, 0163-2116 (Print) 0163-2116 (Linking)

Tjalsma, H., Scholler-Guinard, M., Lasonder, E., Ruers, T.J., Willems, H.L., Swinkels, D.W., (2006). Profiling the humoral immune response in colon cancer patients: diagnostic antigens from Streptococcus bovis. *Int J Cancer*, Vol. 119, No. 9, pp. 2127-2135, 0020-7136 (Print) 0020-7136 (Linking)

Travers, P., Rosen, F.S., 1997. Immuno biology bookshelf the comprehensive resource on CD-ROM. Current Biology; Garland Pub., [London ; San Francisco] [New York], pp. 1 CD-ROM.

Vogelmann, R., Amieva, M.R., (2007). The role of bacterial pathogens in cancer. *Curr Opin Microbiol*, Vol. 10, No. 1, pp. 76-81, 1369-5274 (Print) 1369-5274 (Linking)

Waisberg, J., Matheus Cde, O., Pimenta, J., (2002). Infectious endocarditis from Streptococcus bovis associated with colonic carcinoma: case report and literature review. *Arq Gastroenterol*, Vol. 39, No. 3, pp. 177-180, 0004-2803 (Print) 0004-2803 (Linking)

Wang, D., Dubois, R.N., (2010). The role of COX-2 in intestinal inflammation and colorectal cancer. *Oncogene*, Vol. 29, No. 6, pp. 781-788, 1476-5594 (Electronic) 0950-9232 (Linking)

Wentling, G.K., Metzger, P.P., Dozois, E.J., Chua, H.K., Krishna, M., (2006). Unusual bacterial infections and colorectal carcinoma--Streptococcus bovis and Clostridium septicum: report of three cases. *Dis Colon Rectum*, Vol. 49, No. 8, pp. 1223-1227, 0012-3706 (Print) 0012-3706 (Linking)

Wilson, W.R., Thompson, R.L., Wilkowske, C.J., Washington, J.A., 2nd, Giuliani, E.R., Geraci, J.E., (1981). Short-term therapy for streptococcal infective endocarditis. Combined intramuscular administration of penicillin and streptomycin. *JAMA*, Vol. 245, No. 4, pp. 360-363, 0098-7484 (Print) 0098-7484 (Linking)

Zarkin, B.A., Lillemoe, K.D., Cameron, J.L., Effron, P.N., Magnuson, T.H., Pitt, H.A., (1990). The triad of Streptococcus bovis bacteremia, colonic pathology, and liver disease. *Ann Surg*, Vol. 211, No. 6, pp. 786-791; discussion 791-782, 0003-4932 (Print) 0003-4932 (Linking)

zur Hausen, H., (2006). Streptococcus bovis: causal or incidental involvement in cancer of the colon? *Int J Cancer*, Vol. 119, No. 9, pp. xi-xii, 0020-7136 (Print) 0020-7136 (Linking)

9

Intestinal Host-Microbiome Interactions

Harold Tjalsma and Annemarie Boleij

Department of Laboratory Medicine, Nijmegen Institute for Infection,
Inflammation and Immunity (N4i) & Radboud University Centre for Oncology (RUCO)
of the Radboud University Nijmegen Medical Centre,
The Netherlands

1. Introduction

A human body contains at least tenfold more bacteria cells than human cells and the most abundant and diverse microbial community (also known as microbiota or microbiome) resides in the large intestine (colon). It is estimated that this colonic microbiome is composed of ~10^{14} bacterial cells, comprising >10^3 species (Dethlefsen *et al.*, 2006; Qin *et al.*, 2010). Intestinal microbiomes differ from individual to individual but remain relatively stable during adult life (Green *et al.*, 2006; Arumugam *et al.*, 2011). The resident microbiome provides the host with core functions that are essential for digestion of food and control of intestinal epithelial homeostasis. Conversely, an increasing body of evidence supports a relationship between infective agents and human colorectal cancer (CRC) by production of DNA damaging metabolites or toxins, and the induction of cell proliferation and pro-carcinogenesis pathways by a subpopulation of the intestinal microbiota. It could be speculated that the intrinsic intestinal microbiome of a certain individual may contain an unfavorable number of disease-inducing bacteria. On the long term, their activities may override the health-promoting activities of the commensal bacterial population. On the other hand, the dramatic physiological alterations that result from colon carcinogenesis itself (Hirayama *et al.*, 2009) disturbs the local intestinal microenvironment and causes (local) shifts in the microbiota composition and provides a portal of infection for certain opportunistic pathogens. The latter phenomenon could explain why some uncommon bacterial infections are often associated with CRC. In this chapter we will discuss the mechanisms by which intestinal bacteria may drive the initiation and progression of sporadic CRC, but also the driving forces of intestinal carcinogenesis on local microbial dysbiosis and the consequences thereof will be reviewed.

2. Intestinal microbiome

The colonic epithelium is the first line of defense against enteric antigens and bacteria. In a healthy colon, the epithelial barrier regulates uptake of nutrients and limits uptake of potential toxic substances and infectious agents (Chichlowski & Hale, 2008). Goblet cells are specialized epithelial cells within the mucosa that produce a viscous mucus layer that covers the intestinal epithelium (Heazlewood *et al.*, 2008). This mucus layer is thick and consists of an inner firmly attached layer, that excludes bacteria from direct contact with the underlying mucosa, and an outer loose mucus layer that mainly functions as lubricant (Atuma *et al.*, 2001). Bacterial colonization of the gastrointestinal tract occurs during the first two years of life. After this period, the microbiota composition is rather stable throughout adulthood (Dethlefsen *et al.*, 2006). Nevertheless, it is likely that the colonic microbiota transiently respond to dietary intake and host physiology (Thompson-Chagoyan *et al.*, 2007). The inter-individual microbiomes differ consistently, however, it is thought that these different marked microbiota may perform similar functions, and genetically complement their host with crucial physiological functions that are not provided by the human genome itself (Candela *et al.* 2010; Gill *et al.*, 2006; Neish, 2009; O'Hara & Shanahan, 2006; Xu *et al.*, 2007). Intestinal microbiome-specific metabolic functions increase energy yield and storage from diet, regulate fat storage and generate essential vitamins, which are primarily due to the fermentation of indigestible dietary polysaccharides (Neish, 2009). It has been shown that mucosa-associated bacteria differ from the community recovered from feces, but are rather uniformly distributed throughout the colon (Green *et al.*, 2006; Macfarlane *et al.*, 2004; Zoetendal *et al.*, 2002). This mucosa-adherent population is less prone to physiological effects, such as dietary changes (Sonnenburg *et al.*, 2004), and prohibits colonization of intruding pathogens (Stecher & Hardt, 2008). Malfunctioning of the host epithelial defense mechanisms, increases the risk for bacterial infection and intestinal inflammation, as seen in patients with inflammatory bowel disease (IBD). Intestinal disease can also be directly triggered by enteropathogenic pathogens, like *Shigella*, *Citrobacter* and *Salmonella* species, that avail of virulence mechanisms that allows them to outcompete the commensal mucosa-associated bacterial population and to breach the mucosal barrier and intestinal innate immune system (Stecher *et al.*, 2007).

3. Bacterial promotion of CRC

The genetic background of the host together with dietary intake, influences the microbial composition in the gut. However progression of CRC itself also influences the gut barrier and micro-environment in the intestine. This dynamic interplay between environment, genetic and microbial influences makes it hard to dissect the exact contribution of the microbiota in the development and progression of CRC. In the next paragraphs, the mechanisms by which the intestinal microbiota could contribute to CRC are further discussed. The significance of the intestinal microbiome on the development of CRC is probably best illustrated by the fact that patients with IBD, which originates from an altered host response to a normal intestinal bacterial population (Round & Mazmanian, 2009), have a high predisposition for CRC (Macfarlane *et al.*, 2005).

3.1 Promotion of tumorigenesis

The effect of intestinal bacteria on CRC development has been studied in the intestinal neoplasia mouse model ($Apc^{min/+}$). This mutant mouse strain carries a heterozygous mutation in the *APC* locus (Moser *et al.*, 1990), meaning that only a single hit in the wild-type allele results in adenoma formation. Studies with germ-free $Apc^{min/+}$ mice revealed that the formation of adenomas was strongly reduced by as much as 50%, compared to mice bred under conventional conditions (Dove *et al.*, 1997; Moser *et al.*, 1990; Su *et al.*, 1992). When such mice were exposed to enterotoxigenic *Bacteroides fragilis* (ETBF), tumors developed more rapidly, whereas mice colonized with non-toxigenic *Bacteroides fragilis*

(NTBF) showed no increased tumor formation compared to conventional mice (Housseau & Sears, 2010).

These data clearly show that the intestinal microbial population has a strong promoting effect on tumor progression in mice that have a genetic predisposition for developing intestinal adenomas and that certain species within the intestinal microbiota contribute more than average to this process.

3.2 Stimulation of TLR signaling

A balanced immune stimulation to commensal and pathogenic bacteria is crucial for a healthy intestinal tract. Toll-like receptors (TLRs) are proteins that activate immune responses towards potentially harmful pathogens upon sensing of pathogenic substances, such as cell wall components. However, chronic overstimulation of these responses may be detrimental by leading to the initiation and progression of CRC (Fukata & Abreu, 2007).

A direct impact of bacteria on the development of CRC through the TLR5/MyD88 pathway was demonstrated in germ-free and gnotobiotic mice. These animal experiments revealed that $MyD88^{-/-}$ knock-out mice that were treated with the carcinogen azoxymethane (AOM) failed to develop colorectal tumors when these mice were subjected to bacteria. In contrast, control mice rapidly developed CRC upon bacterial colonization of their intestinal tract. These results implicate that TLR/MyD88 signaling is a prerequisite for the development of CRC (Uronis et al., 2009). In addition, it was shown that tumors in $Apc^{min/+}$ $MyD88^{-/-}$ mice were significantly smaller than those found in $Apc^{min/+}$ mice (Rakoff-Nahoum & Medzhitov, 2007). Another study showed that $TLR4^{-/-}$ mice were partly protected against the development of neoplasia by tumor-inducing chemical agents (Killeen et al., 2009). Additional evidence was presented that TLR4 signaling can promote colon carcinogenesis by stimulating tumor infiltration of Th17 cells (T-helper cell subset that produces IL-17) through the increased production of pro-inflammatory signals (Su et al., 2010). It can be envisaged that bacterial TLR4 ligands, such as LPS, play an important role in this increased chemotactic activity of tumor cells (Scanlan et al., 2008). Importantly, Th17 cells have directly been implicated in the pathogenesis of Enterotoxigenic Bacteroides fragilis-induced CRC (Housseau & Sears, 2010; Wu et al., 2009). Thus, although TLR signaling is important for the effective clearance of harmful pathogens and can mediate anti-tumor cell responses, chronic TLR activation may tip the delicate balance towards tumor-promoting activities (Rakoff-Nahoum & Medzhitov, 2009).

Altogether, the above mentioned studies indicate that chronic bacterial stimulation of inflammatory pathways at malignant sites promotes, and may even be a prerequisite for, intestinal tumor development.

3.3 Upregulation of COX-2

Cyclooxygenase-2 (COX-2) is one of the key players in the progression of CRC. The expression of COX-2 is highly elevated in colonic tumors and correlated with disease stage and stimulates cell proliferation and pro-inflammatory pathways by the production of prostaglandins (Menter et al., 2010). Human intervention studies have clearly shown that the usage of Non-Steroidal Anti-Inflammatory Drugs (NSAIDS) can reduce CRC risk by as much as 75% (Eaden et al., 2000; Labayle et al., 1991; Thun et al., 1991). Evidence for bacterial involvement in the upregulation of COX-2 during CRC development was gained through animal and in vitro studies. First, superoxide radicals produced by Enterococcus faecalis were shown to upregulate the expression of COX-2 in hybrid hamster cells containing human chromosomes, as well as in macrophages (Wang & Huycke, 2007). Furthermore, macrophages that were pre-treated with a COX-2 inhibitor and subsequently exposed to *E. faecalis* totally inhibited the induction of chromosome instability (CIN) in these hybrid hamster cells. Second, an animal study published by Ellmerich *et al.* (2000b) indicated that *Streptococcus bovis* biotype II.1 (*Streptococcus infantarius*) could also play a role in the progression of CRC through induction of the COX-2 pathway. These investigators employed a rat model in which pre-treatment with azoxymethane (AOM) induced pre-neoplastic aberrant crypt foci (ACF). When such rats were co-exposed to *S. infantarius* or cell wall antigens from this bacterium, the number of ACF increased drastically and also adenomas were found, whereas the latter were totally absent in the control mice treated with AOM alone. In addition, the production of the pro-inflammatory cytokine IL-8 in the mucosa of rats exposed to *S. infantarius* was increased. This finding is in accordance with *in vitro* studies on epithelial Caco-2 cells that release both IL-8 and PGE2 upon incubation with *S. infantarius* (Biarc *et al.*, 2004). Moreover, Abdulamir *et al.* (2010) have recently shown that increased COX-2 and IL-8 expression was associated with the presence of *Streptococcus gallolyticus* (*S. bovis* biotype I) in human colon tumor tissue. However, IL-8 expression was not increased in non-malignant tissue that contained *S. gallolyticus.* Together these studies indicate that COX-2 induction is associated with both tumor development and exposure to bacterial stimulants.

3.4 Toxin-induced promotion of cell proliferation

Enterotoxigenic *Bacteroides fragilis* (ETBF) has been implicated in the promotion of CRC through inflammatory pathways. *B. fragilis* is a normal inhabitant of the gastrointestinal tract, but its enterotoxigenic form is only present in approximately 20% of the healthy population (Sears, 2009). ETBF produces the *B. fragilis* toxin that degrades E-cadherin in epithelial cells, which causes β-catenin to migrate towards the nucleus where it can activate cell proliferation pathways (Wu *et al.*, 2003). Consequently, $APC^{min/+}$ mice colonized with ETBF were shown to suffer from increased tumor burden compared to control mice colonized with non-toxigenic *B. fragilis* (NTBF) strains (Housseau & Sears, 2010; Wu *et al.*, 2009). Importantly, Wu *et al* (2009). showed that this increased tumor burden was mediated through the increased expression of STAT3 that leads to a Th17 response. Importantly, increased tumor formation could be blocked by anti-IL17 therapy. These experiments clearly show that induction of a STAT3/Th17-dependent pathway for inflammation, leads to inflammation-induced cancer by ETBF in a mouse model. Since ETBF is a quite common bacterium in the gastro-intestinal tract, this finding could have major implications for the role of these bacteria in the development of CRC in the human population. This idea is further corroborated by the fact that patients with CRC have indeed increased carriage rates of ETBF compared to NTBF (Toprak *et al.*, 2006). It should be realized that this mechanism of tumor induction could also be associated with other toxigenic intestinal bacterial strains.

3.5 Toxin-induced DNA damage

Certain *E. coli* strains can induce increased mutation rates in eukaryotic cells as demonstrated by Cuevas-Ramos and colleagues (2010). Their experiments showed that *E. coli* strains harboring the *pks* island caused DNA damage in human epithelial cells and in an *ex vivo* mouse intestinal model by the induction of single strand breaks and activation of DNA damage signaling pathways. The *pks* gene cluster codes for nonribosomal peptide synthetases and polyketide synthetases (pks) that synthesize a genotoxin named Colibactin. The *pks* island is commonly present in about 34% of commensal *E. coli* isolates. Upon infection of epithelial cells with physiological concentrations of *pks*+ strains, initial DNA damage occurred. Furthermore, it was shown that cells continued to proliferate in the presence of DNA damage after *E. coli* infection, resulting in an increased mutation frequency (Cuevas-Ramos *et al.*, 2010). These studies suggest that *pks*+ strains of *E. coli* could be involved in the initiation and progression of CRC. As, *E. coli* is generally regarded as a normal commensal inhabitant of the gastro-intestinal tract, Bronowski and co-workers investigated the differences between *E. coli* strains collected from healthy individuals and CRC patients (Bronowski *et al.*, 2008). These experiments showed that a subset of *E. coli* strains recovered from CRC tissue shared pathogenicity islands, encoding an alfa haemolysin and a cytotoxic necrotizing factor, with uropathogenic *E. coli* strains. This suggests that besides Colibactin production, other virulence characteristics may also mediate the tumor promoting capacity of *E. coli pks*+ strains.

3.6 Metabolite-induced DNA damage
Sulfate reducing bacteria use sulfate as energy source by converting it to sulfide and hydrogen sulfide (H_2S) in the human colon. The genotoxic potential of H_2S is in part mediated by oxidative free radicals, which results in increased levels of DNA damage in cultured epithelial cells (Attene-Ramos *et al.*, 2006; Attene-Ramos *et al.*, 2007; Attene-Ramos *et al.*, 2010). Furthermore, exposure to H_2S may disrupt the balance between apoptosis, proliferation and differentiation (Cai *et al.*, 2010; Deplancke & Gaskins, 2003). Interestingly, also COX-2 was shown to be upregulated in epithelial cells after H_2S treatment at physiological concentrations, probably through generation of reactive oxygen species (Attene-Ramos *et al.*, 2010). Increased fecal H_2S concentration was implicated as a risk factor for the development of colonic neoplasia in a clinical study (Kanazawa *et al.*, 1996). Whether these increased H_2S levels originates from increased activity of sulfate reducing bacteria and/or reduced epithelial capacity to degrade H_2S remains to be investigated.

E. faecalis was also found to produce extracellular superoxide in colonic tissue of rats, which is the result of dysfunctional microbial respiration (Huycke *et al.*, 2002). These rats produced up to 25-fold increased concentrations of hydroxylated aromatic metabolites in urine than rats colonized with a closely-related strain. Importantly, superoxide can be converted to hydrogen peroxide, which has the potential to diffuse into epithelial cells and cause DNA damage. In an *in vitro* setup, it was shown that the formation of DNA adducts by *E. faecalis* was mediated by activated COX-2 expression in macrophages that in turn promoted DNA damage in epithelial target cells (Wang & Huycke, 2007; Wang *et al.*, 2008). Since COX-2 induction has a clear clinical association with CRC, this might indicate that superoxide-producing bacteria have a contributing role in disease development. This notion is further underscored by the finding that *E. faecalis* fecal carriage was increased in CRC patients, whereas the number of butyrate producing bacteria was decreased (Balamurugan *et al.*, 2008). However, no clinical evidence has been presented that associates superoxide producing enterococci with adenomas or CRC (Winters *et al.*, 1998). This clearly indicates that, although the *in vitro* data and animal studies strongly suggest that oxygen radicals from bacterial origin could play an important role in CRC initiation or progression, the clinical impact of these findings remains to be properly examined in well-designed clinical studies (Huycke & Gaskins, 2004).

Bacteroides species produce fecapentaenes that are potent mutagens that have been shown to alkylate DNA, which leads to mutagenic adducts. Some evidence points towards a mechanism in which oxygen radicals cause oxidative damage to DNA (Hinzman *et al.*, 1987; Povey *et al.*, 1991; Shioya *et al.*, 1989). Fecapentaenes appear in relatively high concentrations in human feces, however, no significant differences in fecapentaene levels were found in feces from CRC patients and controls (Schiffman *et al.*, 1989). In view of their mutagenic potential, however, fecapentaenes should be regarded as possible bacterial inducers of CRC (de Kok & van Maanen, 2000). For instance, their detrimental effects may locally contribute to the accumulation of mutations in epithelial cells, which is not directly reflected by the increased levels in fecal material.

3.7 Induction of pro-carcinogenic pathways

Some evidence exists that certain intestinal bacteria can also directly induce host epithelial pathways that make cells more susceptible to DNA damage by carcinogenic substances. Maddocks *et al.* (2009) have shown that enteropathogenic *E. coli* can down-regulate mismatch repair genes in colon epithelial cells. It may be envisaged that this impaired expression can lead to a net increased mutation rate upon co-exposure to genotoxic dietary compounds. This study accentuates that bacteria can directly interfere with gene expression in epithelial cells which, under certain conditions, may lead to increased carcinogenesis rates.

4. CRC microbiome

The preceding paragraphs describe the potential mechanisms by which bacteria can play a role in the initiation and progression of CRC. In the following paragraphs, the effects of colonic malignancies on the (local) microbial composition are discussed. It is evident that the dramatic physiological and metabolic alterations that result from colon carcinogenesis itself (Hirayama et al., 2009) will locally disturb the intestinal environment. Consequently, this will cause (local) shifts in microbiota composition as the altered tumor metabolites and intestinal physiology will recruit a bacterial population with a competitive advantage in this specific microenvironment. This is exemplified by the fact that infections with certain opportunistic intestinal pathogens have been associated with CRC for many years (see Section 5). Thus pre-malignant sites seem to constitute a preferred niche for a subset of intestinal bacteria and facilitate their outgrowth and eventually entry into the human body. Importantly, local outgrowth of harmful bacteria could also accelerate tumor progression after disease has been initiated by other factors.

The effect of colonic tumors on the microbiome composition has been investigated by several studies. First, Scanlan *et al.* (2008) investigated the bacterial diversity in healthy, polypectomized patients with increased risk for CRC and CRC patients. These studies showed a significant increased diversity of the *Clostridium leptum* and coccoides subgroups in the CRC patients compared to a healthy control group. Importantly, metabonomic faecal water analysis was able to distinguish CRC and polypectomized patients from healthy individuals, which is indicative for an altered metabolic activity of the intestinal microbiota in these patients. In another study by Maddocks *et al.* (2009) it was shown that the mucosa of adenomas and carcinomas contained increased numbers of *E. coli* compared to colonic mucosa from healthy controls. It was speculated that certain surface antigens on tumor cells, which display homology to surface antigens of fetal origin, may be responsible for the binding of *E. coli* and thus local recruitment of these bacterial strains (Martin *et al.*, 2004; Maddocks *et al.*, 2009; Swidsinski *et al.*, 1998). A similar relation has been described for the opportunistic pathogen *Streptococcus bovis*. This bacterium is thought to selectively colonize malignant and pre-malignant colonic sites by which it can cause systemic infections in susceptible individuals (see Section 5). Some contradicting results on actual *S. bovis* colonization of tumor tissue have, however, been reported. Conventional culturing techniques to determine the carriage rate of *S. bovis* in adenoma, carcinoma and healthy biopsies did not provide clear evidence for the selective colonization of adenomas or carcinomas by this bacterium (Norfleet & Mitchell, 1993; Potter et al., 1998). More recently, Abdulamir and co-workers showed the presence of *Streptococcus gallolyticus* (*S. bovis* biotype I) DNA in carcinoma and adenoma tissue via polymerase chain reaction (PCR)-based techniques, which are more sensitive than conventional culturing techniques. DNA from *S. gallolyticus* was detected in about 50% of the tumor biopsies and in 35% of off- tumor tissue samples from the same patients. Strikingly, however, *S. gallolyticus* DNA was only found in <5% of the colonic tissue samples of healthy control subjects (Abdulamir *et al.*, 2010). More recently, several studies have assessed the bacterial communities in healthy, adenoma and CRC tissue by deep 16S ribosomal DNA sequencing approaches. Shen and colleagues compared the bacterial composition in normal tissue samples from adenoma patients and from individuals without colon abnormalities. The data showed increased levels of proteobacteria and decreased bacteroidetes species in off- tumor tissue samples from adenoma patients (Shen *et al.*, 2010). Interestingly, Sobhani *et al.* (2011) reported that the abundance of Bacteroides was significantly increased in tumor and normal tissue of cancer patients compared to healthy controls. More importantly, the abundance of Bacteroides was higher in tumor tissue of cancer patients than adjacent off-tumor tissue, which was paralleled by an increased IL-17/CD3 immune cell infiltration in the malignant tissues. Another recent study by Marchesi *et al.* (2011), compared differences in healthy and cancerous tissue within cancer patients and found that tumor tissue was overrepresented by species of the genera *Coriobacteridae*, *Roseburia*, *Fusobacterium* and *Faecalibacterium* that are generally regarded as gut commensals with probiotic features. On the contrary, this study found decreased colonization of *Enterobacteriaceae*, such as *Citrobacter*, *Shigella*, *Cronobacter*, and *Salmonella* in adjacent off- tumor mucosa from the same investigated patients.

The development of colorectal tumors is schematically depicted from left to right. Initiation of carcinogenesis is a process in which many factors are involved. As discussed in this Chapter, certain bacterial pathogens, bacterial toxins, or bacterial toxic metabolites (1) may contribute to the initiation and progression of CRC by causing DNA damage, induction of COX-2/IL-8, TLR signalling and/or cell proliferation pathways (2). Consequently, the altered metabolic profile of colon tumor cells and/or differentially expression of bacterial receptor molecules on tumor cells (3) creates a new niche that recruits a different bacterial population (4) of which certain opportunistic pathogens can eventually breach the bowel wall and cause a systemic bacterial infection (5). The latter group of bacteria may play an important signalling function for the early detection of CRC by serological assays.

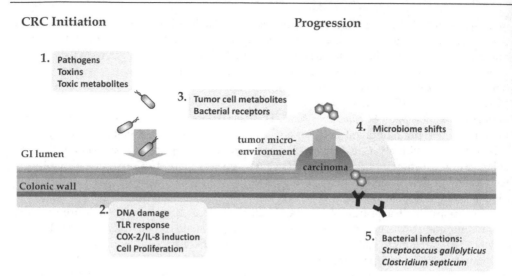

Fig. 1. Host-Microbiome interactions during CRC

5. CRC-associated bacterial infections

5.1 Streptococcus bovis

The most extensively studied bacterium that has a well-appreciated association with CRC concerns *Streptococcus bovis*. McCoy and Mason first reported such a case in 1951 (McCoy & Mason, 1951). In the 1970's this association was re-discovered by Hoppes and Lerner, who reported that 64% of the *S. bovis* endocarditis cases had gastrointestinal disease (Hoppes & Lerner, 1974). A few years later, Klein *et al.* (1977) reported an increased incidence of CRC in patients with *S. bovis* endocarditis. These investigators additionally discovered that fecal carriage of *S. bovis* in CRC patients was increased about 5-fold compared to healthy controls. At the time, these findings led to the recommendation to perform colonic evaluation in patients that were diagnosed with an *S. bovis* infection. Over the years, many studies have confirmed the association between *S. bovis* infection and CRC. In these studies, the prevalence of *S. bovis* infection with underlying CRC ranged from 10 – 100% (median 60%) for patients that underwent colonic evaluation (Boleij *et al.*, 2011b).

5.1.1 Streptococcus bovis biotypes

Based on phenotypic diversity, *S. bovis* was previously divided into three biotypes I, II.1 and II.2. Of these biotypes, biotype I is most often associated with endocarditis, while biotype II is mostly found in cases of bacteremia or liver disease. Strikingly, the association between *S. bovis* biotype I infection and CRC (21- 71%) is much higher then that of *S. bovis* biotype II (11-30%) (Corredoira *et al.*, 2008; Corredoira *et al.*, 2005; Giannitsioti *et al.*, 2007; Herrero *et al.*, 2002; Jean *et al.*, 2004; Lee *et al.*, 2003; Ruoff *et al.*, 1989; Vaska & Faoagali, 2009)(Beck *et al.*, 2008; Tripodi *et al.*, 2004). In fact, the reported incidences of carcinomas and adenomas in *S. bovis* biotype II infected patients are within the range for the normal asymptomatic population (0.3% for carcinomas / 10-25% for adenomas), whereas the rates for *S. bovis* biotype I were significantly increased (Lieberman & Smith, 1991; Lieberman *et al.*, 2000; Spier *et al.*, 2010). The distinct association of these different *S. bovis* biotypes with CRC may have accounted for the wide range of association percentages that have been reported over the years in literature. More importantly, because most studies have not discriminated between *S. bovis* biotypes the association between *S. bovis* biotype I and CRC may have structurally been underestimated. It is important to note that Schlegel *et al.* (2003) suggested renaming *S. bovis* biotype I into *S. gallolyticus* subsp. *gallolyticus*, *S. bovis* biotype II/1 into *S. infantarius* subsp. *coli* or *S. infantarius* subsp. *infantarius* and to rename *S. bovis* biotype II/2 into *S. gallolyticus* subsp. *pasteurianus*. This new nomenclature should be used to better discriminate between the different *S. bovis* subspecies of which *S. gallolyticus* is the only species with an unambiguous association with CRC (Boleij *et al.*, 2011b).

5.1.2 Streptococcus gallolyticus

Recently, some striking differences between *S. bovis* biotypes were revealed that could explain their different association rates with CRC. First of all, *S. gallolyticus* seems to contain distinguished mechanisms to adherence to extracellular matrix (ECM) structures like collagen and fibrinogen (Ellmerich *et al.*, 2000a; Sillanpaa *et al.*, 2008; Sillanpaa *et al.*, 2009). Interestingly, (pre-)malignant colonic sites are characterized by displaced collagen of the lamina propria (Galbavy *et al.*, 2002; Yantiss *et al.*, 2001), through which specifically *S. gallolyticus* may colonize these sites. Besides the ECM components, also other structures at the epithelial surface may play a role in the initial adhesion to enterocytes. For example, Henry-Stanley *et al.* (2003) reported binding of *S. bovis* strains to heparan sulfate proteoglycans, which may be mediated by surface-associated HlpA (Boleij *et al.*, 2009). In an *in vitro* trans-well model containing a differentiated intestinal monolayer, the paracellular translocation efficiency of *S. gallolyticus* was shown to be significantly higher than that of other *S. bovis* biotypes. This could mean that this bacterium has an advantage over other *S. bovis* subspecies to cross an intestinal epithelium, which possibly only occurs at (pre-)malignant sites with reduced barrier function (Boleij *et al.*, 2011a). Recent data suggested that *S. gallolyticus* does not induce a strong pro-inflammatory IL-8 response in epithelial cells in contrast to other *S. bovis* strains, which may be a possibly mechanism by which *S. gallolyticus* stays rather invisible for macrophages in the lamina propria. Furthermore, Hirota *et al.* (1995) discovered that *S. gallolyticus* isolates from endocarditis patients, express human sialyl Lewis[x] antigens on their cell surface unlike other fecal isolates. Mimicking human sialyl antigens, which are naturally present on monocytes and granulocutes, could therefore be a second mechanism of *S. gallolyticus* to remain unnoticed by the human innate immune system. Moreover, sialyl Lewis[x] antigens could make these bacteria more efficient in binding to endothelial cells and invasion into the circulatory system (Hirota *et al.*, 1996). Finally, *S. gallolyticus* was shown to have superior efficiency to form biofilms on collagen I and IV surfaces (Boleij *et al.*, 2011a; Sillanpaa *et al.*, 2008). The latter finding could explain the increased incidence of *S. gallolyticus* as causative agent in infective endocarditis. Based on the current state-of-the-literature (July 2011), the following events in CRC-associated *S. gallolyticus* endocarditis can be envisaged **i)** *S. gallolyticus* specifically adheres to (pre-)malignant colonic sites for instance via binding to displaced collagen of the lamina propria or other tumor cell specific adherence factors; **ii)** *S. gallolyticus* may promote tumor progression by induction of the COX-2 pathway; **iii)** *S. gallolyticus* takes advantage of the distorted structure of the colonic epithelium at (pre-)malignant sites to pass the colonic wall; **iv)** *S. gallolyticus* stays relatively invisible for the innate immune system and can reach the blood stream; **v)** *S. gallolyticus* can cause a secondary infection at sites with high exposure of collagens, such as present at damaged heart values. It should be noted, however, that many of these data were obtained by *in vitro* studies and that it remains to be determined how this relates to the *in vivo* situation.

5.2 Clostridium septicum

In addition to *S. gallolyticus* endocarditis, also *Clostridium septicum* infections have been clinically associated with sporadic CRC (Chew & Lubowski, 2001; Mirza *et al.*, 2009). *C. septicum* is not considered to be part of the normal intestinal microbiota and is a rare cause of bacteremia (<1% of all cases). Hermsen *et al.* (2008) investigated 320 cases of *C. septicum* infections, 42% of which had a gastrointestinal origin. Malignant disease was present in 30-50% of these cases. The underlying mechanism of this association is not known, but it has been speculated that the hypoxic and acidic environment of the tumor specifically favor germination of *C. septicum* spores that enter the gastrointestinal tract via contaminated food (Dylewski & Luterman). A direct involvement of *C. septicum* in the development of CRC has thus far not been investigated, but it is hypothesized that *C. septicum* infections are primarily a consequence of CRC itself. Also *Clostridium perfringens* and *Clostridium butyricum* have been described in relation with CRC (Cabrera *et al.*, 1965; Rathbun, 1968). However, these strains are much less virulent than *C. septicum* and their association with CRC is less evident. Although infections with *C. septicum* are rare, underlying malignancy should be suspected and also in these cases full bowel examination could eventually save patients' lives.

5.3 Helicobacter pylori

Helicobacter pylori has been classified as gastric cancer-causing infective agent by the International Agency for Research on Cancer (IARC) in 1994. Most *H. pylori* strains, however, are non-invasive organism and exist in a non-adherent extracellular mucous environment. A small number of strains adheres to gastric epithelial cells, which most likely involves a number of different surface receptors (Wilkinson *et al.*, 1998). The presence of the pathogenicity island, expressing the cytotoxins VacA and CagA, is an important virulence determinant in these strains (Ekstrom *et al.*, 2001; Huang *et al.*, 2003; Crabtree *et al.*, 1994; Kuipers *et al.*, 1995). It is thought that long-term exposure to these toxins induces gastric inflammation that can eventually lead to gastric carcinomas (Higashi *et al.*, 2002; Fox, 2002). A meta-analysis conducted in 2006 by Zumkeller *et al.* indicated also a slightly increased risk for CRC (factor 1.4) in individuals with a *H. pylori* infection (Zumkeller *et al.*, 2006). Another study showed that CagA status was associated with a significantly increased risk (factor >10) for CRC among hospitalized patients that were *H. pylori* seropositive (Shmuely *et al.*, 2001). Notably, this study again underscores the importance of proper microbiological classification and characterization of cancer-associated infectious agents, since not all *Helicobacter* strains may be associated with CRC. Like has been the case for *S. bovis*, lack of proper distinction between *H. pylori* subspecies could have biased or even underestimated a possible association of this bacterium with this disease (Erdman *et al.*, 2003a,b).

6. CRC Microbiome-based Immunoassays

The occurrence of specific CRC-associated bacterial infections, as discussed in the previous section, paves the way for the development of novel diagnostic tools. In this respect, it is important to realize that *S. gallolyticus* infections occur without clinical symptoms due to its mild virulence (Haimowitz *et al.*, 2005). Clinical manifestation of *S. gallolyticus* infections in otherwise compromised patients (*e.g.* damaged heart valves), may very well only represent the tip of the iceberg of all infections with this bacterium in individuals with (pre-)malignant colonic lesions. This notion has been the incentive to investigate whether a humoral immune response to sub-clinical *S. gallolyticus* infections could aid in the early detection of CRC. Notably, as infectious agents in general induce a more pronounced immune response compared to tumor "self" antigens, CRC-associated bacterial antigens could be instrumental in the immunodiagnosis of this disease (Tjalsma, 2011). Furthermore, several features of circulating antibodies make these attractive targets in diagnostic medicine: **i)** they reflect a molecular imprint of disease-related antigens from all around the human body, **ii)** although an antigen may be present only briefly, the corresponding antibody response is likely to be persistent, **iii)** the half-life of antibodies is about 15 days which minimizes daily fluctuations, **iv)** antibodies are highly stable compared to many other serum proteins making serum-handling protocols less stringent, **v)** the amplification cascade governed by the humoral immune system causes a surplus of circulating antibodies after appearance of the cognate (low-abundance) antigen. Several studies have shown that serum antibody levels against *S. bovis/S. gallolyticus* antigens could discriminate CRC cases from healthy controls (Abdulamir et al., 2009; Darjee & Gibb, 1993; Tjalsma et al., 2006). Interestingly, the humoral immune response to ribosomal protein (Rp) L7/L12 from *S. gallolyticus* was found to be higher in early CRC compared to late CRC stages, whereas this was not paralleled by increased antibody production to endotoxin, an intrinsic cell wall component of the majority of intestinal bacteria (Boleij et al., 2010). This implies that the immune response to RpL7/L12 is not a general phenomenon induced by the loss of colonic barrier function. Furthermore, this observation could point to a temporal relationship between *S. gallolyticus* and CRC, suggesting that late stage tumors may change in such a way that bacterial survival in the tumor microenvironment is diminished. The possibility that disease progression may drive bacteria out of the cancerous tissue is similar to what has been reported for *H. pylori* during gastric cancer progression (Corfield et al., 2000; Kang et al., 2006). A relationship of *S. bovis* with early stages of CRC is underscored by a vast amount of case studies showing that its infection was associated with pre-malignant adenomas. These cases would have remained undiscovered if these patients did not present with an active *S. bovis* infection. Future research should be aimed at development of more specific *S. gallolyticus*-based serological assays to investigate the clinical utility of such tests for the early detection of CRC (Tjalsma et al., 2006, 2008; Tjalsma, 2010). Furthermore, as CRC is a highly heterogeneous disease that is probably accompanied by even more heterogeneous microbiome shifts, accurate diagnosis based on biomarkers from a single bacterial species on the population level is highly unlikely. Therefore, future research should also be aimed at the identification of additional tumor-associated intestinal bacteria that may never have been found to cause clinical infections but do induce a humoral immune response. Furthermore, as discussed in Section 3 of this Chapter, certain mucosa-associated bacteria may be involved in CRC initiation or progression. Invasiveness of these pathogens or exposure to their antigens may elicit IgG responses that are valuable for CRC risk assessment. These individuals may not directly need bowel examination, but could be enrolled in a more strict monitoring program.

7. Conclusions

The development of CRC is a multistep process that may take over 20 years to progress from an adenoma into an advanced carcinoma. The fact that the intestinal microbiome plays an important role in this process is clearly shown by the inflammatory effects of intestinal bacteria, which are essential to develop disease in animal models. Furthermore, accumulating evidence suggests that bacterial production of toxins, toxic metabolites and the direct influences on pro-carcinogenic pathways in host epithelial cells are contributing factors that promote the accumulation of mutations that may eventually lead to carcinomas. However, still many questions remain to be answered. For example, our knowledge on the on the impact of CRC on the local intestinal microbiota and *vice versa*, is still in its infancy. Future research should focus on the detailed mapping of the microbiota in close proximity of early adenomas and carcinomas. These local changes in microbiota may for instance provide clues in the understanding why only 10% of the adenomas progress into carcinomas. Such knowledge could give us new leads for cancer diagnosis, for example by using signaling bacteria, such as *S. gallolyticus* that benefit from the altered tumor environment, as diagnostic targets. Furthermore, this knowledge could provide leads for the selective removal of high-risk bacterial populations by health promoting species, as a new strategy in CRC prevention. Altogether, this Chapter points out that the colonic microbiota should be regarded as an important factor in intestinal carcinogenesis. Further research in this field is crucial to fully understand the etiology of CRC and has a high potential to lead to new diagnostic tools and therapeutic interventions.

8. Acknowledgements

We thank Albert Bolhuis, Dorine Swinkels, Bas Dutilh, Carla Muytjens, Guus Kortman, Ikuko Kato, Julian Marchesi, Philippe Glaser, Rian Roelofs, Shaynoor Dramsi & Wilbert Peters for inspiring discussions. Work in our laboratory was supported by the Dutch Cancer Society (KWF; project KUN 2006-3591) and the Dutch Digestive Diseases Foundation (MLDS; project WO10-53). Correspondence to: Harold Tjalsma, Department of Laboratory Medicine (LGEM 830), Radboud University Nijmegen Medical Centre, P.O. Box 9101, 6500 HB, Nijmegen, The Netherlands; H.Tjalsma@labgk.umcn.nl.

9. References

Abdulamir, A. S., Hafidh, R. R., Mahdi, L. K., Al-jeboori, T. & Abubaker, F. (2009). Investigation into the controversial association of Streptococcus gallolyticus with colorectal cancer and adenoma. *BMC Cancer* 9, 403.

Abdulamir, A. S., Hafidh, R. R. & Abu Bakar, F. (2010). Molecular detection, quantification, and isolation of Streptococcus gallolyticus bacteria colonizing colorectal tumors: inflammation-driven potential of carcinogenesis via IL-1, COX-2, and IL-8. *Mol Cancer* 9, 249.

Arumugam, M., Raes, J., Pelletier, E., Le Paslier, D., Yamada, T., Mende, D.R., Fernandes, G.R., Tap, J., Bruls, T., Batto, J.M., Bertalan, M., Borruel, N., Casellas, F., Fernandez, L., Gautier, L., Hansen, T., Hattori, M., Hayashi, T., Kleerebezem, M., Kurokawa, K., Leclerc, M., Levenez, F., Manichanh, C., Nielsen, H.B., Nielsen, T., Pons, N., Poulain, J., Qin, J., Sicheritz-Ponten, T., Tims, S., Torrents, D., Ugarte, E., Zoetendal, E.G., Wang, J., Guarner, F., Pedersen, O., de Vos, W.M., Brunak, S., & Doré, J. (2011) Enterotypes of the human gut microbiome. *Nature* 473, 174-80.

Attene-Ramos, M. S., Wagner, E. D., Plewa, M. J. & Gaskins, H. R. (2006). Evidence that hydrogen sulfide is a genotoxic agent. *Mol Cancer Res* 4, 9-14.

Attene-Ramos, M. S., Wagner, E. D., Gaskins, H. R. & Plewa, M. J. (2007). Hydrogen sulfide induces direct radical-associated DNA damage. *Mol Cancer Res* 5, 455-459.

Attene-Ramos, M. S., Nava, G. M., Muellner, M. G., Wagner, E. D., Plewa, M. J. & Gaskins, H. R. (2010). DNA damage and toxicogenomic analyses of hydrogen sulfide in human intestinal epithelial FHs 74 Int cells. *Environ Mol Mutagen* 51, 304-314.

Atuma, C., Strugala, V., Allen, A. & Holm, L. (2001). The adherent gastrointestinal mucus gel layer: thickness and physical state in vivo. *Am J Physiol* 280, G922-929.

Balamurugan, R., Rajendiran, E., George, S., Samuel, G. V. & Ramakrishna, B. S. (2008). Real-time polymerase chain reaction quantification of specific butyrate-producing bacteria, Desulfovibrio and Enterococcus faecalis in the feces of patients with colorectal cancer. *J Gastroenterol Hepatol* 23, 1298-1303.

Biarc, J., Nguyen, I. S., Pini, A. & other authors (2004). Carcinogenic properties of proteins with pro-inflammatory activity from Streptococcus infantarius (formerly S. bovis). *Carcinogenesis* 25, 1477-1484.

Boleij, A., Schaeps, R. M. J., de Kleijn, S., Hermans, P. W., Glaser, P., Pancholi, V., Swinkels, D. W. & Tjalsma, H. (2009). Surface-exposed Histone-like protein A modulates adherence of Streptococcus gallolyticus to colon adenocarcinoma cells. *Infec Immun* 77, 5519-5527.

Boleij, A., Roelofs, R., Schaeps, R. M., Schulin, T., Glaser, P., Swinkels, D. W., Kato, I. & Tjalsma, H. (2010). Increased exposure to bacterial antigen RpL7/L12 in early stage colorectal cancer patients. *Cancer* 116, 4014-4022.

Boleij, A., Muytjens, C. M. J., Bukhari, S. I., Cayet, N., Glaser, P., Hermans, P. W., Swinkels, D. W., Bolhuis, A. & Tjalsma, H. (2011a). Novel clues on the specific association of Streptococcus gallolyticus subsp gallolyticus with colorectal cancer. *J Infect Dis* 203, 1101-1109.

Boleij, A., van Gelder, M.M.H.J., Swinkels, D. W., & Tjalsma, H. (2011b). Clinical Importance of Streptococcus gallolyticus infections among colorectal cancer patients: systematic review and meta-analysis. *Clin Infect Dis*, in press.

Bronowski, C., Smith, S. L., Yokota, K., Corkill, J. E., Martin, H. M., Campbell, B. J., Rhodes, J. M., Hart, C. A. & Winstanley, C. (2008). A subset of mucosa-associated Escherichia coli isolates from patients with colon cancer, but not Crohn's disease, share pathogenicity islands with urinary pathogenic E. coli. *Microbiology* 154, 571-583.

Cabrera, A., Tsukada, Y. & Pickren, J. W. (1965). Clostridial Gas Gangrene and Septicemia in Malignant Disease. *Cancer* 18, 800-806.

Cai, W. J., Wang, M. J., Ju, L. H., Wang, C. & Zhu, Y. C. (2010). Hydrogen sulfide induces human colon cancer cell proliferation: role of Akt, ERK and p21. *Cell Biol Int* 34, 565-572.

Candela, M., Maccaferri, S., Turroni, S., Carnevali, P. & Brigidi, P. (2010) Functional intestinal microbiome, new frontiers in prebiotic design. *Int Journal Food Microbiol* 140, 93-101.

Chew, S. S. & Lubowski, D. Z. (2001). Clostridium septicum and malignancy. *ANZ journal of surgery* 71, 647-649.

Chichlowski, M. & Hale, L. P. (2008). Bacterial-mucosal interactions in inflammatory bowel disease: an alliance gone bad. *Am J Physiol Gastrointest Liver Physiol* 295, G1139-1149.

Corfield, A. P., Myerscough, N., Longman, R., Sylvester, P., Arul, S. & Pignatelli, M. (2000). Mucins and mucosal protection in the gastrointestinal tract: new prospects for mucins in the pathology of gastrointestinal disease. *Gut* 47, 589-594.

Corredoira, J., Alonso, M. P., & Coira, A (2008). Characteristics of Streptococcus bovis endocarditis and its differences with Streptococcus viridans endocarditis. *Eur J Clin Microbiol Infect Dis* 27, 285-291.

Corredoira, J. C., Alonso, M. P., & Garcia, J. F. (2005). Clinical characteristics and significance of Streptococcus salivarius bacteremia and Streptococcus bovis bacteremia: a prospective 16-year study. *Eur J Clin Microbiol Infect Dis* 24, 250-255.

Crabtree, J. E., Farmery, S. M., Lindley, I. J., Figura, N., Peichl, P. & Tompkins, D. S. (1994). CagA/cytotoxic strains of Helicobacter pylori and interleukin-8 in gastric epithelial cell lines. *J Clin Pathol* 47, 945-950.

Cuevas-Ramos, G., Petit, C. R., Marcq, I., Boury, M., Oswald, E. & Nougayrede, J. P. (2010). Escherichia coli induces DNA damage in vivo and triggers genomic instability in mammalian cells. *Proc Nat AcadSci USA* 107, 11537-11542.

Darjee, R. & Gibb, A. P. (1993). Serological investigation into the association between Streptococcus bovis and colonic cancer. *J Clin Pathol* 46, 1116-1119.

de Kok, T. M. & van Maanen, J. M. (2000). Evaluation of fecal mutagenicity and colorectal cancer risk. *Mutation Res* 463, 53-101.

Deplancke, B. & Gaskins, H. R. (2003). Hydrogen sulfide induces serum-independent cell cycle entry in nontransformed rat intestinal epithelial cells. *FASEB J* 17, 1310-1312.

Dethlefsen, L., Eckburg, P. B., Bik, E. M. & Relman, D. A. (2006). Assembly of the human intestinal microbiota. *Trends Ecol Evol,* 21, 517-523.

Dove, W. F., Clipson, L., Gould, K. A., Luongo, C., Marshall, D. J., Moser, A. R., Newton, M. A. & Jacoby, R. F. (1997). Intestinal neoplasia in the ApcMin mouse: independence from the microbial and natural killer (beige locus) status. *Cancer Res* 57, 812-814.

Dylewski, J. & Luterman, L. Septic arthritis and Clostridium septicum: a clue to colon cancer. *Cmaj* 182, 1446-1447.

Eaden, J., Abrams, K., Ekbom, A., Jackson, E. & Mayberry, J. (2000). Colorectal cancer prevention in ulcerative colitis: a case-control study. *Alimen Pharmacol Therapeutics* 14, 145-153.

Ekstrom, A. M., Held, M., Hansson, L. E., Engstrand, L. & Nyren, O. (2001). Helicobacter pylori in gastric cancer established by CagA immunoblot as a marker of past infection. *Gastroenterology* 121, 784-791.

Ellmerich, S., Djouder, N., Scholler, M. & Klein, J. P. (2000a). Production of cytokines by monocytes, epithelial and endothelial cells activated by Streptococcus bovis. *Cytokine* 12, 26-31.

Ellmerich, S., Scholler, M., Duranton, B., Gosse, F., Galluser, M., Klein, J. P. & Raul, F. (2000b). Promotion of intestinal carcinogenesis by Streptococcus bovis. *Carcinogenesis* 21, 753-756.

Erdman, S. E., Poutahidis, T., Tomczak, M., Rogers, A. B., Cormier, K., Plank, B., Horwitz, B. H. & Fox, J. G. (2003a). CD4+ CD25+ regulatory T lymphocytes inhibit microbially induced colon cancer in Rag2-deficient mice. *Am J Pathol* 162, 691-702.

Erdman, S. E., Rao, V. P., Poutahidis, T. & other authors (2003b). CD4(+)CD25(+) regulatory lymphocytes require interleukin 10 to interrupt colon carcinogenesis in mice. *Cancer Res* 63, 6042-6050.

Fox, J. G. (2002). The non-H pylori helicobacters: their expanding role in gastrointestinal and systemic diseases. *Gut* 50, 273-283.

Fukata, M. & Abreu, M. T. (2007). TLR4 signalling in the intestine in health and disease. *Biochem Soc Trans* 35, 1473-1478.

Galbavy, S., Lukac, L., Porubsky, J., Cerna, M., Labuda, M., Kmet'ova, J., Papincak, J., Durdik, S. & Jakubovsky, J. (2002). Collagen type IV in epithelial tumours of colon. *Acta Histochem* 104, 331-334.

Giannitsioti, E., Chirouze, C., Bouvet, A. & other authors (2007). Characteristics and regional variations of group D streptococcal endocarditis in France. *Clin Microbiol Infect* 13, 770-776.

Gill, S. R., Pop, M., Deboy, R. T. & other authors (2006). Metagenomic analysis of the human distal gut microbiome. *Science (New York, NY* 312, 1355-1359.

Green, G. L., Brostoff, J., Hudspith, B. & other authors (2006). Molecular characterization of the bacteria adherent to human colorectal mucosa. *J Appl Microbiol* 100, 460-469.

Haimowitz, M. D., Hernandez, L. A. & Herron, R. M., Jr. (2005). A blood donor with bacteraemia. *Lancet* 365, 1596.

Heazlewood, C. K., Cook, M. C., Eri, R. & other authors (2008). Aberrant mucin assembly in mice causes endoplasmic reticulum stress and spontaneous inflammation resembling ulcerative colitis. *PLoS Med* 5, e54.

Henry-Stanley, M. J., Hess, D. J., Erickson, E. A., Garni, R. M. & Wells, C. L. (2003). Role of heparan sulfate in interactions of Listeria monocytogenes with enterocytes. *Med Microbiol Immunol* 192, 107-115.

Hermsen, J. L., Schurr, M. J., Kudsk, K. A. & Faucher, L. D. (2008). Phenotyping Clostridium septicum infection: a surgeon's infectious disease. *J Surgical Res* 148, 67-76.

Herrero, I. A., Rouse, M. S., Piper, K. E., Alyaseen, S. A., Steckelberg, J. M. & Patel, R. (2002). Reevaluation of Streptococcus bovis endocarditis cases from 1975 to 1985 by 16S ribosomal DNA sequence analysis. *J Clin Microbiol* 40, 3848-3850.

Higashi, H., Tsutsumi, R., Fujita, A., Yamazaki, S., Asaka, M., Azuma, T. & Hatakeyama, M. (2002). Biological activity of the Helicobacter pylori virulence factor CagA is determined by variation in the tyrosine phosphorylation sites. *Proc Nat Acad Sci USA* 99, 14428-14433.

Hinzman, M. J., Novotny, C., Ullah, A. & Shamsuddin, A. M. (1987). Fecal mutagen fecapentaene-12 damages mammalian colon epithelial DNA. *Carcinogenesis* 8, 1475-1479.

Hirayama, A., Kami, K., Sugimoto, M., Sugawara, M., Toki, N., Onozuka, H., Kinoshita, T., Saito, N., Ochiai, A., Tomita, M., Esumi, H., & Soga, T. (2009). Quantitative metabolome profiling of colon and stomach cancer microenvironment by capillary electrophoresis time-of-flight mass spectrometry. *Cancer Res* 69: 4918-25.

Hirota, K., Kanitani, H., Nemoto, K., Ono, T. & Miyake, Y. (1995). Cross-reactivity between human sialyl Lewis(x) oligosaccharide and common causative oral bacteria of infective endocarditis. *FEMS Immun Med Microbiol* 12, 159-164.

Hirota, K., Osawa, R., Nemoto, K., Ono, T. & Miyake, Y. (1996). Highly expressed human sialyl Lewis antigen on cell surface of streptococcus gallolyticus. *Lancet* 347, 760.

Homann, N., Tillonen, J. & Salaspuro, M. (2000). Microbially produced acetaldehyde from ethanol may increase the risk of colon cancer via folate deficiency. *Int J Cancer* 86, 169-173.

Hoppes, W. L. & Lerner, P. I. (1974). Nonenterococcal group-D streptococcal endocarditis caused by Streptococcus bovis. *Annals Int Med* 81, 588-593.

Housseau, F. & Sears, C. L. (2010). Enterotoxigenic Bacteroides fragilis (ETBF)-mediated colitis in Min (Apc+/-) mice: a human commensal-based murine model of colon carcinogenesis. *Cell Cycle* 9, 3-5.

Huang, J. Q., Zheng, G. F., Sumanac, K., Irvine, E. J. & Hunt, R. H. (2003). Meta-analysis of the relationship between cagA seropositivity and gastric cancer. *Gastroenterology* 125, 1636-1644.

Huycke, M. M., Abrams, V. & Moore, D. R. (2002). Enterococcus faecalis produces extracellular superoxide and hydrogen peroxide that damages colonic epithelial cell DNA. *Carcinogenesis* 23, 529-536.

Huycke, M. M. & Gaskins, H. R. (2004). Commensal bacteria, redox stress, and colorectal cancer: mechanisms and models. *Exp Biol Med* 229, 586-597.

Itzkowitz, S. H. & Yio, X. (2004). Inflammation and cancer IV. Colorectal cancer in inflammatory bowel disease: the role of inflammation. *Am J Physiology* 287, G7-17.

Jean, S. S., Teng, L. J., Hsueh, P. R., Ho, S. W. & Luh, K. T. (2004). Bacteremic Streptococcus bovis infections at a university hospital, 1992-2001. *J Formosan Med Ass* 103, 118-123.

Jemal, A., Siegel, R., Ward, E., Hao, Y. P., Xu, J. Q. & Thun, M. J. (2009). Cancer Statistics, 2009. *CA-Cancer J Clin* 59, 225-249.

Kanazawa, K., Konishi, F., Mitsuoka, T., Terada, A., Itoh, K., Narushima, S., Kumemura, M. & Kimura, H. (1996). Factors influencing the development of sigmoid colon cancer. Bacteriologic and biochemical studies. *Cancer* 77, 1701-1706.

Kang, H. Y., Kim, N., Park, Y. S., Hwang, J. H., Kim, J. W., Jeong, S. H., Lee, D. H., Jung, H. C. & Song, I. S. (2006). Progression of atrophic gastritis and intestinal metaplasia drives Helicobacter pylori out of the gastric mucosa. *Dig Dis Sci* 51, 2310-2315.

Killeen, S. D., Wang, J. H., Andrews, E. J. & Redmond, H. P. (2009). Bacterial endotoxin enhances colorectal cancer cell adhesion and invasion through TLR-4 and NF-kappaB-dependent activation of the urokinase plasminogen activator system. *Br J Cancer* 100, 1589-1602.

Klein, R. S., Recco, R. A., Catalano, M. T., Edberg, S. C., Casey, J. I. & Steigbigel, N. H. (1977). Association of Streptococcus bovis with carcinoma of the colon. *New Engl J Med* 297, 800-802.

Knasmuller, S., Steinkellner, H., Hirschl, A. M., Rabot, S., Nobis, E. C. & Kassie, F. (2001). Impact of bacteria in dairy products and of the intestinal microflora on the genotoxic and carcinogenic effects of heterocyclic aromatic amines. *Mutation Res* 480-481, 129-138.

Kuipers, E. J., Perez-Perez, G. I., Meuwissen, S. G. & Blaser, M. J. (1995). Helicobacter pylori and atrophic gastritis: importance of the cagA status. *J Nat Cancer Inst* 87, 1777-1780.

Labayle, D., Fischer, D., Vielh, P., Drouhin, F., Pariente, A., Bories, C., Duhamel, O., Trousset, M. & Attali, P. (1991). Sulindac causes regression of rectal polyps in familial adenomatous polyposis. *Gastroenterology* 101, 635-639.

Lee, R. A., Woo, P. C., To, A. P., Lau, S. K., Wong, S. S. & Yuen, K. Y. (2003). Geographical difference of disease association in Streptococcus bovis bacteraemia. *JMed Microbiol* 52, 903-908.

Lieberman, D. A. & Smith, F. W. (1991). Screening for colon malignancy with colonoscopy. *Am J Gastroenterol* 86, 946-951.

Lieberman, D. A., Weiss, D. G., Bond, J. H., Ahnen, D. J., Garewal, H. & Chejfec, G. (2000). Use of colonoscopy to screen asymptomatic adults for colorectal cancer. Veterans Affairs Cooperative Study Group 380. *New Engl J Med* 343, 162-168.

Macfarlane, S., Furrie, E., Cummings, J. H. & Macfarlane, G. T. (2004). Chemotaxonomic analysis of bacterial populations colonizing the rectal mucosa in patients with ulcerative colitis. *Clin Infect Dis* 38, 1690-1699.

Macfarlane, S., Furrie, E., Kennedy, A., Cummings, J. H. & Macfarlane, G. T. (2005). Mucosal bacteria in ulcerative colitis. *Brit J Nutr* 93 Suppl 1, S67-72.

Maddocks, O. D., Short, A. J., Donnenberg, M. S., Bader, S. & Harrison, D. J. (2009). Attaching and effacing Escherichia coli downregulate DNA mismatch repair protein in vitro and are associated with colorectal adenocarcinomas in humans. *PloS One* 4, e5517.

Marchesi, J. R., Dutilh, B. E., Hall, N., Peters, W. H. M., Roelofs, R., Boleij, A. & Tjalsma, H. (2011). Towards the human colorectal cancer microbiome. *PloS One* 6:e20447.

Martin, H. M., Campbell, B. J., Hart, C. A., Mpofu, C., Nayar, M., Singh, R., Englyst, H., Williams, H. F. & Rhodes, J. M. (2004). Enhanced Escherichia coli adherence and invasion in Crohn's disease and colon cancer. *Gastroenterology* 127, 80-93.

McCoy, W. & Mason, J. M. (1951). Enterococcal endocarditis associated with carcinoma of the sigmoid; report of a case. *J Med Ass Alab* 21, 162-166.

Menter, D. G., Schilsky, R. L. & DuBois, R. N. (2010). Cyclooxygenase-2 and cancer treatment: understanding the risk should be worth the reward. *Clin Cancer Res* 16, 1384-1390.

Mirza, N. N., McCloud, J. M. & Cheetham, M. J. (2009). Clostridium septicum sepsis and colorectal cancer - a reminder. *World J Surg Oncol* 7, 73.

Moser, A. R., Pitot, H. C. & Dove, W. F. (1990). A dominant mutation that predisposes to multiple intestinal neoplasia in the mouse. *Science* 247, 322-324.

Neish, A. S. (2009). Microbes in gastrointestinal health and disease. *Gastroenterology* 136, 65-80.

O'Hara, A. M. & Shanahan, F. (2006). The gut flora as a forgotten organ. *EMBO reports* 7, 688-693.

Povey, A. C., Schiffman, M., Taffe, B. G. & Harris, C. C. (1991). Laboratory and epidemiologic studies of fecapentaenes. *Mutation Res* 259, 387-397.

Qin, J., Li, R., Raes, J., Arumugam, M., Burgdorf, K.S., Manichanh, C., Nielsen, T., Pons, N., Levenez, F., Yamada, T., Mende, D.R., Li, J., Xu, J., Li, S., Li, D., Cao, J., Wang, B., Liang, H., Zheng, H., Xie, Y., Tap, J., Lepage, P., Bertalan, M., Batto, J.M., Hansen, T., Le Paslier, D., Linneberg, A., Nielsen, H.B., Pelletier, E., Renault, P., Sicheritz-Ponten, T., Turner, K., Zhu, H., Yu, C., Li, S., Jian, M., Zhou, Y., Li, Y., Zhang, X., Li, S., Qin, N., Yang, H., Wang, J., Brunak, S., Doré, J., Guarner, F., Kristiansen, K., Pedersen, O., Parkhill, J., Weissenbach, J., (2010). A human gut microbial gene catalogue established by metagenomic sequencing. *Nature* 464, 59-65.

Rakoff-Nahoum, S. & Medzhitov, R. (2007). Regulation of spontaneous intestinal tumorigenesis through the adaptor protein MyD88. *Science* 317, 124-127.

Rakoff-Nahoum, S. & Medzhitov, R. (2009). Toll-like receptors and cancer. *Nat Rev Cancer* 9, 57-63.

Rathbun, H. K. (1968). Clostridial bacteremia without hemolysis. *Arch Int Medicine* 122, 496-501.

Round, J. L. & Mazmanian, S. K. (2009). The gut microbiota shapes intestinal immune responses during health and disease. *Nat Rev Immunol* 9, 313-323.

Ruoff, K. L., Miller, S. I., Garner, C. V., Ferraro, M. J. & Calderwood, S. B. (1989). Bacteremia with Streptococcus bovis and Streptococcus salivarius: clinical correlates of more accurate identification of isolates. *J Clin Microbiol* 27, 305-308.

Rutter, M., Saunders, B., Wilkinson, K. & other authors (2004). Severity of inflammation is a risk factor for colorectal neoplasia in ulcerative colitis. *Gastroenterology* 126, 451-459.

Scanlan, P. D., Shanahan, F., Clune, Y., Collins, J. K., O'Sullivan, G. C., O'Riordan, M., Holmes, E., Wang, Y. & Marchesi, J. R. (2008). Culture-independent analysis of the gut microbiota in colorectal cancer and polyposis. *Environl Microbiol* 10, 789-798.

Schiffman, M. H., Van Tassell, R. L., Robinson, A. & other authors (1989). Case-control study of colorectal cancer and fecapentaene excretion. *Cancer Res* 49, 1322-1326.

Sears, C. L. (2009). Enterotoxigenic Bacteroides fragilis: a rogue among symbiotes. *Clin Microbiol Rev* 22, 349-369.

Sellon, R. K., Tonkonogy, S., Schultz, M., Dieleman, L. A., Grenther, W., Balish, E., Rennick, D. M. & Sartor, R. B. (1998). Resident enteric bacteria are necessary for development of spontaneous colitis and immune system activation in interleukin-10-deficient mice. *Infect Immun* 66, 5224-5231.

Shen, X. J., Rawls, J. F., Randall, T. & other authors (2010). Molecular characterization of mucosal adherent bacteria and associations with colorectal adenomas. *Gut Microbes* 1, 138-147.

Shioya, M., Wakabayashi, K., Yamashita, K., Nagao, M. & Sugimura, T. (1989). Formation of 8-hydroxydeoxyguanosine in DNA treated with fecapentaene-12 and -14. *Mutation Res* 225, 91-94.

Shmuely, H., Passaro, D., Figer, A., Niv, Y., Pitlik, S., Samra, Z., Koren, R. & Yahav, J. (2001). Relationship between Helicobacter pylori CagA status and colorectal cancer. *Am J Gastroenter* 96, 3406-3410.

Sillanpaa, J., Nallapareddy, S. R., Singh, K. V., Ferraro, M. J. & Murray, B. E. (2008). Adherence characteristics of endocarditis-derived Streptococcus gallolyticus ssp. gallolyticus (Streptococcus bovis biotype I) isolates to host extracellular matrix proteins. *FEMS Microbiology Lett* 289, 104-109.

Sillanpaa, J., Nallapareddy, S. R., Qin, X. & other authors (2009). A collagen-binding adhesin, Acb, and 10 other putative MSCRAMM and pilus family proteins of Streptococcus gallolyticus subsp. gallolyticus (S. bovis biotype I). *J Bact* 191, 6643-6653.

Sobhani, I., Tap, J., Roudot-Thoraval, F., Roperch, J. P., Letulle, S., Langella, P., Corthier, G., Tran Van Nhieu, J. & Furet, J. P. (2011). Microbial dysbiosis in colorectal cancer (CRC) patients. *PloS One* 6, e16393.

Sonnenburg, J. L., Angenent, L. T. & Gordon, J. I. (2004). Getting a grip on things: how do communities of bacterial symbionts become established in our intestine? *Nature immunol* 5, 569-573.

Spier, B. J., Walker, A. J., Cornett, D. D., Pfau, P. R., Halberg, R. B. & Said, A. (2010). Screening colonoscopy and detection of neoplasia in asymptomatic, average-risk, solid organ transplant recipients: case-control study. *Transpl Int* 23, 1233-1238.

Stecher, B., Robbiani, R., Walker, A. W. & other authors (2007). Salmonella enterica serovar typhimurium exploits inflammation to compete with the intestinal microbiota. *PLoS Biol* 5, 2177-2189.

Stecher, B. & Hardt, W. D. (2008). The role of microbiota in infectious disease. *Trends Microbiol* 16, 107-114.

Su, L. K., Kinzler, K. W., Vogelstein, B., Preisinger, A. C., Moser, A. R., Luongo, C., Gould, K. A. & Dove, W. F. (1992). Multiple intestinal neoplasia caused by a mutation in the murine homolog of the APC gene. *Science* 256, 668-670.

Su, X., Ye, J., Hsueh, E. C., Zhang, Y., Hoft, D. F. & Peng, G. (2010). Tumor microenvironments direct the recruitment and expansion of human Th17 cells. *J Immunol* 184, 1630-1641.

Swidsinski, A., Khilkin, M., Kerjaschki, D., Schreiber, S., Ortner, M., Weber, J. & Lochs, H. (1998). Association between intracpithelial Escherichia coli and colorectal cancer. *Gastroenterology* 115, 281-286.

Takada, H., Hirooka, T., Hiramatsu, Y. & Yamamoto, M. (1982). Effect of beta-glucuronidase inhibitor on azoxymethane-induced colonic carcinogenesis in rats. *Cancer Res* 42, 331-334.

Thompson-Chagoyan, O. C., Maldonado, J. & Gil, A. (2007). Colonization and impact of disease and other factors on intestinal microbiota. *Dig Dis Sci* 52, 2069-2077.

Thun, M. J., Namboodiri, M. M. & Heath, C. W., Jr. (1991). Aspirin use and reduced risk of fatal colon cancer. *The New Engl J Medicine* 325, 1593-1596.

Tjalsma, H., Scholler-Guinard, M., Lasonder, E., Ruers, T. J., Willems, H. L. & Swinkels, D. W. (2006). Profiling the humoral immune response in colon cancer patients: diagnostic antigens from Streptococcus bovis. *Int J Cancer* 119, 2127-2135.

Tjalsma, H., Schaeps, R. M. & Swinkels, D. W. (2008). Immunoproteomics: From biomarker discovery to diagnostic applications. *Proteomics Clin Appl* 2, 167-180.

Tjalsma, H. (2010). Identification of biomarkers for colorectal cancer through proteomics-based approaches. *Exp Rev Proteomics* 7, 879-895.

Tjalsma, H. (2011).Hybrid multiplex assays for the early detection of colorectal cancer: a perspective. *Clin Lab Int* 35, 10-12.

Toprak, N. U., Yagci, A., Gulluoglu, B. M., Akin, M. L., Demirkalem, P., Celenk, T. & Soyletir, G. (2006). A possible role of Bacteroides fragilis enterotoxin in the aetiology of colorectal cancer. *Clin Microbiol Infect* 12, 782-786.

Uronis, J. M., Muhlbauer, M., Herfarth, H. H., Rubinas, T. C., Jones, G. S. & Jobin, C. (2009). Modulation of the intestinal microbiota alters colitis-associated colorectal cancer susceptibility. *PloS One* 4, e6026.

Vaska, V. L. & Faoagali, J. L. (2009). Streptococcus bovis bacteraemia: identification within organism complex and association with endocarditis and colonic malignancy. *Pathology* 41, 183-186.

Wang, X. & Huycke, M. M. (2007). Extracellular superoxide production by Enterococcus faecalis promotes chromosomal instability in mammalian cells. *Gastroenterology* 132, 551-561.

Wang, X., Allen, T. D., May, R. J., Lightfoot, S., Houchen, C. W. & Huycke, M. M. (2008). Enterococcus faecalis induces aneuploidy and tetraploidy in colonic epithelial cells through a bystander effect. *Cancer Res* 68, 9909-9917.

Wilkinson, S. M., Uhl, J. R., Kline, B. C. & Cockerill, F. R., 3rd (1998). Assessment of invasion frequencies of cultured HEp-2 cells by clinical isolates of Helicobacter pylori using an acridine orange assay. *J Clin Pathol* 51, 127-133.

Winters, M. D., Schlinke, T. L., Joyce, W. A., Glore, S. R. & Huycke, M. M. (1998). Prospective case-cohort study of intestinal colonization with enterococci that produce extracellular superoxide and the risk for colorectal adenomas or cancer. *Am J Gastroenterol* 93, 2491-2500.

Wu, S., Morin, P. J., Maouyo, D. & Sears, C. L. (2003). Bacteroides fragilis enterotoxin induces c-Myc expression and cellular proliferation. *Gastroenterology* 124, 392-400.

Wu, S., Rhee, K. J., Albesiano, E. & other authors (2009). A human colonic commensal promotes colon tumorigenesis via activation of T helper type 17 T cell responses. *Nature medicine* 15, 1016-1022.

Xu, J., Mahowald, M. A., Ley, R. E. & other authors (2007). Evolution of symbiotic bacteria in the distal human intestine. *PLoS Biology* 5, e156.

Yantiss, R. K., Goldman, H. & Odze, R. D. (2001). Hyperplastic polyp with epithelial misplacement (inverted hyperplastic polyp): a clinicopathologic and immunohistochemical study of 19 cases. *Mod Pathol* 14, 869-875.

Zoetendal, E. G., von Wright, A., Vilpponen-Salmela, T., Ben-Amor, K., Akkermans, A. D. & de Vos, W. M. (2002). Mucosa-associated bacteria in the human gastrointestinal tract are uniformly distributed along the colon and differ from the community recovered from feces. *Appl Environ Microbiol* 68, 3401-3407.

Zumkeller, N., Brenner, H., Zwahlen, M. & Rothenbacher, D. (2006). Helicobacter pylori infection and colorectal cancer risk: a meta-analysis. *Helicobacter* 11, 75-80.

Part 4

Study Reports

10

Fluorescent Biomarker
in Colorectal Cancer

E. Kirilova[1], I. Kalnina[1], G. Kirilov[1] and G. Gorbenko[2]
[1]*Daugavpils University, Daugavpils,*
[2]*N. Karazin University of National Academy of Sciences, Kharkov,*
[1]*Latvia*
[2]*Ukraine*

1. Introduction

Patients with gastrointestinal cancer exhibit a poorly functioning immune system that is characterized, in part, by decreases in T-lymphocyte proliferation (Greenstein, et al., 1991; Milasiene et al., 2007) and reduced $CD4^+:CD8^+$ ratios (Arista et al., 1994; Franciosi et al., 2002). In different pathologies (including these and other types of cancers), membrane damage in immune cells (and other cell types) often evolves as a consequence of alterations that are induced in cell-associated lipids and proteins in the affected patients (Gryzunov and Dobretsov, 1994, 1998; Rolinsky et al., 2007). It is now widely accepted that the dynamics (actual rate of occurrence - not only incidence) of these changes, along with the types of alterations in structure(s) of the immune system cells' lipids/proteins themselves, play a critical role in the maintenance of the immune status of any given organism (Lakowicz, 2000).

As a result of the potential importance of changes in the structural integrity of cells of the immune system, it is important for clinicians to receive information on the biophysical status of these cells via quick, reliable, reproducible methods. In this regard, fluorescent probes have shown to be excellent tools for use in such protocols (Lakowicz, 2000, 2006). The work reported here, which built upon earlier findings reported by our laboratories, investigated the possibility of using the fluorescent probe ABM (an amine derivative of benzanthrone) for the detection of structural/functional alterations in blood plasma albumin and among immunocompetent cells in patients with select types of pathologies, i.e,. cancers. Such an analysis has a great potential for use not only for helping to comprehend mechanisms of immunomodulation associated with the induction/progression of malignancies, but might also have the potential to serve as a very important prognostic indicator of long-term survival among patients with such pathologies.

In the work reported here, ABM fluorescence intensity in blood plasma and following combination with cell suspensions from colorectal cancer patients was examined in the context of the host's immunological parameters and state of cancer progression. For study patients with colorectal cancer were examined: 1) 1 day before and 10 days after their surgical treatment (Stages II-III) (Kalnina et al., 2009); 2) as disease worsened (Stages IIa, IIIb, IV) (Kalnina et al., 2010b); 3) advanced cancer patients, they were divided into two groups in accordance of its survival rate (0-6 months and > 24 months) (Kalnina et al., 2011). Apart from the aforementioned potential benefits from these types of studies to clinicians in general, this type of research is very important in Latvia itself. This is because, in the context of oncological diseases seen among the Latvian population (as recently as in 2006), colorectal cancers rank third in incidence, only surpassed by lung cancers and urogenital tumors.

2. ABM: Distribution and spectral characteristics in cells and blood plasma

A new fluorescent probe, a derivative of 3-aminobenzanthrone (ABM) at the Daugavpils University, Daugavpils, Latvia.

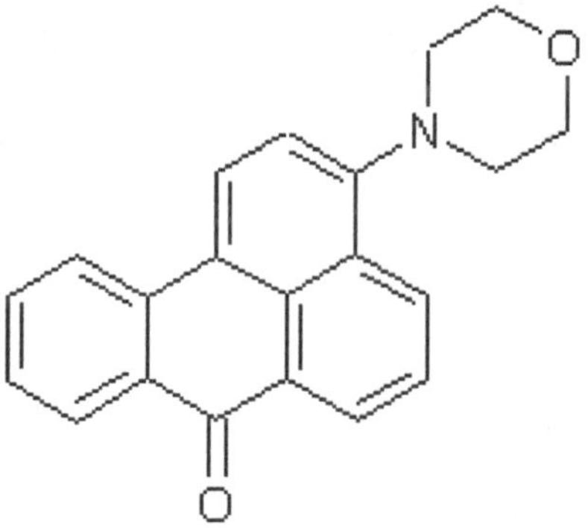

Fig. 1.Chemical Structure of probe ABM

Synthesis and properties of probe ABM were described in (Kalnina et al., 2004, 2007, 2009, 2010a; Kirilova et al., 2008).

3. ABM binding with blood plasma albumin

3.1 ABM binding with blood plasma albumin before and after surgical treatment

In the colorectal cancer patients, the ABM emission spectra maximum (i.e., at 650 nm) — after combination with the patients' blood plasma — was not altered in comparison to that seen with the plasma from the healthy control volunteers. In contrast, with respect to fluorescence intensity, before their individual surgical treatments, the average ABM intensity in the patients' blood plasma was decreased compared to that seen with the samples from the healthy donors. Specifically, the fluorescence associated with samples from the colorectal cancer group (Figure 2) were decreased by 23.0%. At 10 days after their operations, the average ABM fluorescence intensity in the samples from the colorectal cancer group were decreased further by 13.9%.

The average intensity values of the plasma samples from the cancer patients were significantly ($P < 0.05$) different from the control volunteers' average value. Whether these observations tracked actual changes in the levels of plasma albumin were also investigated. The results (data not shown) indicate that plasma albumin concentrations ($\mu g/\mu L$) pre-surgery in the patient group (71.73 ± 1.34) were below those in the plasma of the health controls (83.41 ± 1.16). This meant that the pre-surgery values for albumin only indicated levels in colorectal group samples that were ≈ 14% below control, while the samples' fluorescence intensity was correspondingly lower than the control value by 23.0% . The plasma albumin concentrations after surgery seemed to be insignificantly impacted. Specifically, these value was in colorectal cancer patients samples 68.48 ± 1.78 (in $\mu g/\mu L$, mean ± SD).

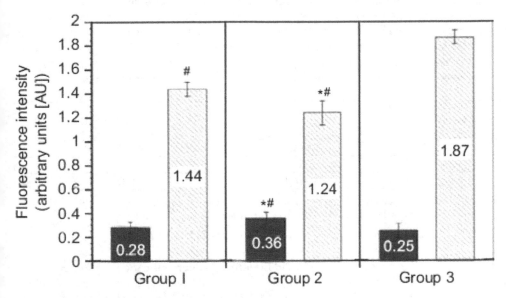

Fig. 2. ABM fluorescence intensity in lymphocytes and in plasma from "Colorectal group" patients. Colorectal cancer patients only (Stage II–III) (n = 10). Group number in figure is used to reflect from whom/when samples were isolated [i.e., Group 1: pre-surgery; Group 2: post-surgery; and Group 3: from healthy donors (control group; n = 14)]. Solid bar in each set: ABM fluorescence in lymphocytes; hatched bar in each set: ABM fluorescence in plasma. All intensity values are shown in AU (arbitrary units; mean ± SE). At $P < 0.05$, *value significantly different from pre-surgical value and/or #significantly different from control group value.

It is of interest to note that while the post-surgery albumin values in these patients samples were ≈18% below control levels, their corresponding fluorescence intensity were now even more depressed relative to that of the controls by ≈ 34%. These results strongly suggest that the noted changes in ABM fluorescence post-surgery in the cancer patients were most likely attributable to some change in the protein(s) themselves rather than due to post-surgery complications (i.e., bleeding or other mechanisms affecting blood volume/composition). To ascertain whether these results (different ABM spectral characteristics) could be explained, in part, by altered structural characteristics of the plasma albumin in the cancer patients, the average binding constant (Ka) values were determined using the Klotz graphical method. These analyses revealed that the average Ka values for the pre-surgery samples from the colorectal patient group decreased strongly from the respective constant associated with the control group (i.e., 1.0 X 10^5 M−1, colorectal cancer group; 1.8 X 10^5 M−1, healthy control group). These values represent decrements of from 28% to 45% in the binding of ABM to albumin in the plasma of these patients; the reason for the decrement remains to be fully determined. Interestingly, even though the fluorescence intensity values decreased further for the patients following their surgical procedures, the average Ka values for the samples from the patients increased relative to corresponding preoperative values (i.e., 1.3 X 10^5 M−1).

3.2 ABM binding with blood plasma albumin as a function of stage

The average ABM fluorescence intensity in patient's blood plasma was decreased compared to that seen with healthy donors. Specifically, the fluorescence intensity associated with samples from colorectal cancer patients (Table 1) was decreased by 23% (average value of 1.44 fluorescence units for those at Stage IIA-IIIB) and 42% (average value of 1.09 units for those at Stage IV) relative for the healthy controls(an average value of 1.87 units).

Group	Stage	F (PI)[a]
1	IIA-IIIB	[#][*]1.44±0.12
2	IV	[*]1.09±0.11
3	Controls	1.87±0.13

[a]F (PI) = fluorescence intensity in blood plasma; Values shown are in mean (± SE).
Value (p<0.05) significantly different from that of [*] control or [#] Group 2 patients.

Table 1. Spectral characteristics of ABM in blood plasma of colorectal cancer patients

3.3 ABM spectral characteristics in blood plasma of advanced cancer patients

The average ABM fluorescence intensity in the patients (Group 1 and Group 2) blood plasma was decreased (i.e., by 37.4% and 24.1%, respectively) as compared to that seen in healthy donors (Table 2). In Group 2 average intensity significantly (p<0.05) differs from Group 1 value and also control group value by 10.6 % and 31.7 %, respectively. Total albumin (TA) concentration in Group 1 and Group 2 patients was decreased (relative to control value) by 23.5% and 16.1%, respectively. Effective albumin (EA) concentration was decreased by 40.0% and 27.7%, respectively. The lowest value EA/TA in these patients plasma reached 0.61 (Group 1), and 0.66 (Group 2); (donor group 0.79-0.81).

Group	Survival rate (months)	F (PI)	EA	TA	EA/TA
1	0-6	1.17 ± 0.14	39.0 + 1.1	63,80 + 1.02	0,61
2	> 24	1.42 ± 0.09	47.0 + 1.2	70,80 + 1.14	0,66
Control		1.87 ± 0.13	65.0 + 1.3	83,4 + 1.16	0,78
P<0.05 between groups		1-2, 1-3, 2-3	1-2, 1-3, 2-3	1-2, 1-3, 2-3	

F (PI) = fluorescence intensity in blood plasma;. Values shown are in mean (± SE).
EA- "healthy" albumin equivalent in patients plasma, g/L
TA- total albumin concentration, g/L
EA/TA- reserve of albumin binding capacity

Table 2. Spectral parameters and binding sites čaracteristics of ABM in blood plasma of advanced cancer patients

4. ABM binding with lymphocytes

4.1 ABM binding with lymphocytes before and after surgical treatment

In the colorectal cancer patients, the ABM emission spectra maximum (i.e., at 650 nm) after combination with the patients' lymphocytes (as with their plasma) was not altered in comparison to that seen with the cells from the healthy control volunteers. Surprisingly, the average ABM fluorescence intensity value noted from colorectal patients group was actually 12.0% greater than the control level (Figure 3); however, even with this increase, the value was not significantly different from the average control value. In contrast to what was observed with the plasma samples, the average ABM fluorescence intensity values noted with the cells from patients at 10 days after their operations were greater than the values seen with the control volunteers' cells by 44%. In comparison to the pre-operative values, these average ABM fluorescence intensity values at 10 days after the patients' operations had increased by 28.6%.

COLORECTAL CANCER PATIENTS (Stage II-III) (n=10)					
	CD16+%	aCD16+	CD4+:CD8+	CD38+%	Lymphocytes (%)
b1	‡15.95±2.18	‡314.18±39.27	‡1.27±0.10	‡3.40±1.20	28.00±1.30
2	*‡7.93±1.43	*‡144.75±22.44	*‡1.50±0.13	*‡12.70±3.40	*‡23.50±2.20
3(Controls)	12.50±1.10	389.00±24.11	1.88±0.16	24.60±1.60	28.00±1.30

a Values shown are in terms of absolute numbers (mean ± SE).
b Indicates when or from whom samples were isolated: (1) before surgical treatment; (2) after surgical treatment; and (3) healthy donors (control group; n=14).
* Value significantly different from pre-surgical value (P<0.05); ‡significantly different from control group value (P<0.05).

Table 3. Peripheral blood lymphocyte subpopulation counts in the distinct subsets of the study's cancer patients.

4.2 ABM binding with lymphocytes as a function of stage

In general, among the gastrointestinal cancer patients examined here, the ABM emission spectra maximum (i.e., at 650 nm) after combination of the probe with the patients' lymphocytes was not altered in comparison to that seen with the cells from the healthy control volunteers (spectral data not shown). The ABM fluorescence intensity in the samples from colorectal patient group in Stages IIA-IIIB was not significantly different from the average control value (0.28 vs. 0.25 fluorescence units, respectively; Fig.3). In contrast, there was a significant reduction in ths parameter among the cells from the cancer patients in Stage IV (a decrease of 44%; (0.14 vs. 0.25 units).

4.3 ABM spectral characteristics in lymphocytes of advanced cancer patients

The ABM fluorescence intensity in the samples from advanced cancer patients (Group 1) was not different from the average value (0.25 vs. 0.25) fluorescence units, respectively: (Table 4). In contrast, there was a significant increase in this parameter among the cells from the cancer patients Group 2 as compared with Group 1 (by 80.8%) and healthy donors (by 112%) (0.25 vs. 0.52 units).

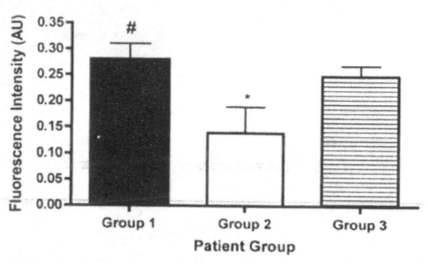

Fig. 3. ABM fluorescence intensity in lymphocytes from colorectal cancer patients as a function of stage. 1) Stage IIA-IIIB (black fill); 20 Stage IV (clear fill); 3) healthy donors (control group; stripped fill). All values are shown as mean (-+SE). At p< 0.05, values significantly different from that of "control patients, Group 2 patients.

5. Lymphocyte count and subpopulations

5.1 Lymphocytes count and subpopulations before and after surgical treatment

The absolute number of CD3+ cells and CD16+ natural killer cells; the relative percentages of all lymphocytes, CD16+ and CD38+ cells; as well as the CD4+:CD8+ ratio in the blood samples of the healthy volunteers and of the cancer patients, before and after each underwent their operations, were determined. The results among the patients in the "colorectal" group (Table 3) indicate that, before surgery, the numbers of CD16+ cells, the relative percentage of CD38+ cells, and the CD4+:CD8+ ratio were each significantly decreased (i.e., by 19.2%, 86.2%, and 32.4%, respectively) as compared to corresponding control subject values. Somewhat unexpectedly, relative percentages of CD16+ cells in this group were actually significantly greater (by 27.6%)—and the relative percentage of lymphocytes no different—than in the blood of the control volunteers. Within this same group, after surgery, the number and percentages of CD16+ cells, as well as the percentages of all lymphocytes, were each significantly reduced (i.e., by 53.9%, 50.3%, and 16.1%, respectively) relative to corresponding pre-surgery levels. Again, the relative percentage of CD38+ cells and the CD4+:CD8+ ratio increased (by 27.4% and 18.1%, respectively) compared to pre-surgical values, but again did not reach control levels (i.e., still were 48.4 and 20.2% lower, respectively).

5.2 Lymphocytes count and subpopulations as a function of stage

On the other hand, there were significant changes in the relative percentages of CD4+ cells at almost every stage in both cancer groups (Fig. 4). Among colorectal cancer patients, the percentages of CD4+ cells decreased 25.5 and 38.3% from control levels as the stages progressed (actual values: 28.6%, Stage IIA-IIIB; 23.7%, Stage IV; and, 38.4%, controls). Patients with Stage IV colorectal cancer yielded any statistically significant shift from control subject levels of CD8+ cells (an increase of ≈38%, i.e., shift from 19.5% to 26.9%).

The levels of lymphocytes (both total and the CD4+ and CD8+ sub-populations) in the blood samples of the cancer patients and healthy volunteers were also assessed here. The results show that among the patients in both cancer groups, the relative percentages of lymphocytes were moreover not significantly altered relative to the control levels irrespective of disease stage (Figures 4 and 5). Of all the patients, only those in Stage IV had lower blood lymphocyte levels that approached or reached statistical significance. Among the Stage IV colorectal cancer patients, levels were decreased 18.5% (a shift from 28.0% [control] down to ≈22.8%);

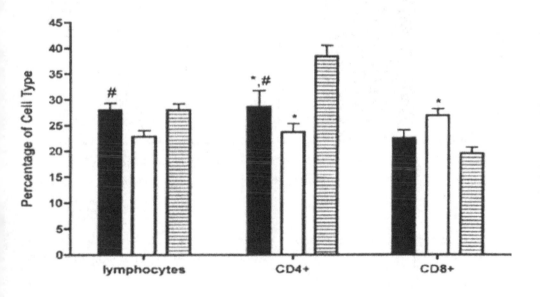

Fig. 4. Lymphocyte counts (as percentage %) and T-lymphocyte subpopulation Levels (as % of all lymphocytes present) in cancer patients as a function of stage. 1) Stage IIA-IIIB (black fill); 2) Stage IV (clear fill); 3) healthy donors (control group; striped fill).

Because shifts in CD4+:CD8+ ratios are often used as indices of altered host immune status, these values were also calculated from the patients' blood samples. The results show that among the colorectal cancer patients (Fig 5.), the CD4+:CD8+ ratios were all significantly lower than those for the healthy control subjects and became significantly further lower as the stage worsened. Specifically, the ratios dropped to 1.27 and 0.88 (shifts of 32.4% and 53.2%) at Stages IIA-IIIB and IV, respectively, from the 1.88 value for the controls.

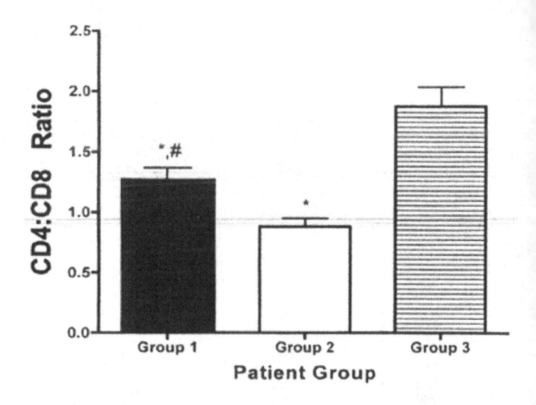

Fig. 5. T-lymphocyte subpopulation ratios in cancer patients as a function of stage.
1) Stage IIA- IIIB (black fill); 2) Stage IV (clear fill); 3) healthy donors (control group; striped fill).

5.3 Lymphocytes count and subpopulations in advanced cancer patients

Among the patients in both advanced cancer groups, the relative number of lymphocytes were significantly decreased (i.e.by 52.6% and 39.6%, respectively) as compared to corresponding control values. It is necessary to note that relative number of lymphocytes in Group 2 is significantly higher than in the Group 1 patients, but lower than the control value (see Table 4). In patients with advanced cancer and metastases there is reduction in both numbers of lymphocytes and proportions of CD4+/CD8+ T-lymphocytes which are thought to play an important role in cell-mediated immunity. The results indicate that in Group 1 and Group 2 patients the ratio CD4+/CD8+ was significantly reduced (i.e. by 58.5% and 47.9%, respectively) relative to corresponding control level. Actual values of Group 1 and Group 2 - 0.78, 0.98, respectively from the 1.88 control value. It is of interest to note that in Group 2 this parameter stay significantly higher as compared with results in Group 1, but did not reached control value.

Group	Survival rate, months	F(Ly), a.u.	Ly (%)	CD4+(%)	CD8+(%)	CD4+/CD8+
1	0-6	0,25±0,03	13,31±1,16	20,93±1,13	27,00±1,39	0,78±0,09
2	>24	0,53±0,11	16,95±1,18	26,14±1,32	26,70±1,31	0,98±0,08
3 Control		0,25±0,03	28,00±1,30	38,40±2,10	19,50±1,20	1,88±0,16
p<0.05, between groups		1-2;2-3	1-2;1-3;2-3	1-2;1-3;2-3	1-3;2-3	1-2;1-3;2-3

F(Ly) - fluorescence intensity in lymphocytes
Values shown are in mean (±SE)

Table 4. ABM fluorescence intensity in lymphocytes. Peripheral blood lymphocytes subpopulation counts in advanced cancer patients

6. Examination of relationship between ABM fluorescence and blood lymphocyte profiles

Pre-operation, in the colorectal patient group, the ABM fluorescence intensity was found to correlate with the relative number of CD38+ cells (r = +0.956). After the operations, both the CD4+:CD8+ ratio and relative number of CD38+ cells in patients blood was observed to be increased.

In colorectal cancer group, the ABM fluorescence intensity in blood plasma and the lymphocytes was found to correlate with CD4+:CD8+ ratios (in all stages of cancer) and the percentage (%) of lymphocytes/ subtypes in their blood. The degree of any relationship between cancer progression/staging, lymphocyte levels, and fluorescence among the lymphocytes was less obvious. Specifically, in terms of disease progression, cell levels and fluorescence intensity weakly tracked together (i.e., r = +0.512) for the colorectal patients. .

With respect to associations between the plasma albumin fluorescence measurements and each of the individual lymphocyte-associated endpoints measured (except for cell fluorescence itself), many of the same patterns as noted above were evident. Once again, in terms of disease progression, although cell levels and albumin fluorescence intensity weakly tracked together (i.e., r = +0.513) among the colorectal patients.

In both groups of advanced cancer the ABM fluorescence intensity in blood plasma and lymphocytes was found to correlate to with CD4+/CD8+ ratios. In advanced cancer groups (in contrast to other groups) there is direct (not inverse) correlation between lymphocytes count and ABM fluorescence intensity. There seemed to be a good relationship between total lymphocyte (and subpopulation) levels and ABM fluorescence in both groups of patients. There is also good associations between the plasma albumin fluorescence measurements and each of the individual lymphocyte/albumin associated endpoints measured "effective" and total albumin concentration, reserve of albumin binding capacity.

7. Discussion

The novel fluorescent probe ABM (an amino derivative of benzanthrone) localizes deep within the phospholipids bilayer of lymphocytes membrane. Thus, in studies with lymphocytes, it can be concluded that changes in the spectral parameters of ABM (i.e., shifts in magnitude of fluorescence or actual wavelength associated with normal maximal fluorescence [i.e., Fmax]) could reflect modifications in one/ more interdependent (i.e., inter-related) properties of the cells. These could include the lymphocytes' (1) outer membrane physicochemical state, (2) membrane microviscosity,
(3) proliferative activity, (4) lipid metabolism, and/or (5) phenotypical profile. As seen in the studies mentioned here, while the noted changes in the studied parameters (i.e., fluorescence behavior) could be useful in reflecting alterations in lymphocytes of the cancer patients in each subgroup (at both pre- and post-surgical stages), they may also ultimately be of use as potential indicators of alteration in cellular immunity in these individuals. Follow-up studies are underway to see whether this concept can be validated. We also sought to ascertain whether shifts in ABM binding with plasma albumin could potentially be utilized as a part of an overall preliminary immunodiagnostic screening test in cancer patients. The choice to examine albumin, among the myriad of constituents in plasma, is that this protein is practically the single source of ABM binding and subsequent fluorescence in plasma (Gryzunov and Dobretsov, 1994, 1998). Our earlier studies showed that within plasma, albumin is nearly alone in binding with ABM with a very high level of selectivity (Kalnina et al., 1996, 2004, 2007). The distribution of ABM fluorescence (intensity) within fractions of human plasma was seen to be albumin >>> globulins >> non-specific binding by other components (i.e., 90%, ≈ 5%, < 1%, respectively). These widely disparate binding results were confirmed in studies wherein exogenous globulin was added to plasma samples and there was no shift in fluorescence intensity or Fmax. Clearly, only significant shifts in albumin levels or alterations/ conformational changes in albumin itself seemed to have a major impact on these ABM fluorescence endpoints. In the present study, the differences in total albumin concentrations, **pre- and post-surgery**, among the cancer patients in each group did not seem to correlate well with the relative changes in ABM fluorescence (relative to values in control subjects' plasma). This apparent "extra diminution" in fluorescence strongly suggested that there was either a novel competition for probe by other substances in the patients' plasma or that the albumin in these patients had undergone modification(s) that affected its ability to bind ABM. The fact there were substantive changes in binding constant (Ka) values lends support to the latter viewpoint. However, this finding in and of itself does not outright preclude the possibility of the former event having occurred as well.These shifts in ABM binding constants in the plasma samples from the cancer patients, as noted earlier, could be due to a generic decreased binding by/conformational changes in their albumin molecules. Structural or functional alterations of albumin could be manifest as "shifts" away from normal "main" binding sites with high affinity for the probe to other binding sites with far lower affinities and specificities. Such shifts would be in agreement with the observations of Togashi and Ryder (2006) that albumin molecules are known to contain different binding sites (i.e., classes) for various probes. As Petitpas et al. (2001b, 2003) noted, albumin normally carries a variety of endogenous ligands like nonesterified fatty acids, bilirubin, and thyroxine; however, this protein can also bind an impressive array of drug molecules, including warfarin, ibuprofen, and indomethacin, as well as their metabolites (Petitpas et al., 2001a). It seems very likely

that patients in the groups in the present study had ingested painkillers (both prescribed and retail) during the course of their disease; thus, a presence of these drugs/ metabolites on their albumin could have contributed to the noted shifts in ABM fluorescence /Ka values. Our future studies will endeavor to recruit non-cancer patients with a "similar" history of painkiller intake in order to ascertain whether this was a main reason underlying our observations (regarding the albumin outcomes) or if there is something more inherently unique to the patient's cancer-bearing status that influenced the measured endpoints. This second standpoint is not without foundation. In oncopathology, the blood plasma content of two important unsaturated fatty acids (i.e., oleic acid and arachidonic acid) is increased, and these natural constituents also increasingly occupy binding sites on albumin (Gryzunov and Dobretsov, 1994, 1998). Both are observed to occupy binding sites distributed across the protein that happen to also be bound by medium or long-chain saturated fatty acids. The resulting restrictions imparted on the binding configurations of the protein would then account for shifts in the binding affinities at the primary sites between polyunsaturated fatty acids and their saturated or mono-unsaturated counterparts (Petitpas et al., 2001). It remains to be determined whether these alterations in fatty acid composition/binding also result in conformational changes in the albumin that impact upon ABM binding to its major (high selectivity) binding sites. As noted earlier, changes in fluorescence parameters of the cancer patients' lymphocytes could be reflective of changes in one/more inherent characteristics of their cells. In these studies, at least two, that is, proliferative activity and phenotypical character, could readily, albeit indirectly, be evaluated by examining changes in lymphocyte populations (i.e., their numbers) themselves. While the flow cytometry studies did indicate significant changes in lymphocyte (and subpopulation) levels among the cancer patients, unfortunately, the studies failed to yield overall lymphocyte (or subtype) population patterns that paralleled the concurrent changes in ABM fluorescence (i.e., Table 1 vs. Figure 2, example of this "lack of comparativeness"). Among all the subpopulation endpoints reported, only those of "CD38+%" and the "CD4+:CD8+ ratios" approached reflecting trends seen with the patients' fluorescence measurements. Specifically, the pre-surgery levels of each of these cytometric values were "maximally" reduced relative to the control subjects' values; post-surgery, these two values were increased, but in contrast to the fluorescence levels, these values did not reattain (or surpass) counterpart control levels. In light of the cancer patients' post-surgical (1) persistent lower numbers of lymphocytes (both total and within subclasses) and (2) fluorescence values that were uniformly significantly greater than in control subjects' cells, we surmise some factor(s) about these patients' lymphocytes (i.e., some undefined phenotypical characteristics) can cause amplification of the ABM fluorescent response. The fact that this "disconnect" between these two parameters is most predominant during the post-operative period strongly suggests that these as yet-undefined modifying factors in the cancer patients might be related to their general immune response to the surgical procedure. Our future studies will need to recruit non-cancer patients with a "similar" history of surgical intervention/protocols (such as among patients suffering enterocolitis, undergoing local biopsies for non-cancer disorders, etc.) to ascertain whether the surgical procedure itself was a main reason for our observations (regarding the "disconnect") or whether, as with the albumin findings, there is something more inherently unique to a cancer-bearing status that influenced the measured endpoints. As expected, the CD4+:CD8+ ratios were seen to be increased in the cancer patients after they had undergone their respective operation. This would be expected as it is well accepted that CD4+ helper cells stimulate and CD8+ (suppressor and cytotoxic) cells inhibit the immune response during the healing process. While that explanation for any potential changes in the phenotypic characteristics of these patients' lymphocytes is somewhat straightforward, what is less clear is the basis for the post-surgical increase in CD38+% values and why, to begin with, they are lower than in the control groups. This is because, most often, increased levels of CD38+ cells are associated with patients suffering with lymphocytic leukemias than with the solid tumors (such as those associated with gastrointestinal cancers (Kalnina et al., 2009). In general, CD38 is expressed primarily on B-lymphocytes and T-lymphocytes, as well as stem/germ cells, the CD38 ligand is an ADP-ribosyl cyclase enzyme that regulates the activation and growth of these lymphoid (as well as myeloid) cells . The data in the current study clearly show no evidence of any B-lymphocyte-based leukemia (Kalnina et al., 2009) (i.e., CD16+ cell levels were lower in patients' pre- and post-surgery blood samples than in controls) among the cancer patients. Thus, we conclude that the increase in CD38+ cell levels is more probably due to an increased presence of CD38+ T-lymphocytes. We conclude from our findings that the increase in CD38+ cell levels post-surgery was not likely due to absolute increases in T-lymphocytes, but in their activities. Such an outcome would be in keeping with the changes in the fluorescence values for these lymphocytes. For this premise to be valid, apart from showing that there are increases in relative levels of CD38-bearing T-lymphocytes due to activation during the post-surgery healing process, there still needs to be an explanation as to why these cells' levels were initially lower in the patients than in the controls. One potential explanation is in the biology of the tumors themselves, that is, they are solid tumors of the gastrointestinal system that impact on a wide variety of local cell types, including the endothelium. This particular cell type in the gut is of interest here in that there appears to be a critical relationship among endothelial cells, CD38 expression, and activation of T-lymphocytes (i.e., CD4+CD45RA+ cells. It is plausible that normal interactions between T-lymphocytes and endothelium are likely "interrupted" simply as a result of changes in accessibility (secondary to alterations in gut architecture as tumor grew). A lack of lymphocyte– endothelium interactions could help explain why there was a diminution in CD38+ cell levels before surgery; during the post-surgery recovery, angiogenic processes (i.e., during microvasculature repair/reformation at wound site) would allow for an increase in these particular cell–cell interactions—in particular, with a population of endothelial cells in very active states during the reparative processes. Future histopathology studies using biopsied samples from the gastrointestinal tracts of patients with cancers and those that underwent biopsies for non-cancer-based reasons (see earlier comments) should be useful in allowing us to verify the degree of these hypothesized cell–cell interactions. Apart from potential changes in lymphocyte-endothelium interactions as contributing factors for the reductions (vs. controls) in CD38+ cell levels—and their "recoveries" after surgical removal of the tumor—in the cancer patients, there are other possible reasons for these two observations. Among these, specifically, is the fact that patients with colorectal/gastrointestinal cancers (especially those at more advanced stages) tend to have significant levels of circulating interleukin (IL)-4 . This is critical in that it has been shown, at least with B-lymphocytes, that exposure of these cells to IL-4 reduced the amount of CD38 antigen on and in these cells; no evidence was obtained for accelerated breakdown, shedding, or internalization of CD38 molecules, or for the accumulation of CD38 molecules in the cell interior, due to IL-4 (Kalnina et al., 2009). In our ongoing studies, we will analyze patients' blood samples for IL-4 both pre- and post-surgery to see whether its levels reflect the observed changes in the CD38+ lymphocytes and their fluorescence responses (indicative of phenotypic changes likely related to activation) in the presence of ABM. The results of the ABM studies presented here show that, as might be expected, the presence of solid tumors and surgical interventions can affect the functional activity of lymphocytes. These results are in agreement with previously- performed investigations to characterize the outer cell membrane of lymphocytes of cancer patients, patients with autoimmune disease (i.e., rheumatoid arthritis), and workers who had been contaminated during the clean up at Chernobyl (Kalnina et al., 2004, 2010a, Zvagule, 2010). Likewise, the observed changes in the ABM spectral parameters in blood plasma are probably coupled with alterations in cellular mechanisms of immune regulation in the patients here. Ongoing studies are seeking to answer this very question.

The studies here showed that spectral characteristics (fluorescence intensity) differed among the various patient sub-groups. These findings suggest likely physical (structural) and functional alterations in the patients' cells were a **function of cancer stage.** It is known that ABM fluorescence intensity can change in accordance with environment polarity and, consequently, in relation to plasma membrane microviscosity (that in turn correlates with cell lipid metabolism). There are various pathological states (i.e., cancer) in which the lipid composition and specific fatty acid content in lymphocyte membranes and blood plasma are disturbed (Kalofoutis et al., 1996). For example, colorectal cancer patients have abnormal plasma and erythrocyte fatty acid levels, as well as of their polyunsaturated metabolites (Robinson et al., 2001). Ultimately, in lymphocytes, because membrane physicochemical status and cell lipid metabolism play pivotal roles in signal transduction pathway(s) activities important in maintaining cell function (Kim et al., 1999), it would not be unexpected that disturbances in these parameters could result in altered immunocompetence in hosts with these affected cells. Fluorescence intensity of ABM in lymphocytes suspension tended to decrease with progression of cancer. Shifts in magnitude of ABM fluorescence could reflect modifications in one/more interdependent properties of cells (Kalnina et al., 2007). As seen in the studies mentioned here, at least two parameters are responsible for this phenomenon. In this studies, at least two, that is proliferative activity and phenotypical character could readily, albeit indirectly, be evaluated by examining changes in lymphocytes populations (ie., their numbers) themselves. While the flow cytometry studirs did indicate significant changes in lymphocytes (and sunpopulations) levels among the cancer patients, unfortunately, the studies failed to yield overall lymphocyte (or subtipe) population patterns that paralleled the concurrent changes in ABM fluorescence example of this "lack of comparativeness"). The studie of Milasiene (Milasiene et al., 2007) also suggest that immunosuppression covers many aspects of the complex immune system, and therefore, we have many unexpected findings.

The studies here also revealed significant changes in ABM fluorescence associated with the plasma (re: albumin) of the cancer patients. The choise to examine albumin, among the myriad of constituents in plasma, is that this protein is practically the single source of ABM binding and subsequent fluorescence in plasma. We know form earlier studies that plasma albumin binds ABM with a very high selectivity (Kalnina et al., 1996, 2004, 2007, 2009, 2010b, Zvagule et al., 2010) and that only very significant shifts in plasma albumin levels or structural changes in albumin itself seemed to impact on ABM fluorescence. In the previous study (Kalnina et al., 2009) the differences in total albumin concentrations in patients groups did not seem to correlate well with the relative changes in ABM fluorescence (relative to values of control subjects plasma). The fluorescent method reveal the "effective" concentration of albumin (equivalent of "healthy" albumin in blood plasma). The total concentration of albumin is conservative. In general, serious alterations in plasma albumin levels are often reflective of poor outcomes in cancer patients (Seve et al., 2007). As noted above, the changes in patient plasma albumin levels ($\approx$14-18% below control) were far less than the recorded shifts in ABM intensities and it seemed these measures were "picking up" changes beyond those that could solely be attributed to a change in total albumin status. The additional 'binding shifts' seen with the cancer patients' plasma samples could be due, in part, to decreased binding by/conformational changes in their albumin. There are several ways in which tumor-and/or treatment-associated agents can bind to albumin and cause allosteric modifications that lead to structure and function changes: (1) tumor cells release a variety of bioactive proteins/peptide fragments - sequestration by carrier proteins (like albumin) protect these materials from clearance (and amplify their circulating levels; Kazmierczak et al., 2006); (2) plasma content of select key unsaturated fatty acids (i.e., oleic and arachidonic acids) is increased - these then increasingly occupy binding sites on albumin (Gryzunov and Dobretsov, 1994, 1998; Petitpas et al., 2001b); and, (3) an array of drugs, e.g., ibuprofen, indomethacin, etc. (and their metabolites) commonly ingested by cancer patients readily bind with albumin (Petitpas et al., 2001a, 2003). As was the case with lymphocytes, the shifts in cancer patient plasma ABM fluorescence intensity were related to disease stage. While moderate alterations in albumin-ABM signals were already noted at early (Stages II) phases of cancer, the effects were amplified as cancer evolved to Stages III-IV. It is likely that as cancer progressed, the levels of pathological/pharmacological metabolites in the patient's blood increased and their albumin could not ultimately bind them all. One consequent structural/functional alteration induced in the albumin could be a shift in ABM binding away from normal primary high affinity sites to others with lower affinities/specificities. Such shifts would be in agreement with the observations of Togashi and Ryder (2006) and Rolinski et al. (2007) who noted that albumin molecules contained different binding sites (i.e., classes) that differed in affinity, quantum yield, and degrees of polarization (i.e., higher mobility of bound probe and increased accessibility by water) for ABM and various other probes. The results of the current investigation also seemed to reflect what was predicted to occur based upon electron spin resonance (ESR) spectroscopy studies that measured structural and functional changes in serum albumin of patients with other cancers (Kazmierczak et al., 2006). Specifically, analyses of ESR spectra (using spin probes) revealed substantial differences in spectrum variables when samples from patients were compared with those from healthy hosts. For example, the increasing width of the spectral line in samples from the cancer patients indicated an alteration in albumin conformation that limited the movement of the spin probe at a binding site, as well as changes in the albumin capacity to bind spin probe, polarity of spin probe binding site, and probe mobility (Kazmierczak et al., 2006). While increased binding of tumor-/treatment-associated agents (leading to the sequelea outlined above) could be a means by which changes in albumin-ABM fluorescence evolved here, there are other means by which the albumin ability to bind the probe may have been altered. While we demonstrated here there were changes in ABM fluorescence after inter-actions with lymphocytes (and plasma albumin) obtained from gastrointestinal cancer patients, another major question that needed addressing was whether there were actual biologic/immunologic modifications associated with these alterations. As noted earlier, changes in fluorescence parameters of patient lymphocytes could reflect changes in one/more inherent characteristics of these cells, including their phenotypical character. While the flow cytometry studies identified significant alterations in lymphocyte (and sub-populations) levels among all the cancer patients, variations in total lymphocyte levels never *clearly and consistently* paralleled the corresponding changes in ABM fluorescence for the gastric cancer subjects. In contrast, there seemed to be a good relationship between these endpoints in the colorectal patients. For now, it remains unclear why there should be a divergence in these patterns based on the cancer type itself.

The observed changes in ABM intensity in the lymphocytes might be useful to reflect current CD4+ and/or CD8+ status in the pacients. In this regard, the same (as above) disease-related differences in the relationships were apparent between changes in ABM fluorescence and those in CD4+ levels in the patients. The noted shifts in CD4+ levels were expected; cancer- related CD4+ cell deficiency is a frequent finding in digestive system cancer patients (Franciosi et al, 2002). In our previous investigations, CD4+:CD8+ ratios tended to parallel ABM fluorescence levels (i.e., lowest among patients who manifested decreased fluorescence in their lymphocyte suspensions (Kalnina et al, 2007, 2009, 2010a,2010b). In those earlier studies, CD4+:CD8+ ratios gradually decreased as CD8+ levels increased with progression of cancer stage (Wang et al., 2004; Kalnina et al., 2007). In the studies here, the shifts seem to depend more on decreases in CD4+ levels as each disease became metastatic. These outcomes would be in keeping with the studies by Tancini et al. (1990) and (McMillan et al. (1997) that indicated that decreases in CD4+:CD8+ ratios in gastric cancer patients mainly depended on increases in CD8+ T-cytotoxic cells in patients with early stage disease whereas it was due to decreases in CD4+ T-helper cells in those with metastases (later stage disease). Thus, at least clearly for colorectal cancer patients, our results suggest that measures of ABM fluorescence intensity values for lymphocytes (and to a lesser extent, for plasma albumin) could potentially be used in clinical immunological screenings (instead of more expensive routine tests) to provide a snapshot of immune status in these cancer patients. Whether the utility of these measures could/would extend to human disease states remains to be determined.

8. Conclusion

Fluorescence behaviour of ABM could be useful to reflecting alterations in lymphocytes in each subgroup and they may ultimately be of use as potential indicators of alterations in cellular immunity in individuals. We also sought to ascertain whether shifts in ABM binding with plasma albumin could be potentially utilized as part of an overall preliminary immunodiagnostic screening test in cancer patients. Taken together it would appear that progression of cancer is associated with changes of immune function and more specifically a reduction in absolute number of CD4 + T-lymphocytes and either an increase or not change in the absolute count of CD8+ T-lynphocytes. Study suggests that higher number of absolute lymphocytes count and ratio CD4+: CD8+ have beneficial effect on overall survival of patients with advanced tumor. Overall survival depends also on quantitative parameters of cellular immunity of cancer patients. Thus, immune status of the immune system of patients with advanced tumor before treatment is important for its survival. The immunosuppression and metastatic spread are interconnected. The low plasma albumin level also were identified as bad independent marker of prognosis. Fluorescent based method is pertinent to pathway profiling, target validation, and clinical diagnosis, prediction of therapeutic effacy, and monitoring of treatment outcomes. ABM fluorescence intensity values for plasma albumin and lymphocytes (as reflection of their functional activity) might be useful tool in the evolution of the immune status of pacients. Taken together, all the results showed that measures of ABM spectral characteristics could potentially be a useful tool to estimate the immune status of gastrointestinal patients. Compared to many commonly used diagnostic protocols, this fluorescence based method is less expensive and not very time consumming, technically simple and 100 times more sensitive than standard absorbance based methods.

9. Acknowledgments

This work was supported by European Structural Funds, Project Nr. 2009/0205/1!DP/1.1.1.2.0/09/APIA/VIAA/152

10. References

Arista, M, Callopoli, A., Franceschi, L., Santini, A., Schiratti, M., Conti, L., Fillippo, F., and Gandolfo, G. M. 1994. Flow cytometric study of lymphocytes subsets in patients at different stages of colorectal carcinoma. *Dis. Colon Rectum* 37:S30-34.

Duncan, D. B. 1970. Query multiple comparison methods for comparison methods for comparing regression coefficient. *Biometrics* 26:141-143.

Franciosi, C., Bravo, A., Romano, F., Fumagalli L., Cerea, K., Conti, M., Rovelli, F., and Uggeri, F. Immunodeficiency in radically operable gastric cancer patients. 2002. *Hepato-gastroenterology* 49:857-859.

Greenstein, A., Pecht, M., Kaver, I., Trainin, N., and Braf, Z. 1991. Characterization of peripheral blood T-cell subpopulation of bladder cancer patients. *Urol. Res.* 19: 219-222.

Gryzunov, Y. A., and Dobretsov, G. E. (Eds.). 1994. *Plasma Albumin in Clinical Medicine.* Moscow: Irius Publishers.

Gryzunov, Y.A., and Dobretsov, G.E. (Eds) . 1998. *Plasma Albumin in Clinical Medicine* (Book2). Moscow: GEOTAR

Kalnina, I., and Meirovics, I. 1999. A new fluorescent probe, ABM: Properties and application in clinical diagnostics. *J. Fluorescence* 9:27-32.

Kalnina, I., Bruvere, R., Gabruseva , N., Zvagule, T., Heisele, O., Volrate, A., Feldmane, G., and Meirovics, I. 2004. Phenotypical characteristics of leukocytes of Chernobyl clean-up workers from Latvia: Use of fluorescent probe ABM. *Biol. Memb.* 21:72-78.

Kalnina, I., Klimkane, L., Kirilova, E., Toma, M. M., Kizane, G., and Meirovics, I. 2007. Fluorescent probe ABM for screening gastrointestinal patient's immune state. *J. Fluoresccence* 17:619-625.

Kalnina, I., Bruvere, R., Zvagule, T., Gabruseva, N., Klimkane, L., Kirilova, E., Meirovics, I., and Kizane, G. 2010a. Fluorescent probe ABM and estimation of immune state in patients with different pathologies. *J. Florescence* 20::9-17.

Kalnina, I., Kirilova, E., Klimkane, L., and Kirilov, G. 2009. Altered characteristics of albumin in blood of gastrointestinal cancer patients: Correlation with changes in lymphocytes populations. *J. Immunotoxicol.* 6:293-300.

Kalnina, I., Kurjane. N., Kirilova, E., Klimkane, L., Kirilov, G., Zvagule, T. 2010b. Correlation of altered plasma albumin characteristics and lymphocyte populations to tomor stage in gastrointestinal cancer patients. *Cancer Biomarkers* 7(2): 91-99.

Kalnina I., Kirilova E., Klimkane L., Kirilov G., Gorbenko G. 2011. Fluorescent biomarker in gastrointestinal and advanced tumor. 2 nd Intrernational Conference on Cancer Immunotherapy and Immunomonitoring (CITIM 2011) ; May 2-5, Budapest, Hungary, p.82.

Kalofoutis, A., Nicolaidou-Politis, V., and Bouloukos, A. 1996. Significance of lymphocyte fatty acid changes in renal failure. *Nephron* 73: 704-706.

Kazmierczak, S. C, Gurachevsky, A., Matthes, G., and Muravsky, V. 2006. Electron spin resonance spectroscopy of serum albumin: A novel new test for cancer diagnosis and monitoring. *Clin. Chem.* 52:2129-2134.

Kim, C. W., Choi, S. H., Chung, E. I., Lee, M. J., Byun, E. K., Ryu, M. N., and Bang Y. I. 1999. Alterations of signal transducing molecules and phenotypical characteristics in peripheral blood lymphocytes from gastric carcinoma patients. *Pathology* 67:123-128.

Kirilova, E. M., Kalnina, I., Kirilov G. 2008. Spectroscopic study of benzanthrone 3-N-derivatives as new hydrophobic fluorescent probes for biomolecules. *J. Fluorescence* 18: 645-648.

Lakowicz, J. R. (Ed.) 2000. *Protein Fluorescence. Vol. 6.* New York: Plenum Press.

Lakowicz J.R. Principles of fluorescence spectroscopy (3rd ed.) Springler Verlag. New York, 2006.

McMillan, D. C., Fyffe, G. D, Wotherspoon, H. A, Cooke, T. G, and McArdle, C. S. 1997. Prospective study of circulating T-lymphocyte subpopulations and disease progression in colorectal cancer. *Dis. Colon Rectum* 40:1068-1071.

Milasiene, V., Stratilatovas, E., and Norkiene, V. 2007. The importance of T-lymphocyte subsets on overall survival of colorectal and gastric cancer patients. *Medicina (Kaunas)* 43:548-554.

Petitpas, I., Bhattacharya, A. A., Twine, S., East, M., and Curry, S. 2001a. Crystal structure analysis of warfarin binding to human serum albumin: Anatomy of drug site I. *J. Biol. Chem.* 276:22804-22809.

Petitpas, I., Grune T., Bhattacharya, A., and Curry, S. 2001b. Crystal structures of human serum albumin complexed with monounsaturated and polyunsaturated fatty acids. *J. Mol. Biol.* 314:955-960.

Petitpas, I., Petersen, C. E., Ha, C. E., Bhattacharya, A. A., Zunszain, P. A., Ghuman, J., Bhagavan, N. V., and Curry, S. 2003. Structural basis of albumin-thyroxine interactions and familial dysalbuminemic hyperthyroxinemia. *Proc. Natl. Acad. Sci. USA* 100:6440-6445.

Robinson L. E., Clandinin M. T., and Field C. I. 2001. R3230 AC Rat mammary tumor and dietary long-chain (n=3) fatty acids change immune cell composition and function during mitogen activation. *J. Nutr.* 131:2001-2027.

Rolinski, O. J., Martin, A., and Birch, D. J. 2007. Human serum albumin and quercetin interactions monitored by time resolved fluorescence evidence of enhanced discrete rotamer conformations. *J. Biomed. Optics* 12:34013.1-34013.7.

Seve, P., Ray-Coquard, I., Trillet-Lenoir, V., Sawyer, M., Hanson, J., Brousolle, C., Negrier, S., Dumontet, C., and Mackey J. R. 2007. Low serum levels and liver metastasis are powerful prognostic markers for survival in patients with carcinomas of unknown primary site. *Cancer* 109:2623-2624.

Tancini, G., Barni, S., Rescaldani, R., Fiorelli, G., Vivani, S., and Lissoni, P. 1990. Analysis of T-helper and suppressor lymphocyte subsets in relation to the clinical stage of solid neoplasma *Oncology* 47:381-384.

Togashi, D. M., and Ryder, A. G. 2006. Time-resolved fluorescence studies on bovine albumin denaturation process. *J. Fluorescence* 16:153-160.

Wang, X. X., Su W. L., and Zhu, W. X. 2004. Correlation of the changes of T-lymphocyte phenotype to tumor stage and operative pattern of gastric cancer. *Al Zhena* 23:1065-1068.

Zvagule T., Kalnina, I., Kurjane, N., Bruvere, R., Gabruseva, N., and Skesters, A. 2010. Long-term effects of low doses of ionizing radiation on Chernobyl clean-up workers from Latvia. *Intern. J. Low Rad.* 7(1) : 20-31.

11

Tumor Infiltrating Lymphocytes as Prognostic Factor of Early Recurrence and Poor Prognosis of Colorectal Cancer After Radical Surgical Treatment

Vaclav Liska[1], Ondrej Daum[2], Petr Novak[1], Vladislav Treska[1],
Ondrej Vycital[1], Jan Bruha[1], Pavel Pitule[1] and Lubos Holubec[3]
[1]*Department of Surgery,*
[2]*Institute of Pathology,*
[3]*Department of Oncology, Charles University Prague,*
Medical School and Teaching Hospital Pilsen,
Czech Republic

1. Introduction

Sixty percent of patients with colorectal cancer (CRC) are afflicted with distant metastases (liver or lung metastatic process) or a local relapse of malignancy (Bird et al., 2006). The possibilities of surgical and oncological treatment of this disease offer us a large spectrum of treatments including the combination of surgical procedures and consecutive oncological treatments. In the case of radical surgical therapy we can consider the curative access. The main medical problem of CRC is the high rate of recurrences after radically performed surgical therapy. The operability of recurrence is only about 30% in the case of local relapse and 20% in the case of distant metastases (Coleman et al., 2008; Kobayashi et al., 2007). The second dominant problem is the early recurrence of CRC after radical surgical treatment, when the patients undergo a difficult and exhausting procedure with a high risk of perioperative complications without any significant differences in overall survival against modern palliative therapy (Van den Eynde & Hendlisz, 2009).

Contemporary clinical and histopathological prognostic factors (staging, grading, etc.) used for the detection of patients with a high risk of relapse and a short overall survival rate and for the indication of adjuvant oncological treatment after radical surgery are not sufficient. Tumor infiltrating lymphocytes (TIL) were described as a good prognostic factor for patients with a high risk of relapse. They are critical indicators of efficient antitumor immunological response. Their number, type and morphology of TIL cells determine resulting tumor prognosis (Atreya & Neurath, 2008; Galon et al., 2006). They could be connected also with the suppression of micrometastatical disease after radical surgery (Gajowski et al., 2006; Pages et al., 2005). We can recognize either the type of immune cells or distinguish their morphological aspects (infiltration of any part of tumor or surrounding of tumor or tributary lymph nodes) (Talmadge et al., 2007).

We detail only short overview of their types and function. We recommend the readers with deeper interest in these problems to find comprehensive reviews in the cited papers (Jochems et al., 2011; Ohtani 2007). From this view we find CD8+ and CD4+ T lymphocytes (Fig. 1a & Fig. 1b), natural killer cells (Fig. 1c), dendritic cells (Fig. 1d), macrophages, etc. The exact function of these cells is under current discussion. We only know that they play main role in controlling tumor development and growth. CD8+ T lymphocytes within cancer cell nests of colorectal cancer have significant impact on the survival of patients. They contain the cytolytic enzyme granzyme-B. In case of increased proliferating activity of CD8+ T lymphocytes we observe their activated and cytotoxic phenotype that is significantly associated with the absence of early metastatic events (vascular emboli, lymphatic invasion or perineural invasion of tumor cells) and with a decreased rate of cancer recurrence (Atreya & Neurath, 2008, Pages et al., 2010). A high density of memory T lymphocytes within colorectal cancer tissue was more frequently observed in patients without early detectable signs of metastatic events and was associated with both improved disease free interval (DFI) and prolonged overall survival (OS) (Galon et al., 2006; Pages et al., 2005).

Natural killer cells (NK cells) mediate an effective lysis of cancer cells but the mechanism of detection of cancer cells is different from CD8+ T lymphocytes (Cooper et al., 2009). NK cells are mainly involved in the innate immune response and do not recognize specific tumor associated antigen on the surface of cancer cells as CD8+ T lymphocytes. NK cells lyse the cancer cells that are opsonized by surface antibody. NK cells also respond to other signals as cytokines produced by antigen presenting cells, which allow them to mediate early host responses against pathogen (Moretta et al., 2006). Decreased preoperative number of NK cells was associated with increased frequency of postoperative recurrence of colorectal cancer (Atreya & Neurath, 2008; Cooper et al., 2001). Their crucial role in the elimination of haematological malignancies, primary and secondary tumors has been recognized (Lucas et al., 2007; Ljunggren & Malmberg, 2007, Stojanovic & Cerwenka, 2011). In the last year there are some signs that NK-cells have the capacity for memory-like responses, a property that was previously thought to be limited to adaptive immunity, but in this view the discussion still continues (Cooper et al., 2009).

Dendritic cells are considered to be most potent antigen presenting cells. They play key role in activation, stimulation and recruitment of T lymphocytes. They can also induce antigen-specific unresponsiveness or immune tolerance. Immature dendritic cells enter tumor tissue, uptake and process its antigens. Then after they migrate to lymph nodes, undergo maturation and interact with T-lymphocytes that are able to recognize presented antigen and so T-lymphocytes play effector role of this tumor-specific immunity (Atreya & Neurath, 2008; Pages et al., 2005; Sandel et al., 2005; Steinman et al., 2003).

Macrophages are important producers of different factors that have function during tumor progression and also during tumor progression control. Their function is not fully understand, but it was described that the number of tumor infiltrating macrophages correlates with overall survival of colorectal cancer patients (Atreya & Neurath, 2008; Pollard, 2004; Forssell et al., 2007). It seems that several types of tumor infiltrating macrophages influence the balance between pro- and anti-tumor properties of immune system (Forssell et al., 2007).

From the morphologic view we can observe TIL in the specific portions of tumor and so we detect lymphocytic infiltration intratumoral (ITL – intratumoral lymphocytes) (Fig.

2a),intrastromal (ISL – intrastromal lymphocytes) (Fig. 2b), peritumoral (PTL – peritumoral lymphocytes) (Fig. 2c) and Crohn-like reaction (Crohn-like PTL)(Fig. 2d). We can also describe reactive histological changes in tributary lymph nodes (LN reactions). It means follicular hyperplasia (LN-FH) (Fig. 3a.), sinus histiocytosis (LN-SH) (Fig. 3b.) and the presence of granulomas (LN-GR) (Fig. 3c) (Ogino et al, 2009; Pages et al., 2005).

The aim of this study was to analyze the relationship of contemporary clinical and histopathological factors and TIL to determine patients with a high risk of poor overall survival and tendency to early recurrence of malignancy with shortened disease free interval (DFI) after radical surgery for CRC.

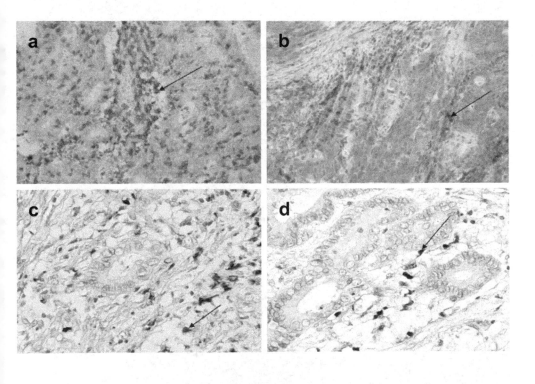

Fig. 1. Examples of tumor infiltration by immune cells: a) CD8+ T lymphocytes; b) CD4+ T lymphocytes; c) Natural killer cell (CD 57 staining) and d) Dendritic cells (S 100 staining).

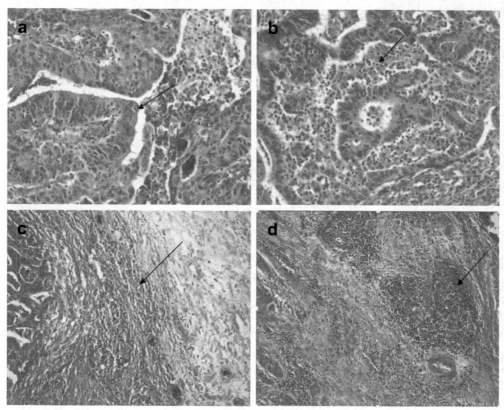

Fig. 2. Different localisation of TIL within the tumor tissue: a) intratumoral lymphocytes; b) intrastromal lymphocytes; c) peritumoral lymphocytes and d) Crohn-like peritumoral lymphocytes. All sections stained with hematoxylin-eosin.

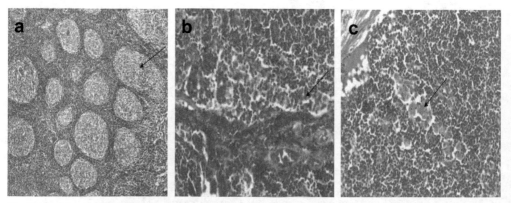

Fig. 3. Reactive histological changes in tributary lymph nodes: a) follicular hyperplasia; b) sinus histiocytosis and c) presence of granulomas. All sections stained with hematoxylin-eosin.

2. Methods

We analyzed 150 patients who underwent radical surgical procedure for CRC between the years 2004-2007 at the Department of Surgery, Medical School and Teaching Hospital in Pilsen, Charles University in Prague. We selected only patients who were operated on electively – our aim was to decrease the risk of inflammation that is often connected with the acute operation of CRC and does not depend on the immune reaction against a tumor but could be evoked by the distension of the bowel. We also excluded patients who had risk of understaging (for example low number of analysed lymph nodes) and patients with a synchronous metastatic process. The inclusion standard was also the entire follow-up of patients during the whole postoperative period to increase the number of patients with a diagnosed early recurrence of CRC.

The following clinical parameters were statistically analysed in relation to the disease free interval (DFI) and the overall survival (OS): staging, grading, preoperative leukocytosis, type of surgical procedure (radical vs. palliative), postoperative complications and postoperative oncological treatment.

2.1 Histology

We examined three different sections of each tumor and also sections of all found lymph nodes. Tissue for light microscopy was fixed in 4% formaldehyde and embedded in paraffin using routine procedures. Five micrometer-thick sections were cut from the tissue blocks and stained with hematoxylin-eosin.

The type and grade of all tumors were determined according to WHO 2000 guidelines. The stage of tumors was established according to UICC 2002 guidelines. We evaluated endovascular (VI), endolymphatic (LI) and perineural infiltration (PI) by cancer cells (0 – none, 1 – yes). Lymphocytic infiltration was detected as intratumoral (ITL – intratumoral lymphocytes), intrastromal (ISL – intrastromal lymphocytes), peritumoral (PTL – peritumoral lymphocytes) and Crohn-like reaction (Crohn-like PTL), and scaled as none (0), mild (1), moderate (2) and severe (3). Reactive histological changes in lymph nodes (LN reactions) were detected as follicular hyperplasia (LN-FH), sinus histiocytosis (LN-SH) and the presence of granulomas (LN-GR), and all these parameters were quantified in the same manner as lymphocytic infiltration.

2.2 Immunohistochemistry

For immunohistochemical investigations the following primary antibodies were used: CD4 (clone 4B12, 1:50, Vector Laboratories, Burlingame, CA, USA) and CD8 (clone C8/144B, 1:50, Dako, Glostrup, Denmark). Microwave pretreatment was used in both cases. The primary antibodies were visualized using the supersensitive streptavidin-biotin-peroxidase complex (Biogenex, San Ramon, CA). Appropriate positive and negative control slides were employed. The density of intratumoral infiltration by lymphocytes was evaluated in five High power microscopical fields (HPF) and expressed as the number of immunopositive cells per HPF.

2.3 Statistical evaluation

Statistical analysis was processed by the statistical software Statistica 9.0. The mean, median, standard deviation (SD), minimum, maximum, quartiles, frequencies and other basic statistical measurements were computed in given groups and subgroups of patients corresponding to studied clinical and histopathological parameters.

The relationships between the variables were described by Spearman rank correlation coefficients.

The analyses of Overall survival (OS) and Disease free interval (DFI) were performed by Kaplan-Meier´s survival functions. The influence of given covariates (clinical and histopathological factors) was tested by the Log-Rank test and Wilcoxon test. The Cox regression hazard model, hazard ratio (HR) and 95% confidence interval (CI) for HR were computed for the evaluation of given clinical and histopathological factors to OS or DFI. Multivariate analysis was performed by the use of classification and regression trees (CART). The Cox regression hazard model (stepwise regression) was applied to find the predictors in CART.

3. Results

The statistical analysis of the studied cohort of patients after surgical treatment for colorectal cancer demonstrated an acceptable distribution of basic statistical description parameters (gender ratio 93:57 (male vs. female)). 1, 3 and 5 years overall survival was 92.2%, 76.5% and 70.2% and 1, 3 and 5 year DFI was 85.3%, 64.3% and 49.4%.

The Spearman rank correlation coefficient did not prove any stronger correlation than a moderate correlation at endolymphatic invasion (LI) and lymph node infiltration by metastatic process (Spearman rank correlation coefficient 0.56, p<0,05). All the other studied factors were independent factors or factors with a low correlation.

Statistical analysis proved lymph node infiltration by metastatic process as statistically significant for the prognosis of overall survival (p<0.05) and N2 status of lymph nodes increased the risk of shorter overall survival 9.3x (Fig. 4.).

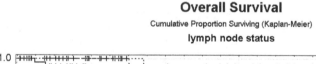

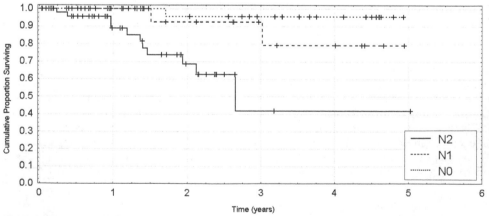

Fig. 4. Statistical analysis proved the lymph node infiltration by a metastatic process as statistically significant for the prognosis of overall survival (p<0.05), and the N2 status of lymph nodes increased the risk of a shorter overall survival 9.3x.

Endovascular infiltration (VI) was proved as a negative prognostic factor of shorter overall survival (Fig.5.). Patients with positive histopathological findings of VI have 3.1x increased risk for shorter overall survival. The presence of peritumoral lymphocytes (PTL) (Fig.6.) and of Crohn-like PTL (Fig.7.) was proved as a positive prognostic factor of OS. Patients with a positive histopathological finding of PTL and Crohn-like PTL have a decreased risk for shorter overall survival (2.3x and 2.3x respectively). Lymph node follicular hyperplasia (LN-FH) was verified as a positive prognostic factor for longer overall survival (Fig.8.). The statistical significance of LN-FH increased also with the raised density of infiltration. LN-FH positivity decreased the risk of shorter overall survival 3.3times.

The severity of CD8+ lymphocytic infiltration was proved by the Cox regression hazard model as a positive prognostic factor enlarging overall survival (cut off 30 cells/HPF). The severity of CD4+ lymphocytic infiltration was proved as a significant factor for the prognosis of overall survival (cut off 4cells/HPF) with 2.5x increased hazard ratio in patients over the cut off (Fig.9.). Statistical analysis did not confirm the statistical significance of CD8/CD4 ratio.

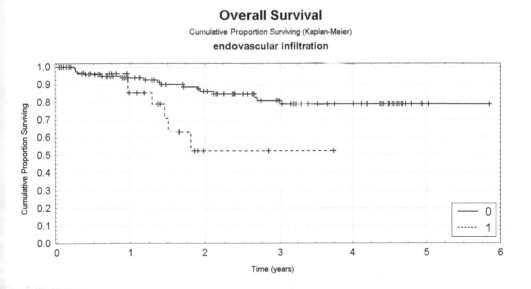

Fig. 5. Endovascular infiltration by cancer cells (VI) was proved as a statistically significant factor for the prognosis of overall survival (p<0.05). The patients with a positive histopathological finding of VI have 3.1x higher risk ratio for shorter overall survival.

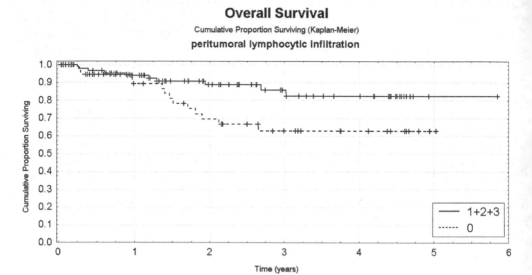

Fig. 6. Presence of peritumoral lymphocytes (PTL) was proved as a statistically significant positive factor for the prognosis of overall survival (p<0.05). The patients with a positive histopathological finding of PTL have 2.3x lower risk ratio for a shorter overall survival.

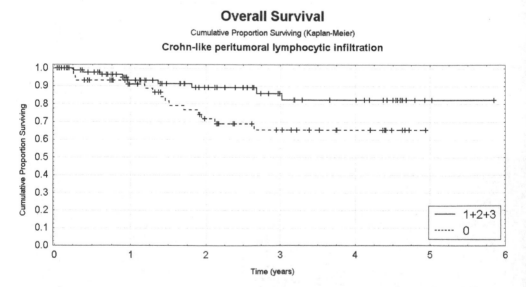

Fig. 7. Presence of Crohn-like PTL was proved as a statistically significant positive factor for the prognosis of overall survival (p<0.05). The patients with a positive histopathological finding of PTL have 2.3x lower risk ratio for a shorter overall survival.

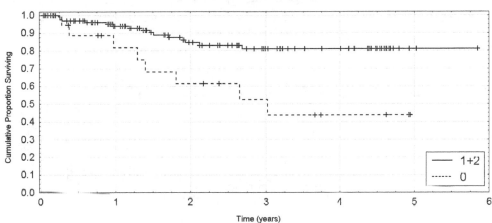

Overall Survival

Cumulative Proportion Surviving (Kaplan-Meier)

lymph nodes follicular hyperplasia

Fig. 8. Lymph node follicular hyperplasia (LN-FH) was verified as a positive prognostic factor for a longer overall survival (p<0.05). The statistical significance of LN-FH increased also with the raised density of infiltration. LN-FH positivity decreased the risk of a shorter overall survival 3.3x.

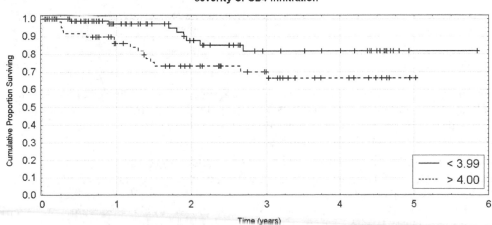

Overall Survival

Cumulative Proportion Surviving (Kaplan-Meier)

severity of CD4 infiltration

Fig. 9. Severity of CD4+ lymphocytic intratumoral infiltration was proved as a significant factor for the prognosis of overall survival (cut off 4cells/HPF) with a 2.5x increased hazard ratio in patients over the cut off (p<0.05).

The Multivariate Cox Regression Hazard Model proved the combination of the severity of lymph node infiltration by metastatic process and LN-FH as the best prognostic factors for the prediction of the risk of shorter overall survival. This situation is demonstrated in the Classification and Regression Tree (CART)(p<0.05) (Fig.10.). All other studied parameters were not proved as statistically significant for the prognosis of overall survival.

Classification and Regression Tree

Overall Survival

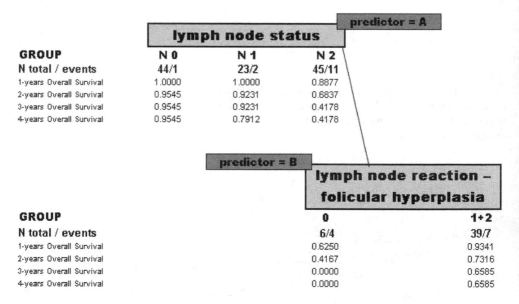

GROUP	N 0	N 1	N 2
N total / events	44/1	23/2	45/11
1-years Overall Survival	1.0000	1.0000	0.8877
2-years Overall Survival	0.9545	0.9231	0.6837
3-years Overall Survival	0.9545	0.9231	0.4178
4-years Overall Survival	0.9545	0.7912	0.4178

predictor = A — lymph node status

predictor = B — lymph node reaction – folicular hyperplasia

GROUP	0	1+2
N total / events	6/4	39/7
1-years Overall Survival	0.6250	0.9341
2-years Overall Survival	0.4167	0.7316
3-years Overall Survival	0.0000	0.6585
4-years Overall Survival	0.0000	0.6585

Fig. 10. Multivariate Cox Regression Hazard Model proved the combination of the severity of lymph node infiltration by a metastatic process and LN-FH as the best prognostic factors for the prediction of risk of a shorter overall survival (p<0.05). This situation is demonstrated in the Classification and Regression Tree (CART).

Perineural infiltration (PI) was proved as a negative prognostic factor of an earlier recurrence (Fig.11.). Patients with a positive histopathological finding of PI have 3.8x increased risk for shorter DFI.

The severity of CD8+ lymphocytic infiltration was proved by the Cox regression hazard model as a positive prognostic factor enlarging DFI (cut off 30cells/HPF) (Fig.12.). Patients over the cut off have 2.2x increased risk of an early recurrence. The severity of CD4+ lymphocytic infiltration was not proved as a significant factor for the prognosis of DFI. Statistical analysis did not confirm the statistical significance of the CD8/CD4 ratio.

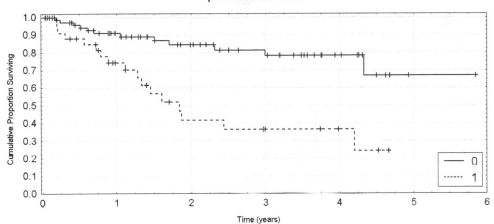

Disease Free Interval

Cumulative Proportion Surviving (Kaplan-Meier)

perineural infiltration

Fig. 11. Perineural infiltration (PI) was proved as a negative prognostic factor of an earlier recurrence (p<0.05). Patients with a positive histopathological finding of PI have a 3.8x increased risk for shorter DFI.

Statistical analysis proved lymph node infiltration by a metastatic process as statistically significant for the prognosis of DFI and N2 status of lymph nodes increased the risk of shorter DFI 5x (Fig. 13.).

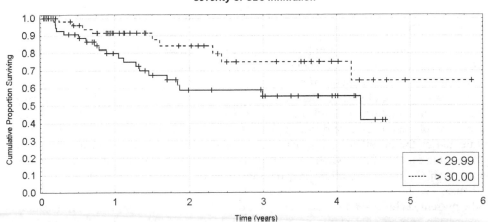

Disease Free Interval

Cumulative Proportion Surviving (Kaplan-Meier)

severity of CD8 infiltration

Fig. 12. Severity of CD8+ lymphocytic intratumoral infiltration was proved as a positive prognostic factor enlarging DFI (cut off 30 cells/HPF) by the Cox regression hazard model (p<0.05). Patients over the cut off have a 2.2x increased risk of an early recurrence.

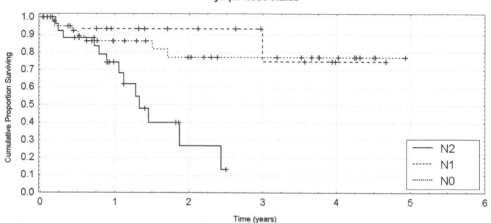

Fig. 13. Statistical analysis proved lymph node infiltration by a metastatic process as statistically significant for the prognosis of DFI, and a N2 status of lymph nodes 5x increased the risk of a shorter DFI (p<0.05).

The Multivariate Cox Regression Hazard Model proved the combination of the severity of the lymph node infiltration by a metastatic process and the severity of CD8 positivity of infiltrating lymphocytes as the best prognostic factors for the prediction of risk of early recurrence (p<0.05). This situation is demonstrated in the Classification and Regression Tree (CART) (Fig. 14). All other studied parameters were not proved as statistically significant for the prognosis of DFI.

4. Discussion

The role of the adaptive immunological response in controlling the growth and relapse of CRC remains controversial and contemporary studies have not answered all the questions about the prognosis of patients after radical surgical treatment of CRC (Galon et al., 2006; Ohtani, 2007; Van den Eynde & Hendlisz, 2009). We analysed our large cohort of patients of CRC with consideration to detect the negative and also positive prognostic factors of early recurrence of the disease and the poor overall survival after radical surgery. It was stimulated by the unsatisfactory situation and some dilemmas in the indication of surgical and oncological treatment, when early recurrence depreciates our effort to radical surgery with a high risk of complications and the long time of the decreased quality of life of our patients.

In the presented clinico-pathological study we demonstrated that lymph node infiltration by a metastatic process, N2 status of lymph nodes, VI, and extent of CD4+ lymphocytic intratumoral infiltration as negative prognostic factors of OS. In contrary PTL, Crohn-like PTL, LN-FH, and severity of CD8+ lymphocytic intratumoral infiltration were proved as positive prognostic factors of the overall survival.

Classification and Regression Tree

Disease Free Interval

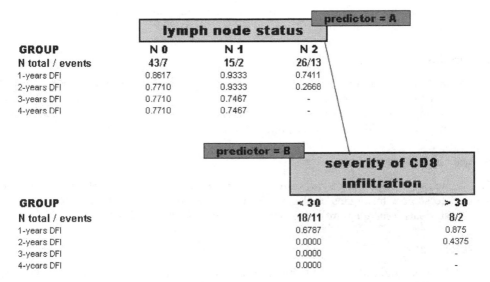

GROUP	N 0	N 1	N 2
N total / events	43/7	15/2	26/13
1-years DFI	0.8617	0.9333	0.7411
2-years DFI	0.7710	0.9333	0.2668
3-years DFI	0.7710	0.7467	-
4-years DFI	0.7710	0.7467	-

GROUP	< 30	> 30
N total / events	18/11	8/2
1-years DFI	0.6787	0.875
2-years DFI	0.0000	0.4375
3-years DFI	0.0000	-
4-years DFI	0.0000	-

Fig. 14. Multivariate Cox Regression Hazard Model proved the combination of the severity of lymph node infiltration by a metastatic process and the severity of CD8 positivity as the best prognostic factors for the prediction of risk of an early recurrence ($p<0.05$). This situation is demonstrated in the Classification and Regression Tree (CART).

The combination of the severity of the lymph node infiltration by a metastatic process and LN-FH were proved as the best prognostic factors for the prediction of risk of a shorter overall survival by the Multivariate Cox Regression Hazard Model.

We also demonstrated PI, lymph node metastatic infiltration and the N2 status of lymph nodes as negative prognostic factors of an earlier recurrence, and the severity of CD8+ lymphocytic intratumoral infiltration as a positive prognostic factor enlarging DFI. The combination of the severity of the lymph node infiltration by a metastatic process and the severity of CD8+ lymphocytic intratumoral infiltration were proved as the best prognostic factors for the prediction of the risk of an early recurrence by the Multivariate Cox Regression Hazard Model.

Our results support the hypothesis that the adaptive immunological response in tumor tissue and its reaction in regional lymph nodes can influence the behavior of CRC and so affect the prognosis of patients (Atreya & Neurath, 2008; Galon et al., 2006). CD4 and CD8 positivity of ITL was demonstrated as a key histopathological sign of tumor-specific immune response that could reflect the contemporary clinical situation and a tendency to relapse (CD4+) or the larger overall survival (CD8+) (Chiba et al. 2004; Koch et al., 2006, Pages et al., 2010).

We assessed several types of tumor infiltrating lymphocytes and clearly identified their relationships to relapse and the overall survival as positive or negative prognostic factors in contrary to previous publications that evaluated only the infiltration of the tumor but not the quality and type of infiltration (Ogino et al., 2009).

Tumor infiltration by lymphocytes seems to be a promising prognostic factor reflecting the risk of patients to early recurrence or poor overall survival. Future work has to be focused on the molecular-biological background of tumor infiltration by lymphocytes to understand their pathophysiological functions (Pages et al., 2005, Zbar, 2004).

5. Conclusion

Tumor infiltrating lymphocytes seem to be promising prognostic factors that could find their use in colorectal surgery and consecutive oncological treatment as an indicator of the type or combinations of therapies reflecting the risk of patients to early recurrence or poor overall survival. The TIL status corresponds to immune control of cancer progression.

6. Acknowledgment

This article was supported by research project MSM 0021620819 (Replacement of and support to some vital organs) and grant IGA MZ CR 10230 and IGA MZ CR 12025 and specific students research grant of Charles University SVV-2011- 262 806.

7. References

Atreya, I., & Neurath, M. F. (2008). Immune cells in colorectal cancer: prognostic relevance and therapeutic strategies. *Expert Review of Anticancer Therapy*, Vol.8, No.4, (April 2008), pp. 561-572, ISSN 1473-7140

Bird, N. C., Mangnall, D., & Majeed, A. W. (2006). Biology of colorectal liver metastases: a review. *Journal of Surgical Oncology*, Vol.94, No.1, (July 2006), pp. 68-80, ISSN 0022-4790

Chiba, T., Ohtani, H., Mizoi, T., Naito, Y., Sato, E., Nagura, H., Ohuchi, A., Ohuchi, K., Shiiba, K., Kurokawa, Y. & Satomi, S. (2004). Intraepithelial CD8+ T-cell-count becomes a prognostic factor after a longer follow-up period in human colorectal carcinoma: possible association with suppression of micrometastasis. *British Journal of Cancer*, Vol.91, No.9, (November 2004), pp. 1711-1717, ISSN 0007-0920

Coleman, M. P., Quaresma, M., Berrino, F., Lutz, J. M., De Angelis, R., Capocaccia, R., Baili, P., Rachet, B., Gatta, G., Hakulinen, T., Micheli, A., Sant, M., Weir, H. K., Elwood, J. M., Tsukuma, H., Koifman, S., Silva, E., Francisci, S., Santaquilani, M., Verdecchia, A., Storm, H. H., Young, J. L. & CONCORD Working Group. (2008). Cancer survival in five continents: a worldwide population-based study (CONCORD). *The Lancet Oncology*, Vol.9, No.8, (August 2008), pp. 730-756, ISSN 1470-2045

Cooper, M. A., Fehniger, T. A., & Caliguiri, M. A. (2001). The biology of human natural killer – cell subsets. *Trends in Immunology*, Vol.22, No.11, (November 2001), pp. 633-640, ISSN 1471-4906

Cooper, M. A., Colonna, M., & Yokoyama, W. M. (2009). Hidden talents of natural killers: NK cells in innate and adaptive immunity. *Embo reports*, Vol.10, No.10, (October 2009), pp. 1103-1110, ISSN 1469-221X

Forssell, J., Oberg, A., Henriksson, M. L., Stenling, R., Jung, A., & Palmquist, R. (2007). High macrophage infiltration along the tumor front correlates with improved survival in colon cancer. *Clinical Cancer research*, Vol.1, No.13, (March 2007), pp. 1472-1479, ISSN 1078-0432.

Gajewski, T. F., Meng, Y., Harlin, H. (2006). Immune suppression in the tumor microenvironment. *Journal of Immunotherapy*, Vol.29, No.3, (May-June 2006), pp. 233-240, ISSN 1524-9557

Galon, J., Costes, A., Sanchez-Cabo, F., Kirilovsky, A., Mlecnik, B., Lagorce-Pagès, C., Tosolini, M., Camus, M., Berger, A., Wind, P., Zinzindohoué, F., Bruneval, P., Cugnenc, P. H., Trajanoski, Z., Fridman, W. H. & Pagès, F. (2006). Type, density, and location of immune cells within human colorectal tumors predict clinical outcome. *Science*, Vol.313, No.5795, (September 2006), pp. 1960-1964, ISSN 0036-8075

Jochems C, Schlom J. (2011). Tumor-infiltrating immune cells and prognosis: the potential link between conventional cancer therapy and immunity. *Exp Biol Med (Maywood)*. Vol. 236, No.5 (May 2011), pp. 567-79, ISSN 1535-3702

Kobayashi, H., Mochizuki, H., Sugihara, K., Sugihara, K., Morita, T., Kotake, K., Teramoto, T., Kameoka, S., Saito, Y., Takahashi, K., Hase, K., Oya, M., Maeda, K., Hirai, T., Kameyama, M., Shirouzu, K. & Muto T. (2007). Characteristics of recurrence and surveillance tools after curative resection for colorectal cancer: a multicenter study. *Surgery*, Vol.141, No.1, (January 2007), pp. 67-75, ISSN 0039-6060

Koch, M., & Beckhove, P. (2006). Op den Winkel J et al. Tumor infiltrating T lymphocytes in colorectal cancer: Tumor-selective activation and cytotoxic activity in situ. *Annals of Surgery*, Vol.244, No.6, (December 2006), pp. 986-992, ISSN 0003-4932

Ljunggren, H.G., & Malmberg, K.J. (2007). Prospects for the use of NK cells in immunotherapy of human cancer. *Nature Reviews. Immunology*, Vol.7, No.5, (May 2007), pp. 329-339, ISSN 1474-1733

Lucas, M., Schachterle, W., Oberle, K., Aichele, P., & Diefenbach, A. (2007). Dendritic cells prime natural killer cells by trans-presenting interleukin 15. *Immunity*, Vol.26, No.4, (April 2007), pp. 503-517, ISSN 1074-7613

Moretta, L., Ferlazzo, G., Bottino, C., Vitale, M., Pende, D., Mingari M. C., & Moretta, A. (2006). Effector and regulatory events during natural killer-dendritic cell interaction. *Immunological Reviews*, Vol.214, No.1, (December 2006), pp. 219-228, ISSN 0105-2896

Ogino, S., Nosho, K., Iraha, N., Meyerhardt, J. A., & Baba, Y. (2009). Lymphocytic reaction to colorectal cancer is associated with longer survival, independent of lymph node count, microsatellite instability, and CpG island methylation phenotype. *Clinical Cancer Research*, Vol. 15, No. 20, (October 2009), pp. 6412-6420, ISSN 1078-0432

Ohtani, H. (2007). Focus on TILs: prognostic significance of tumor infiltrating lymphocytes in human colorectal cancer, *Cancer immunity*, Vol. 7, (February 2007), pp. 4, ISSN 1424-9634

Pagès, F., Berger, A., Camus, M., Costes, A., Molidor, R., Mlecnik, B., Kirilovsky, A., Nilsson, M., Damotte, D., Meatchi, T., Bruneval, P., Cugnenc, P. H., Trajanoski, Z., Fridman, W. H., & Galon, J. (2005). Effector memory T cells, early metastasis, and survival in colorectal cancer. *The New England Journal of Medicine*, Vol.353, No.25, (December 2005), pp. 2654-2666, ISSN 0028-4793

Pagès, F., Galon, J., Die-Nosjeanu, M. C., Tartour, E., & Sautes-Fridman, C. (2010). Immune infiltration in human tumors: a prognostic factor that should not be ignored. *Oncogene*, Vol.29, No.8, (February 2010), pp. 1093-1102, ISSN 0950-9232

Pollard, J. W. (2004). Tumor-educated macrophages promote tumour progression and metastasis. *Nature Reviews. Cancer*, Vol.4, No.1, (January 2004), pp. 71-78, ISSN 1474-175X

Sandel, M. H., Dadabayev, A. R., Menon, A. G., Morreau, H., Melief, C. J., Offringa, R., van der Burg, S. H., Janssen-van Rhijn, C. M., Ensink, N. G. , Tollenaar, R. A., van de Velde, C. J., & Kuppen, P. J. (2005). Prognostic value of tumor-infiltrating dendritic cells in colorectal cancer: role of maturation status and intratumoral localization. *Clinical Cancer Research*, Vol.11, No.7, (April 2005), pp. 2576-2582, ISSN 1078-0432

Steinman, R. M., Hawiger, D., & Nussenzweig, M. C. (2003). Tolerogenic dendritic cells. *Annual review of immunology*, Vol.21, pp. 685-711, ISSN 0732-0582

Stojanovic, A., & Cerwenka, A. (2011). Natural Killer cells and solid tumors. In: *Journal of Innate Immunity*, 10.6.2011, Available from: <http://content.karger.com/produktedb/produkte.asp?doi=325465>.

Talmadge, J. E., Donkor, M., & Scholar, E. (2007). Inflammatory cell infiltration of tumors: Jekyll or Hyde. *Cancer and Metastasis Reviews.* Vol.26, No.3-4, (December 2007), pp. 373-400, ISSN 0167-7659

Van den Eynde, M., & Hendlisz, A. (2009) Treatment of colorectal liver metastases: a review. *Reviews on Recent Clinical Trials,,* Vol.4, No.1, (January 2009), pp. 56-62, ISSN 1574-8871

Zbar, A. P. (2004) The immunology of colorectal cancer. *Surgical Oncology*, Vol.13, No.2-3, (August-November 2004), pp. 45-53, ISSN 0960-7404

Permissions

The contributors of this book come from diverse backgrounds, making this book a truly international effort. This book will bring forth new frontiers with its revolutionizing research information and detailed analysis of the nascent developments around the world.

We would like to thank Dr Rajunor Ettarh, for lending his expertise to make the book truly unique. He has played a crucial role in the development of this book. Without his invaluable contribution this book wouldn't have been possible. He has made vital efforts to compile up to date information on the varied aspects of this subject to make this book a valuable addition to the collection of many professionals and students.

This book was conceptualized with the vision of imparting up-to-date information and advanced data in this field. To ensure the same, a matchless editorial board was set up. Every individual on the board went through rigorous rounds of assessment to prove their worth. After which they invested a large part of their time researching and compiling the most relevant data for our readers. Conferences and sessions were held from time to time between the editorial board and the contributing authors to present the data in the most comprehensible form. The editorial team has worked tirelessly to provide valuable and valid information to help people across the globe.

Every chapter published in this book has been scrutinized by our experts. Their significance has been extensively debated. The topics covered herein carry significant findings which will fuel the growth of the discipline. They may even be implemented as practical applications or may be referred to as a beginning point for another development. Chapters in this book were first published by InTech; hereby published with permission under the Creative Commons Attribution License or equivalent.

The editorial board has been involved in producing this book since its inception. They have spent rigorous hours researching and exploring the diverse topics which have resulted in the successful publishing of this book. They have passed on their knowledge of decades through this book. To expedite this challenging task, the publisher supported the team at every step. A small team of assistant editors was also appointed to further simplify the editing procedure and attain best results for the readers.

Our editorial team has been hand-picked from every corner of the world. Their multi-ethnicity adds dynamic inputs to the discussions which result in innovative outcomes. These outcomes are then further discussed with the researchers and contributors who give their valuable feedback and opinion regarding the same. The feedback is then collaborated with the researches and they are edited in a comprehensive manner to aid the understanding of the subject.

Apart from the editorial board, the designing team has also invested a significant amount of their time in understanding the subject and creating the most relevant covers. They scrutinized every image to scout for the most suitable representation of the subject and create an appropriate cover for the book.

The publishing team has been involved in this book since its early stages. They were actively engaged in every process, be it collecting the data, connecting with the contributors or procuring relevant information. The team has been an ardent support to the editorial, designing and production team. Their endless efforts to recruit the best for this project, has resulted in the accomplishment of this book. They are a veteran in the field of academics and their pool of knowledge is as vast as their experience in printing. Their expertise and guidance has proved useful at every step. Their uncompromising quality standards have made this book an exceptional effort. Their encouragement from time to time has been an inspiration for everyone.

The publisher and the editorial board hope that this book will prove to be a valuable piece of knowledge for researchers, students, practitioners and scholars across the globe.

List of Contributors

Rajunor Ettarh
Department of Structural and Cellular Biology, Tulane University School of Medicine, New Orleans, USA

Spaska Stanilova
Trakia University, Medical Faculty, Department of Molecular Biology, Immunology and Medical Genetics, Bulgaria

Amanda Ewart Toland
The Ohio State University, USA

Rodney J. Scott, Stuart Reeves and Bente Talseth-Palmer
The Centre for Information Based Medicine, The School of Biomedical Sciences and Pharmacy, University of Newcastle, United Kingdom

Rodney J. Scott
Division of Genetics, Hunter Area Pathology Service, United Kingdom

Bente Talseth-Palmer
Hunter Medical Research Institute, United Kingdom

N. Britzen-Laurent, M. Stürzl and E. Naschberger
Division of Molecular and Experimental Surgery, Department of Surgery, University Medical Center Erlangen, Erlangen, Germany

V.S. Schellerer and R.S. Croner
Department of Surgery, University Medical Center Erlangen, Erlangen, Germany

Hytham K. S. Hamid
Department of Surgery, Waterford Regional Hospital, Waterford, Ireland

Yassin M. Mustafa
Department of Internal Medicine, Howard University Hospital, Washington D.C., USA

Lucia Fini, Fabio Grizzi and Luigi Laghi
Laboratory of Molecular Gastroenterology and Department of Gastroenterology, IRCCS Istituto Clinico Humanitas, Rozzano, Milan, Italy

A.S. Abdulamir, R.R. Hafidh and F. Abu Bakar
Institute of Bioscience, University Putra Malaysia, Serdang, Selangor, Malaysia

A.S. Abdulamir
Microbiology Department, College of Medicine, Alnahrain University PO, Baghdad, Iraq

R.R. Hafidh
Microbiology Department, College of Medicine, Baghdad University, Iraq

Harold Tjalsma and Annemarie Boleij
Department of Laboratory Medicine, Nijmegen Institute for Infection, Inflammation and Immunity (N4i) & Radboud University Centre for Oncology (RUCO) of the Radboud University Nijmegen Medical Centre,
The Netherlands

E. Kirilova, I. Kalnina and G. Kirilov
Daugavpils University, Daugavpils, Latvia

G. Gorbenko
N. Karazin University of National Academy of Sciences, Kharkov, Ukraine

Vaclav Liska, Petr Novak, Vladislav Treska, Ondrej Vycital, Jan Bruha and Pavel Pitule
Department of Surgery, Medical School and Teaching Hospital Pilsen, Czech Republic

Ondrej Daum
Institute of Pathology, Medical School and Teaching Hospital Pilsen, Czech Republic

Lubos Holubec
Department of Oncology, Charles University Prague, Medical School and Teaching Hospital Pilsen,
Czech Republic

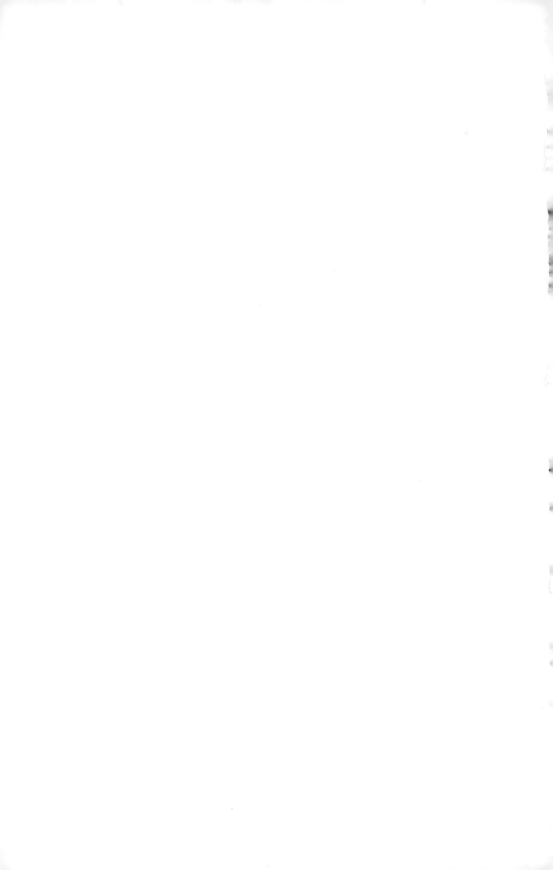